WITHDRAWN
UTSA LIBRARIES

DATE DUE

GAYLORD			PRINTED IN U.S.A.

D1571850

FROM MORALITY TO MENTAL HEALTH

PRACTICAL AND PROFESSIONAL ETHICS SERIES

Published in conjunction with the Association for Practical
and Professional Ethics

General Editor
Robert Audi, University of Notre Dame

Published in the Series:

Practical Ethics:
A Collection of Addresses and Essays
Henry Sedgwick
With an Introduction by Sissela Bok

Thinking Like an Engineer:
Studies in the Ethics of a Profession
Michael Davis

Deliberative Politics:
Essays on Democracy and Disagreement
Edited by Stephen Macedo

Conflict of Interest in the Professions
Edited by Michael Davis and Andrew Stark

Meaningful Work:
Rethinking Professional Ethics
Mike W. Martin

From Morality to Mental Health:
Virtue and Vice in a Therapeutic Culture
Mike W. Martin

FROM MORALITY TO MENTAL HEALTH

Virtue and Vice in a Therapeutic Culture

Mike W. Martin

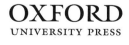

OXFORD
UNIVERSITY PRESS

2006

OXFORD
UNIVERSITY PRESS

Oxford University Press, Inc., publishes works that further
Oxford University's objective of excellence
in research, scholarship, and education.

Oxford   New York
Auckland   Cape Town   Dar es Salaam   Hong Kong   Karachi
Kuala Lumpur   Madrid   Melbourne   Mexico City   Nairobi
New Delhi   Shanghai   Taipei   Toronto

With offices in
Argentina   Austria   Brazil   Chile   Czech Republic   France   Greece
Guatemala   Hungary   Italy   Japan   Poland   Portugal   Singapore
South Korea   Switzerland   Thailand   Turkey   Ukraine   Vietnam

Published by Oxford University Press, Inc.
198 Madison Avenue, New York, New York 10016

www.oup.com

Oxford is a registered trademark of Oxford University Press

Library of Congress Cataloging-in-Publication Data

Martin, Mike W. 1946–
　From morality to mental health : virtue and vice in a therapeutic culture / Mike W. Martin
　　p.　cm.—(Practical and professional ethics series)
　Includes bibliographical references and index.
　ISBN-13: 978-0-19-530471-8
　ISBN-10: 0-19-530471-3
　1. Mental illness.　2. Ethics.　3. Virtues.　4. Vices.　5. Psychotherapy—Moral and
　ethical aspects.　I. Title.　II. Series.

　RC458.M265 2006
　362.2'04—dc22　　2005051812

9 8 7 6 5 4 3 2 1

Printed in the United States of America
on acid-free paper

For Shannon—
generous, loving healer

PREFACE

The therapeutic trend in ethics is the tendency to approach moral matters in terms of mental health, for example by pathologizing vices (alcoholism as a disease), psychologizing virtues (self-respect as self-esteem), and liberalizing attitudes (sex as good, guilt as suspect). The trend unfolded throughout the twentieth-century, although its roots extend to Plato and the Stoics. At its worst, the trend is a confused and dangerous attempt to replace morality with therapy. At its best, the trend integrates moral and therapeutic understanding to yield creative solutions to otherwise intractable problems. In this book I develop an integrated, moral-therapeutic perspective centered on three themes: (1) sound morality is healthy; (2) we are responsible for our health; (3) moral values are embedded in mental health and psychotherapy.

Part I connects Plato's virtue-oriented ethics with psychiatrists' definition of mental disorders. It also explores Freud's and Nietzsche's therapeutic critiques of sick forms of morality. I show how moral virtues overlap and interweave with the criteria for positive mental health—that is, psychological well-being in addition to the absence of mental disorders. Here, as throughout the book, I reject any general dichotomy between moral and therapeutic attitudes.

Part II develops a conception of responsibility for mental health and applies it both to therapist-client relationships and to moral accountability within society. I take seriously the criticism that the therapeutic trend in ethics fosters evasion of responsibility, but I recast the criticism as a caution rather than a basis for opposing the trend. I also respond to the concern that responsibility for mental health leads to blaming victims of mental illness.

Part III discusses responsibilities for health in connection with alcoholism, pathological gambling, serious crime, unjustified violence, and visceral bigotry. In each instance, I make sense of how the same pattern of conduct can be both wrongdoing and sickness. The aim is to show why expansive definitions of mental disorders do not provide automatic excuses for harming others.

Part IV shifts the focus to positive health and personal meaning. I explore the confluence of morality and mental health in pursuing meaningful lives. Topics include depression, self-deception, and philosophical counseling, as well as love, work, and philanthropy.

For their helpful comments on earlier essays from which I draw, I thank David Adams, Peggy Battin, Carolyn Brodbeck, Elliot D. Cohen, Herbert Fingarette, Laurence Finsen, Judge Dennis Fuchs, Donald L. Gabard, Pieranna Garavaso, S. Nassir Ghaemi, Vivian Gill, Ishtiyaque Haji, Sally Iberg, Kathie L. Jenni, Bruce Landesman, Thomas Magnell, Jeffrey Murphy, Jerome Neu, Tim O'Keefe, Gary Shepherd, Stephen Schandler, Laurie Shrage, Robert Solomon, Dale Turner, Margaret Urban Walker, and Virginia Warren. I also thank my students at Chapman University for their stimulus and their helpful ideas. Chapman University provided a semester sabbatical that helped in completing the book. Chapman librarians Gina Wilkinson and Claudia Horn provided highly professional research support. Two anonymous reviewers for Oxford University Press provided invaluable help, as did Cynthia Garver, Jennifer R. Kowing, and especially my editor Peter Ohlin.

I am grateful to the journal editors who permitted me to use published material, in revised form, and to the organizers and audience members of colloquia where versions of chapters were read.

"Alcoholism as Sickness and Wrongdoing," *Journal for the Theory of Social Behaviour*, 29 (1999): 109–131. An earlier version was presented at the University of Redlands (December 1997).

"Depression: Illness, Insight, and Identity," *Philosophy, Psychiatry and Psychology*, 6, no. 4 (1999): 271–286.

"Depression and Moral Health," *Philosophy, Psychiatry and Psychology*, 6, no. 4 (1999): 295–298.

"Moral Health: Responsibility in Therapeutic Culture," *Journal of Value Inquiry*, 34 (2000): 27–43.

"Sick Love and Virtue: Eros in a Therapeutic Culture," Conference on Sex and Love in the New Millennium, California Polytechnic University, Pomona (April 2000).

"Are Bigots Sick?" Midwest Philosophy Colloquium, University of Minnesota, Morris (September 2000).

"Responsibility for Health and Blaming Victims," *Journal of Medical Humanities*, 22, no. 2 (2001): 95–114.

"Ethics as Therapy: Philosophical Counseling and Psychological Health," *International Journal of Philosophical Practice*, 1 (2001). Available at http://www.ijpp.net/

"From Drug Wars to Faith-Based Therapy," Center on Philanthropy, Indiana University, Indianapolis (October 2001).

"On the Evolution of Depression," *Philosophy, Psychiatry and Psychology*, 9, no. 3 (2002): 255–259.

"America's Therapeutic Trend in Ethics: From Moral Character to Mental Disorders," and "Voluntary Service and the Therapeutic Motif," presented as a Lincoln Visiting Scholar at Arizona State University (October 2002).

"America's Therapeutic Trend in Ethics," Conference on Drugs and Justice, University of Utah (April 2003).

"Responsibility for Mental Disorders and Addictions: America's Therapeutic Trend in Ethics," Conference on "Ethics Gone Mad: Morality and Mental Illness," California Polytechnic University, Pomona (May 2004).

Above all, I thank my wife Shannon for daily conversations on these topics over many years, for her insights, and for her love.

CONTENTS

FROM MORALITY TO
MENTAL HEALTH

INTRODUCTION

The Therapeutic Trend

Today we blend and blur morality and mental health. Alcoholics are sick, yet they are punished when their disease manifests itself as drunk driving or child abuse. Addicts using illegal drugs are criminals, but their punishment is likely to be therapy supervised by judges. Character faults have become personality disorders, including most of the seven deadly sins: pride and envy are narcissism; gluttony is an eating disorder; sloth is a dependent personality disorder; acting out in anger is an impulse control disorder; greed is acquisitive desire disorder; and although lust is celebrated in our era of (therapy-supported) sexual liberation, misdirected lust is a psychosexual disorder such as fetishism or voyeurism—and too little lust is hypoactive sexual desire disorder.[1] In addition to pathologizing wrongdoing, we psychologize virtue. Thus, self-respect becomes self-esteem, integrity becomes psychological integration, and responsibility becomes maturity. Health-oriented attitudes permeate schools, workplaces, families, and religions. And moral advice and understanding are sought from psychologists rather than philosophers, therapists rather than theologians.

What is going on? Are we replacing morality with therapy, in confused and dangerous ways? Or are we integrating morality and mental health to find creative approaches to otherwise intractable problems? We are doing some of both. To maintain our moral bearings in a therapeutic culture, we need to understand how morality and mental health are related—not just in the abstract, but with regard to practical concerns such as love and work, self-respect and self-fulfillment, guilt and depression, crime and violence, and alcoholism and other addictions.

The therapeutic trend in ethics, or the *therapeutic trend* for short, is the tendency to approach moral matters in terms of mental health (or more generally in terms of holistic, biopsychosocial, conceptions of health). The tendency has many variations, but they cluster under two umbrellas: replacement and integrative projects. *Replacement projects* renounce morality, or radically dilute it, and replace it with therapy. These projects are confused and alarming, but they constitute a minority movement. Most of the therapeutic trend consists of *integrative projects* which understand morality and mental health as complementary, overlapping, and interwoven. Integrative projects take many forms, some superficial and others insightful. For the most part, the therapeutic trend is best understood as a promising and multifaceted integrative project.

I set forth an integrated, moral-therapeutic perspective centered on three themes: (1) sound morality is healthy; (2) we are responsible for our health, mental as well as physical; and (3) moral values permeate psychotherapy and conceptions of mental health. Before sketching these themes, and anchoring them in virtue ethics and pragmatism, let us gain a fuller sense of what is at stake by considering a few controversies.

Immoral or Ill?

President Bill Clinton's escapade with Monica Lewinsky provoked its share of therapeutic commentary, usually with something less than clinical detachment. Clinton's enemies derided him as a sexually disordered, pathological liar.[2] More gently, cartoonist Jules Feiffer diagnosed him as emotionally immature—a developmental failure of arrested adolescence.[3] Jerome D. Levin, a psychiatrist specializing in addictions, was initially outraged at Clinton, but his moral indignation subsided when he discerned symptoms of the "Clinton Syndrome"—a sexual disorder characterized by low self-esteem and excessive need for emotional reassurance, caused by being raised in a dysfunctional family. "There is no mystery why Bill Clinton would have gotten into a virtually suicidal relationship with Monica Lewinsky. His legacy as an adult child of an alcoholic (ACOA) compelled him to fill the emptiness of his childhood and to repeat the addictive pattern of both his biological and his adoptive parents; his relationship with Lewinsky revived a longstanding behavioral pattern; she fulfilled a complex nexus of unconscious needs."[4] When Hillary Clinton voiced similar ideas, however, she was attacked for rationalizing her husband's immorality. At least in the political arena, it seems that Clinton was either sick or salacious, but not both.[5]

A similar clash of moral and therapeutic attitudes shapes debates about drugs. When Washington, D.C., Mayor Marion Barry was caught on videotape smoking crack cocaine, and when Los Angeles City Councilman Mike Hernandez was arrested for cocaine possession, most observers took it as obvious that their irresponsible conduct rendered them unfit for public office. Spokespersons for the therapeutic community, however, praised their courage in seeking treatment and portrayed them as role models for people struggling with substance dependency disorders.[6] For half a century, the therapeutic community has understood addictions as mental disorders and sought to reshape law and public policy in that direction. Therapists' influence was dramatically illustrated when California's Proposition 36 took effect on July 1, 2001. Prior to then, California's Three Strikes Law mandated lifetime prison sentences for a third-felony possession of cocaine. Since then, most of the same criminals could choose therapy over jail, a choice nearly everyone makes! Some opponents of Proposition 36 favor the even tighter integration of morality and therapy within drug courts, where judges contribute to therapy and therapists contribute to law enforcement. Despite these integrations, we have difficulty acknowledging that addictions to illegal drugs are both mental disorders and morally objectionable habits.

Shifting to prescription drugs, we eagerly embrace pharmacological solutions to behavioral and emotional problems. Ritalin is readily dispensed for attention-deficit and hyperactivity disorders, which involve behaviors traditionally subject to moral discipline by parents and teachers. Prozac and its alternatives are the primary response to depression, if not to everyday low moods. Paxil is pre-scribed for shyness, which is medicalized as social anxiety disorder (or social phobia). Of greater concern, cosmetic surgery and other medical procedures are widely used for Asian-looking eyes, Jewish-looking noses, skin lightening and hair straightening to modify African-American features, thereby reinforcing ethnic stereotypes of beauty. The lines between enhancing and eroding au-tonomy are increasingly blurred.[7]

Far greater controversy surrounds homosexuality. Until 1973, the American Psychiatric Association (APA) listed homosexuality as a mental disorder. Then it changed its mind and affirmed homosexual orientations and activities as normal sexual expression. The swift reversal occurred largely because of pro-tests by gay rights activists who rejected the APA position as homophobic, provoking a vote among its members to decide whether homosexuality is a disorder—an unprecedented and precedent-setting approach to an allegedly scientific matter.[8] The event dramatically illustrates how moral values, along with scientific research, shape conceptions of mental health and mental disor-ders. Conversely, it illustrates how therapeutic outlooks can advance moral understanding by challenging bigotry and overthrowing ignorance. Even the widespread adoption of the medical-sounding term "homophobia," to refer to irrational fear and hatred of homosexuals, has advanced acceptance of gays and lesbians.

Finally, recall the scandal of child-abusing priests, which became a public crisis in 2002, even though it was identified much earlier.[9] Discussions of the crisis blended the languages of sin and sickness. Both the Roman Catholic Church and its critics struggled to sort out the issues of celibacy, homosexuality, homophobia, misogyny, pedophilia, and sex abuse crimes. Some called for abandoning the celibacy rule for priests (and nuns), viewing it as a medieval excrescence that epitomized the church's unhealthy attitudes about sex.[10] Others focused on the church's unhealthy culture of secrecy and patriarchy. Most agreed the Catholic Church had taken naïve half-measures in sending pedo-philes into therapy and then reinstating them in positions of authority where they could assault again. In defending itself, the church blamed psychiatrists for giving them bad advice about the prospects of curing child abusers, illustrating the dramatic influence of therapy on religion. There were also concerns that some cases involved inaccurate repressed memories ("False Memory Syndrome"), echoing Freud's initial assertion and subsequent denial of the veracity of childhood-incest memories.

These controversies are froth on a sea of change, but they suffice to illustrate our cultural ambivalence about how morality and mental health are related. Whether the issue concerns public events or private lives, we are easily ensnared in a *morality-therapy paradox*: Moral and therapeutic perspectives often apply to the same things, and yet they seem at odds. The apparent incompatibility can be expressed as a *morality-therapy dichotomy*: behavioral, emotional, and personality problems are either moral or therapeutic matters, but not both. Individuals are immoral or ill, sinners or sick, depraved or dysfunctional—but not with regard to the same things in the same respects. This morality-therapy dichotomy prevents us from understanding how Clinton's conduct was both irresponsible and sick, how destructive addictions are both wrongdoing and pathology, how medication and discipline might both be appropriate for a hyperactive child, how moral values largely determine whether homosexuality or homophobia is unhealthy, and how child abuse is both evil and ill. To make sense of such complexities, we need to unravel the morality-therapy paradox by dissolving the morality-therapy dichotomy.

Integrating Morality and Therapy

Morality and therapy do seem quite different. Morality is about responsible and irresponsible agents, right and wrong conduct, good and bad character, guilt and shame, blame and punishment, dignity and integrity. Therapy is about healthy and sick organisms, well-being and impairment, fitness and dysfunction, disease and suffering, treatment and healing, maturity and integration. These differences seem to generate oppositions at key junctures. In particular, we often assume that sickness excuses from wrongdoing. Again, moral guilt and blame seem opposed to therapeutic helping and healing. And morality seems oriented to other people, whereas health is self-oriented.

In emphasizing these differences, critics of the therapeutic trend object to its elevation of self-fulfillment over moral community, self-esteem over obligations to others, and a victim mentality over personal responsibility. They also worry about the excessive power given to psychiatrists to rewrite morality. These concerns need to be taken seriously, but the critics underestimate the positive side of the therapeutic trend. They fail to appreciate how intimately morality and mental health are connected.

Three themes bridge morality and mental health. First, *sound morality is healthy*. This does not mean that morality is subordinate to a nonmoral psychological standard, if only because health itself is moral-laden (per the third theme). Instead, it means that justified moral attitudes tend to manifest, promote, and overlap with mental health. Warranted moral views are psychologically realistic in their demands and aspirations. They do not cause excessive guilt, depression, anxiety, compulsions, anger, and hatred; more positively, they tend to promote well-being and self-fulfillment.

This theme presupposes that moral outlooks take different forms, some healthier than others. Those therapists who pursue replacement projects begin by reducing morality to its least palatable form. For example, psychiatrist James Gilligan characterizes morality as punitive, vengeful, obsessed with guilt and blame, and hence a "force antagonistic to life and to love, a force causing illness and death—neurosis and psychosis, homicide and suicide."[11] This reduction of morality to its moralistic excesses impedes understanding, even as it reminds us that blame and guilt are thorny issues in integrating moral and therapeutic understanding. My tack will be to accept blame and guilt as too important to abandon, and yet to insist they are not the heart of morality and to attend to their liability to excess.

For their part, critics of the therapeutic trend stereotype therapy as self-absorbed and idealize morality as entirely community-oriented. In the 1960s, Philip Rieff introduced the term "therapeutic"—as in "the therapeutic" outlook, attitude, ethos, sensibility, motif, or gospel—as a term of cultural criticism in condemning the therapeutic trend for fostering self-absorption and self-ishness.[12] Despite his penetrating insight, Rieff blurred the moral significance of self-fulfillment and authenticity, and he underestimated the importance of re-lationships and community to therapeutic perspectives. So did his followers.

An essential step toward an integrated, moral-therapeutic view is to reclaim the word "therapeutic" by restoring it to its original meaning of "pertaining to health." We also need to widen health and therapy to include not only treating maladies but also preventing mental disorders and promoting positive health—that is, well-being beyond the mere absence of pathology. (In this vein, some psychologists now speak of "positive therapy."[13]) We need to explore mental health as integral to morally desirable social functioning, caring relationships, and flourishing communities.

Second, *we are responsible for our health*, both mental and physical. This does not mean, of course, that we have complete control over our health. Instead, it means we are obligated to take prudent measures to care for our health within limits set by our resources, opportunities, other obligations, and personal as-pirations. It implies developing healthy habits and seeking help when problems grow beyond our immediate control. Responsibility for health pertains to all aspects of sickness, including its cause, cure, consequences, and the condition itself.

It follows that sickness does not automatically excuse wrongdoing. This is a dangerous truth. When misunderstood, it reinforces negative stereotypes of people who have severe mental illnesses, and it neglects society's responsibility to adopt sound public health policies. Nevertheless, if we accept the ongoing expansion of health-oriented approaches to moral matters (as I do), we should also take seriously responsibilities to prevent disorders, to cope with them once they arise, and to avoid using them as excuses for wrongdoing. Those responsibilities must be understood contextually in assessing when and how far sickness excuses or mitigates responsibility.

Third, *moral values are embedded in mental health and psychotherapy*. According to most contemporary definitions, health is biopsychosocial; it has three interwoven aspects: biological (bodily), psychological (mental), and social. My primary interest is psychological or mental health. Mental health is a matter of degree: superlative mental well-being; adequate functioning; suboptimal well-being and functioning; and mental disorders, from mild to severe. In all these degrees, mental health is moral-laden. In particular, moral values are presupposed in *negative definitions* of mental health as the absence of mental disorders. That is because definitions of mental disorders invariably allude to standards of normal functioning, sometimes explicitly as in definitions of antisocial personality disorder (sociopathy) and other times tacitly as in definitions of substance abuse disorders (and other addictions). More directly, moral values are embedded in *positive definitions* of mental health as well-being, effective functioning, adaptive behavior, normalcy, growth, and maturity—in addition to the absence of disorders. Specific health concepts are also moral-laden. For example, self-esteem largely overlaps with the virtue of self-respect, and self-control is both a moral and a therapeutic value.

There is no consensus about how to define mental health.[14] I discuss alternative definitions where relevant, but I frequently return to the definition of mental disorders in the American Psychiatric Association's *Diagnostic and Statistical Manual of Mental Disorders* (*DSM*), currently in its fourth edition with a text revision.[15] One reason for this emphasis is the cultural significance of the *DSM* in shaping attitudes, standardizing reimbursement for services by psychotherapists, and guiding the funding of research. Another reason is that the *DSM*'s "descriptive" approach to defining disorders by reference to actual behavior and emotions, rather than to causes, is helpful in integrating morality and therapy. It facilitates, for example, understanding the same behavior pattern of behavior that defines drug abuse as both a mental disorder and a morally bad habit.

Because moral values partly define mental health and disorders, moral values permeate therapeutic goals and procedures. Psychotherapy takes hundreds of different forms, all of them moral-laden and moral-guided. Properly understood, the nonjudgmental stance of therapists is an ethical requirement aimed at helping clients while respecting their autonomy. It is not an invitation for society to abandon moral judgments and to use sickness as an excuse for wrongdoing. Again, when therapists ask "How do you feel about that?," they elicit, not ignore, their clients' moral values—for nowhere are values more exactly revealed than in emotions.[16] Insofar as mental health and disorders embed moral judgments, we should be wary of allowing health professionals to make those judgments for us.

These three themes—sound morality as healthy, responsibility for health, and mental health as moral-laden—function in several ways in this book. Their primary role is to provide a framework for an integrated, moral-therapeutic perspective, which I apply to a host of practical issues. The themes invite interdisciplinary understanding of moral issues by bringing to bear the resources of psychiatry, psychology, sociology, and other sciences. In another role, the themes are interpretive tools used to elucidate and evaluate what is taking place in American society and elsewhere. The themes highlight desirable social tendencies while aiding in identifying possible abuses. They are deployed in defending my claim that the therapeutic trend, overall, is primarily an integrative project. Despite many distortions and disguises, the main transformations taking place in American society are not replacements of morality but, instead, transformations within morality itself—for example, downplaying or limiting negative emphases (guilt, blame, punishment), accenting positive attitudes (love, compassion, forgiveness), and embracing therapeutic techniques to bring about moral improvement.

To be sure, the therapeutic trend is morally ambiguous. It contains a vast array of therapeutic outlooks, moral perspectives, and attempted integrations and replacements regarding specific issues. Sometimes it encourages individuals to accept greater responsibility for their wrongdoing by seeking and cooperating with therapeutic help. Other times it fosters a victim mentality and encourages the idea that sickness is an automatic excuse for wrongdoing. And as already noted, questions about guilt and blame disrupt any smooth interface between helping and holding responsible. These are but a few of the complications I seek to elucidate.

Pragmatism and Virtue Ethics

As a moral framework, I draw especially on pragmatism and virtue ethics. The following comments on these ethical traditions are brief, but they suffice to indicate that the therapeutic trend has deeper moral roots than critics of the therapeutic trend appreciate.

One such critic, historian Eva Moskowitz, traces "America's therapeutic gospel" to mid-nineteenth-century beliefs in faith healing and "scientific spirituality."[17] In the late 1850s, Phineas P. Quimby proselytized for a Spiritual Science of "mental therapeutics," later called "mind cure"—essentially counseling techniques, positive attitudes, and self-improvement aimed at happiness. Then, in 1881, Mary Baker Eddy founded Christian Science based on the beliefs that evil is illusory and sickness is the product of spiritual failure. These developments inspired a nondenominational movement during the 1890s called "New Thoughters" which castigated traditional religion for promoting pessimism and anxiety. New Thoughters called for a spirituality of optimism and mental health. The legacy of Spiritual Science and New Thoughters is familiar in New Age movements, but it also enters into mainstream medicine under the headings alternative medicine, complementary medicine, and the placebo effect.

As Moskowitz defines it, America's therapeutic gospel is that "happiness should be our supreme goal," that "our problems stem from psychological causes," and that "the psychological problems that underlie our failures and unhappiness are in fact treatable." She documents the influence of the therapeutic gospel throughout the twentieth century in thinking about work, crime, education, the feminist movement, self-help groups, and talk shows such as those by Phil Donahue and Oprah Winfrey. In doing so, she denigrates the gospel for offering simplistic solutions to complex problems. Worse, she charges, the therapeutic gospel "robs us of the ability to make serious moral judgments" by replacing right and wrong with self-esteem and self-fulfillment.[18]

Moskowitz loads the deck against the therapeutic trend by singling out its most superficial manifestations. At the same time, she concludes with a surprising gesture toward an integrated perspective: "We need a politics and a therapeutics that are not mutually exclusive. But this appears difficult if not impossible to achieve."[19] I believe her pessimism is unwarranted; we are making more progress than ideological battles over the therapeutic trend suggest. The present point, however, is that Moskowitz overlooks the deeper roots of the therapeutic trend, including the health-oriented spirituality of Ralph Waldo Emerson, Walt Whitman, and other nineteenth-century Enlightenment thinkers who deserve as much attention as faith-based thinkers. Above all, they include the twentieth-century pragmatists, most notably William James and John Dewey.

William James, who is educated as a physician and is equally creative in philosophy and psychology, interweaves ethical and therapeutic ideas throughout his writings. His sympathetic reflections on the nineteenth-century origins of America's therapeutic trend contrast sharply with those of Moskowitz. In *The Varieties of Religious Experience*, James devotes a chapter to "the religion of healthy-mindedness"—the disposition to see things as good and to adopt an optimistic outlook. Ultimately, James finds healthy-mindedness less profound than the "sick soul's" encounter with evil, and he suggests that excessive optimism can itself be pathological.[20] Nevertheless, he interprets the mind-cure gospel "as having dignity and importance" in expressing part of the truth: "the systematic cultivation of healthy-mindedness as a religious attitude is therefore consonant with important currents in human nature."[21] James's moral-therapeutic outlook is optimistic without being Pollyannaish, and in other writings he used "healthy-mindedness" to refer to affirming what is good rather than affirming everything as good.[22] His faith in human capacities to effect positive change probably emerged from his struggles in overcoming his depression in his mid-twenties. In addition, James emphasizes good habits,[23] an idea prominent in my discussion of alcoholism, pathological gambling, and other addictions.

John Dewey, the pragmatist whom I cite most often, expands James's emphasis on healthy habits in connection with my themes—healthy morality, responsibility for health, and moral-laden mental health. Like James, Dewey is creative in both psychology and philosophy. He understands virtues and vices as habits, and he considers character to be "the interpenetration of habits." Because each of us is a combination of good and bad habits, "all character is speckled."[24] And because habits have a "propulsive power," bad habits can gain control of us and lead to acts we are ashamed of. Yet, "when we are honest with ourselves we acknowledge that a habit has this power because it is so intimately a part of ourselves. It has a hold upon us because we are the habit."[25] Intelligent habits need to replace destructive ones.

Individual responsibility for bad habits, however, must be understood in conjunction with citizens' collective responsibilities for maintaining a decent society. Dewey calls for psychological realism: the need to tailor moral demands to what can reasonably be expected of human beings in light of their social circumstances. He also highlights future-oriented responsibilities and downplays guilt, blame, and unrealistic ideals that "involve human nature in unending civil war."[26] Nevertheless, Dewey takes seriously personal responsibility for health, and he leaves room for reasonable blame and self-blame oriented toward growth.[27] The self that grows is defined in relation to others and to communities. In this way, psychological growth is a moral process, and maturity is a moral achievement.

Dewey repeatedly cautions against dichotomies that limit our resources for solving problems. He calls for "doing away once for all with the traditional distinction between moral goods, like the virtues, and natural goods like health."[28] Far from standing in opposition to health and the therapies which promote it, morality is "concerned with the health, efficiency and happiness of a development of human nature."[29] Conversely, mental health provides essential capacities for moral agency, and healthy habits partly define moral character.

Sound moral outlooks are healthy in that they are defined by personal growth. Morality degrades into a "pathology of goodness" when it is reduced to prohibitions and blaming (rather than to growth of individuals and institutions), priggish self-righteousness (rather than responsible engagement in the world), fanaticism (rather than balanced moral reasoning), and the sentimental disengagement of ethics from the practical world (rather than psychological realism about personal agency and environmental influences). These unhealthy forms of morality are countered by the scientific understanding of human nature. We must continuously apply "a fund of growing knowledge" that enables us to "locate the points of effective endeavor" and to "state problems in such forms that action could be courageously and intelligently directed to their solution."[30]

Dewey does not attempt to derive morality from psychology, unlike some humanistic psychologists.[31] Much less does he reduce morality to psychological tendencies of power and bias, unlike postmodern pragmatists who challenge the possibility of objective moral reasoning. He insists we are capable of intelligent moral reasoning that results in morally reasonable conduct. Moral reasoning is not the application of simple rules. Instead, it consists in reasonably integrating moral values within situations of conflict and doubt—including about what it means to be healthy.[32]

Like all concepts, "health" serves practical purposes. Dewey urges that we stop defining health abstractly, as an ideal or static state. Instead, we should think of it as an ongoing process, interwoven with all our endeavors and relationships in seeking a meaningful life. Rather than the noun "health," we should make prominent the adjective "healthy" and the adverb "healthily." In turn, healthy living should be understood contextually, for "how to live healthily or justly is a matter which differs with every person."[33] Moreover, there is no fixed self, no unchanging soul, but, instead, a mixture of habits requiring continual integration and balancing. Healthy living is a dynamic process in response to particular stresses, frailties, and other challenges to growth.[34] This process requires not only curing ailments but also healthy living that brings "simple and spontaneous joy, vigor and achievement."[35]

James, Dewey, and other pragmatists pave the way for integrating moral and therapeutic perspectives around an ideal of *moral health*—mental well-being based on moral integrity.[36] They were not the first to do so, however. The roots of the therapeutic trend reach back to classical Greek and Roman ethics of character–virtue ethics. In particular, Plato argues that virtue and mental health are identical, as are vice and psychopathology (see chapter 1).[37] Then, the Stoics and Epicureans developed moral-therapeutic views in order to cope in a deeply troubled world. Today, virtue ethics is undergoing a renaissance in which many philosophers seek to integrate morality and psychological understanding.

For example, Lawrence Becker revives the Stoics' therapeutic-oriented ethics. He envisions a conception of psychological health that "will include effective powers of deliberation and choice, and the disposition to use them. It will include curiosity, abundant agent energy, a developed self-concept, and a disposition to regularize, to seek consistency and integration within and among one's endeavors."[38] Psychological health excludes tendencies that undermine moral agency, such as severe phobias and depression; tendencies such as malice and hostility that undermine social interactions and cooperation; lack of control over impulses; and inability to experience happiness.[39] All these disorders are impairments of basic capacities required for responsible moral agency.

Agreeing with Becker, I argue that the capacities defining psychological health are not mere prerequisites for virtue. Instead, they are partly defined by the virtues, and in turn the virtues embody healthy habits. Moral values also guide definitions of much pathology, including antisocial dispositions, lack of self-control over impulses, and anhedonia. These pathologies are "abnormal" because the normal is understood largely in moral terms. We overlook these connections when we associate virtue with the higher reaches of moral excellence, what Becker calls "moral virtuosity." Yet, basic responsibility itself embodies a level of moral decency that tacitly shapes conceptions of psychological health.

In drawing on virtue ethics and pragmatism I am not implying that other ethical theories lack importance in integrating morality and psychotherapy. Virtue ethics needs to be complemented by theories about obligations and rights which specify much of the content of the virtues. Thus, honesty is the virtue of truthfulness and trustworthiness, but neither of these ideas can be understood without invoking obligations to keep promises and avoid deception.[40] Likewise, pragmatism needs to be complemented by the fuller specifications of moral requirements provided by other ethical theories. In places I invoke additional ethical traditions. For example, I draw on Kant's emphasis on duties to oneself in understanding the virtue of self-respect and in connection with responsibilities for our health. I emphasize human rights in thinking about justice in both punishment and in health care. I discuss Nietzsche as a key thinker who bridges classical virtue ethics and modern psychological understanding. And my thinking is influenced by communitarians such as Charles Taylor and Robert Wuthnow, who are simultaneously critics of some parts of the therapeutic trend and contributors to an integrated, moral-therapeutic perspective. If my approach to ethical theory is ecumenical, it is because I believe that all major moral traditions have insights to offer.

Having linked the therapeutic trend to classical virtue ethics, and before turning to a discussion of Plato, I reaffirm there is something distinctively American about the therapeutic trend, as distinctive as American pragmatism—and American jazz. Neal O. Weiner suggests the contemporary "semi-moral/semi-medical way of thinking about what the self ought to be" constitutes "an original American contribution to popular ethics, the moral equivalent of jazz."[41] Like jazz, integrations of morality and therapy take many forms, some more creative than others, but many of them are important in understanding American society.

Part I
MENTAL HEALTH AND
MORAL VIRTUE

It appears, then, that virtue is as it were the health and comeliness and well-being of the soul, as wickedness is disease, deformity, and weakness.

Plato, *Republic*

The popular medical formulation of morality . . . , "virtue is the health of the soul," would, in order to be useful, have to be changed at least to read, "your virtue is the health of your soul." For there is no health as such, and all attempts to define such a thing have failed miserably.

Friedrich Nietzsche, *The Gay Science*

How to live healthily or justly is a matter which differs with every person. It varies with his past experience, his opportunities, his temperamental and acquired weaknesses and abilities.

John Dewey, *Reconstruction in Philosophy*

I

MORAL SICKNESS

Plato and the Psychiatrists

In the *Republic*, Plato undertakes the most famous integration of morality and mental health: "It appears, then, that virtue is as it were the health and comeliness and well-being of the soul, as wickedness is disease, deformity, and weakness."[1] Plato proposes that the health of the mind consists in exercising the cardinal virtues: practical wisdom in making judgments, courage in confronting dangers, temperance in satisfying appetites, and justice in manifesting inner harmony in desirable conduct. Immorality is the absence of healthy self-governance, whether due to ignorance, cowardice, lack of self-control, or inner chaos. For Plato, "moral health" and "moral sickness" are not mere metaphors. They refer to mental health and pathology as defined by concepts of virtue and vice.

Critics of the therapeutic trend denounce Plato's proposal as a dangerous confusion—dangerous, because equating morality with mental health gives health professionals alarming power in moral matters; confusion, because mental health and virtue are entirely different.[2] I agree that morality and mental health should not be equated, but I affirm Plato's core insight: mental health and moral virtue are significantly interwoven in their meaning and reference. This is true when mental health is defined negatively, as the absence of mental disorders, which is the topic of this chapter. It is even more obvious when mental health is defined positively, as psychological well-being, which is the topic of chapter 2.

Plato's Proposal Revised

To illustrate what Plato means by moral sickness, consider Judge David W. Lanier. For years Lanier abused his authority as a judge and the most powerful political figure in Dyer County, Tennessee, by exploiting vulnerable women during divorce proceedings, child custody disputes, child support hearings, and applications for jobs as his secretary. Sometimes he would grab and fondle his victims; other times he would coerce sex acts from them. He was a compulsive sexual predator with "a sensibility in which sex, hate, and the lust for power were so intertwined as to be indistinguishable."[3] Eventually he was convicted on two felony counts of coerced sex and several additional charges of sexual assault.

Lanier is immoral, and he is sick. That is what Plato would have us say, and that is what we naturally do say. We have difficulty, however, understanding how both ascriptions can be true simultaneously. Calling Lanier sick seems to excuse him, at least somewhat. We are hamstrung by a morality-therapy dichotomy that polarizes responsibility and sickness. We have two choices. We can embrace the morality-therapy dichotomy and regard sickness as an automatic excuse for wrongdoing. Doing so would lead us to oppose the therapeutic trend as threatening moral responsibility. Alternatively, we can renounce the dichotomy and reject the assumption that sickness automatically exempts from responsibility. This choice, which I favor, invites a more sympathetic response to the therapeutic trend, while enjoining care in determining exactly when sickness mitigates responsibility for wrongdoing. It also enables us to view Lanier as both sick and responsible, as surely he is.

Whatever the origin of his impulses to exploit women, Lanier is responsible for restraining those impulses and for changing the attitudes that led to them, if necessary by seeking help. No doubt, once the impulses grew strong he faced special psychological obstacles to acting responsibly. He developed a *moral handicap*—an obstacle to exercising immediate responsible control.[4] Yet, the handicap was self-created. Moreover, his psychopathology is not separable from his immorality, as a cause from its effect. Instead, his sickness *is* his immorality—his entrenched habits of cruelty and exploitation and the motivation underlying them. Hence, calling him sick does not excuse; if anything, it accentuates his wrongdoing. Because moral values define his sickness, it makes sense to speak of "moral sickness."[5] In general, individuals are morally and mentally sick when their wrongdoing becomes extensive, extreme, and entrenched.

If we go beyond Lanier's conduct to diagnose his specific mental disorder and its inner sources, we risk becoming amateur psychiatrists. Even so, common sense and "folk psychology" invite some movement inward, while retaining the primary external reference to wrongdoing. Thus, we quite naturally follow Plato's lead in describing Lanier as divided, distorted, unbalanced, in conflict with himself as a moral agent and judge. Etymologically, "health" means wholeness. It carries additional connotations of balance, effective functioning, integration of diverse desires and functions, and self-regulating mechanisms of rational self-reflection and self-restraint.[6] In contrast, Lanier's eroticized aggression distorts normal desires for sex and power, and it overrides his self-regulative desires in ways that harm both him and his victims.

Caution is needed in transplanting Plato's idea of healthy souls into contemporary discussions of mental health. The Greek word *psyche* translates variously as mind, soul, or living force, and Plato adds connotations of moral character.[7] Nevertheless, Plato's proposal that virtue is the health of the soul is not the mere tautology that virtue is good character. Indeed, Plato integrates morality with a psychological theory that is not altogether alien to us. His tripartite division of the mind into reason, spirited element, and appetites adumbrates Freud's division of the mind into ego, superego, and id.[8] Like Freud, he divides the mind into functional parts in order to make sense of inner conflict. He suggests that the mind, like the body, is healthy when its various parts perform their functions well. To perform a function well is to perform it in accord with relevant virtues. Thus, reason performs its task of rational self-governance when guided by wisdom, based on discerning moral goodness; the appetites perform their function of sustaining life when guided by reason in accordance with temperance; the spirited element—something like a sense of honor and shame—performs its auxiliary function of supporting reason's commands when guided by courage; and the ensuing inner harmony manifested in desirable conduct constitutes justice. The opposite occurs in Lanier; his appetites dominate his reason and sense of honor. His psyche is out of balance and dysfunctional.

To be clear, Plato would not say Lanier is sick simply because he has immoral desires. He is sick because those desires are strong and habitual, so as to render his character disordered. In a passage foreshadowing Freud, Plato writes of "unlawful desires" that "bestir themselves in dreams" and in fantasy "will not shrink from intercourse with a mother or anyone else . . . or any deed of blood."[9] In addition to misdirected lust, he uses examples of compulsive drinkers, overeaters, individuals morbidly preoccupied with death, and megalomaniacs whose lust for power grows beyond all bounds of decency. In each case, the individuals are sick because they allow natural desires to become misdirected or excessive.

We need not explore Plato's psychological theory further. His (and Freud's) idea that human desires, emotions, and functions can be neatly sorted into three categories is too simple. Indeed, we can understand mental conflict as clashing desires, and moral reasoning as a response to that conflict, without partitioning the mind. Furthermore, Plato's belief that immorality always involves inner turmoil is simply false—witness the calm sociopathic murderer or the fanatic religious terrorist. In short, we can follow Plato's lead in conceiving mental health as virtue-structured well-being without embracing his psychological theory.

But should we follow his lead? Not completely. Morality and mental health are not identical, either in meaning or reference. They diverge at four junctures. First, morality and mental health do not overlap with regard to severe brain dysfunctions and neurological disorders over which a person has no control. For example, dementia comprises a large category of organically-caused mental diseases involving severe cognitive defects that undermine moral agency.[10] Advanced Alzheimer's disease literally destroys the mind by causing permanent memory impairment, loss of language mastery, inability to identify persons and objects, and incapacity to act. The idea of lacking virtue has no application here, and blaming hapless victims of such diseases is barbarism.

Second, many mild mental disorders, such as minor phobias, are innocuous and largely irrelevant to morality. Like a cold, a mild case of arachnophobia causes distress, but not enough to threaten moral agency. Some disorders even have morally beneficial consequences, as with many "workaholics," who channel their compulsions in socially useful directions, and persons whose suffering deepens their compassion for others.

Third, shifting to immorality, isolated acts of weakness of will, lapses of judgment, negligence, and maliciousness need not involve psychopathology. An individual who only once drives while intoxicated manifests poor judgment, not sickness. It is otherwise with habitual drunk drivers. As Plato and Alcoholics Anonymous would agree, drug addicts are both sick and morally responsible for the harm they cause. In general, only entrenched or egregious wrongdoing warrants talk of sickness.

Fourth, the higher reaches of virtue—including conscientiousness, heroism, and a nuanced sense of justice—are not the same as superlative mental health. Heroic courage and compassion are more than superlative mental health. Indeed, moral commitment can involve sacrificing aspects of mental health. Courageous whistleblowers, for example, often suffer enormous anxiety and depression in the pursuit of moral ideals. And a person who avoids serious immorality might be mentally healthy while lacking serious moral aspiration.

Morality and mental health are not identical, then. Nevertheless, they extensively overlap and interweave in two key areas: basic habits defining responsible agency, and positive health. I next connect the lack of basic habits of responsible agency with mental disorders, as defined by contemporary psychiatry.

DSM: Distress, Disability, Danger

The most influential definition of mental disorders is found in the American Psychiatric Association's *Diagnostic and Statistical Manual of Mental Disorders* (*DSM*). This authoritative tome standardizes clinical discourse for practical purposes, such as funding clinical research and billing insurance companies and government agencies for services rendered by all types of psychotherapists. The *DSM* defines mental disorders as patterns of overt behavior and states involving unacceptable distress, disability, and increased danger. More fully, a mental disorder is any "behavioral or psychological syndrome or pattern that occurs in an individual and that is associated with present distress (e.g., a painful symptom) or disability (i.e., impairment in one or more important areas of functioning) or with a significantly increased risk of suffering death, pain, disability, or an important loss of freedom."[11]

The scope of the definition is breathtaking. It encompasses virtually all undesirable habits and personality traits that significantly disrupt lives by causing distress, difficulty in functioning, or danger. The scope is further widened because the key notions in the definition are left undefined, including "distress," "disability," and "impairment." The *DSM* adds two important caveats, however. First, a syndrome or pattern must not be an "expectable and culturally sanctioned response to a particular event, for example, the death of a loved one." Thus, grief at the death of a loved one is not a mental disorder, even if it impairs normal functioning for a time. Pathological depression occurs only when the disruption in their lives becomes extreme, relative to social norms. In this way, disorders are in part relative to cultural values.

Not all socially disapproved behaviors are mental disorders, however: The *DSM* does not equate deviancy with disorder. According to the second caveat, objectionable conduct must manifest a dysfunction: "Neither deviant behavior (e.g., political, religious, or sexual) nor conflicts that are primarily between the individual and society are mental disorders unless the deviance or conflict is a symptom of a dysfunction in the individual."[12] The force of this caveat is diminished, however, when "dysfunction" is defined largely in terms of socially unacceptable behavior. This occurs frequently. For example, it occurs explicitly in definitions of antisocial personality disorder (sociopathy), pyromania, and pedophilia; it occurs implicitly in definitions of substance dependency, pathological gambling, and other addictions. In such instances, the *DSM* definitions of mental disorders allude to standards of acceptable and unacceptable conduct, using such terms as "excessive," "inappropriate," "unexpected," and "maladaptive."[13] Directly or indirectly, moral values shape the definitions of most mental disorders.

What exactly is "a dysfunction in the individual"? Because psychiatry is dominated by a biomedical model that seeks to uncover organic causes for mental disorders, we might assume that "dysfunction" means organic impairment, such as chemical malfunctions and brain damage, which make it impossible for a person to function normally. Not so! The *DSM* defines mental disorders descriptively, in terms of how people actually behave, feel, desire, and intend.[14] Impairment and dysfunction refer to difficulties in functioning, without claiming the impossibility of change. Again, the causation of disorders is distinct from their definition, and often it is left open for ongoing research. Regardless of their etiology, mental disorders include any pronounced distress, difficulty in functioning, or serious risk of self-harm (beyond culturally sanctioned behaviors such as fighting in a war).

For example, persons with alcohol dependency disorder are said to be impaired because they systematically abuse alcohol, persistently try but fail to quit drinking, continue to drink despite knowing the damage the alcohol is causing, abandon important activities to obtain and use alcohol, and experience distressful tolerance and withdrawal effects.[15] These patterns of behavior and suffering constitute the impairment and the dysfunction, bypassing speculation about whether the person was unable to do otherwise. Again, several large categories delineate areas that Plato would call lack of practical wisdom and rational self-control: drug abuse, eating disorders such as anorexia and bulimia, kleptomania, pyromania, and pathological gambling. The same is true of the grab-bag category "Impulse-Control Disorder Not Otherwise Specified," where impulse control disorder is not complete incapacitation but simply "the failure to resist an impulse, drive, or temptation to perform an act that is harmful to the person or to others."[16] Judge Lanier might find a home in this last category, if not in "Sexual Disorder Not Otherwise Specified."

Personality disorders have special interest. They, too, are defined in terms of overt patterns of maladaptive behavior, attitude, and emotion. For example, "Antisocial Personality Disorder is a pattern of disregard for, and violation of, the rights of others"; "Narcissistic Personality Disorder is a pattern of grandiosity, need for admiration, and lack of empathy"; "Avoidant Personality Disorder is a pattern of social inhibition, feelings of inadequacy, and hypersensitivity to negative evaluation"; and "Paranoid Personality Disorder is a pattern of distrust and suspiciousness such that others' motives are interpreted as malevolent."[17] Plato would consider personality disorders to be character flaws, and so do most of us.

There is an important corollary to the *DSM*'s separation of definition and etiology, concept and causation. Diagnosing a mental disorder does not automatically exempt an individual from responsibility for causing the disorder, much less for the harm caused by the disorder. Of course, some mental disorders do exempt from responsibility, especially those involving severe brain damage. But the *DSM* definitions leave open the extent of responsibility in a given instance. The *DSM* underscores this point with a prominently-placed Cautionary Statement: "The clinical and scientific considerations involved in categorization of these conditions as mental disorders may not be wholly relevant to legal judgments, for example, that take into account such issues as individual responsibility, disability determination, and competency."[18] At least in intent, the *DSM* is not a book of legal and moral excuses—a point to which I return frequently.

Power to Define

Moral values shape definitions of mental disorders, and yet psychiatrists have the authority to define the disorders, as well as to treat them. This power to define raises concerns about therapeutic tyranny. What if psychiatrists (and other health professionals) abuse their power by making unwarranted value judgments, especially by uncritically incorporating biases that are widespread in society?

Psychiatrists now acknowledge, for example, that unjustified value judgments led to pathologizing homosexuality by including it in the *DSM* prior to 1973. Bigotry was even more obviously involved in "inventing" the nineteenth-century mental illness drapetomania—the desire of slaves to escape from their owners. Clearly, social bias often masquerades as medical expertise.[19] In general, therapeutic tyranny is especially likely when psychiatrists deny or disguise their moral judgments, wrapping themselves in the mantle of morally neutral science.[20] The same concealment of moral presuppositions occurs in health psychology. Over and over again, the therapeutic trend shifts from explicit moral judgments to hidden ones embedded in talk of "disorders," "maladjustment," and "abnormality."[21] This easily leads to abusing power.

Historically, the most flagrant abuses involved coerced confinement and experimentation without informed consent. These abuses arose from the paternalistic assumption that psychiatrists knew best what is good for disordered individuals.[22] Other times the abuses arose because psychiatry served political purposes, as in the former Soviet Union, by defining social dissidents as sick. Anthony Kenny blames Plato for paving the way for this "replacement of judges by doctors" and "redescribing moral phenomena in medical terms," such that "all criminals are [viewed as] sick rather than vicious people."[23] Kenny is most concerned about abuses that occur when the medical establishment is given authority to hospitalize individuals indefinitely. This practice has dramatically diminished since Kenny wrote. If anything, the de-institutional movement went too far in the other direction by abandoning seriously disturbed individuals to homelessness, without providing a support system. Nevertheless, therapeutic tyranny is a perennial concern.

A new concern about psychiatric power is emerging. The medicalizing of moral problems bolsters public demands for the services of psychiatrists and other health professionals. Most of us do not sharply distinguish between disorders, for which health services are officially intended, and "enhancements" to positive health (well-being). Indeed, when hopes for increased happiness are involved, we are eager to redefine problems as health disorders in order to gain access to health services, especially those funded by insurance and health maintenance organizations (HMOs). The *DSM* conception of mental disorders makes this expansion easy, for almost any problem brought to therapists involves significant distress or difficulty in functioning. In addition, profits provide a steady incentive for psychiatrists to be complicit.

These "feedback effects" are not unique to mental disorders, and they apply equally to medical "enhancement technologies."[24] For example, by performing thousands of operations each year in response to requests for cosmetic surgery to alter Jewish-looking noses, Asian-slanted eyes, or small breasts, surgeons reinforce racist and sexist stereotypes of beauty.[25] Nevertheless, psychiatrists play a dramatic role in shaping public values, for better or worse. The authority to establish expansive definitions of mental disorders implicates psychiatrists in expanding what the public counts as psychological matters, thereby encroaching on moral matters. At least in some instances, psychiatrists create, via their authoritative definitions, the illnesses they then cure.[26] Then, to gain access to health care services, the public itself eagerly expands their conception of health, counting many everyday problems as illness.

Critics of the *DSM* trace therapeutic tyranny and collusion to expansive concepts of mental health and mental disorders. Accordingly, they propose to redefine mental disorders more narrowly, so that fewer moral values are involved, as I illustrate in a moment. In my view, the critics' definitions tend to be far too narrow, constricting our understanding of mental health. No definition can prevent therapeutic tyranny. Instead, two things are needed to limit psychiatric power: awareness that mental health is moral-laden, and legal safeguards.

First, as citizens we need to be aware of how value judgments shape psychiatrists' definitions of mental disorders. The abuse of psychiatric power ultimately derives from the illusion that mental disorders can be defined by value-neutral science. But the generic definition of disorders and the specific disorders listed in the *DSM* are value-laden: they combine scientific understanding with moral judgments about harm and "social dysfunction." Rem Edwards observes that "most philosophically minded thinkers who have looked critically at the concepts of 'mental health' and 'mental illness' have found them to be inherently value-laden. This means that evaluative components as well as descriptive elements are inescapably a part of their meaning."[27] What is crucial is to ensure that the relevant values are justified. The *DSM* definition of mental disorders relies on values that are both justified and virtually universal: significant distress, mental dysfunction, and increased risk of death and loss of freedom are bad. For this reason, although the *DSM* definition must be used with great care, it remains useful.[28]

Second, we need reasonable laws and policies that limit psychiatrists' power. These safeguards should be tailored to specific dangers in particular contexts, such as therapeutic contexts, insurance coverage, government funding of health care, and law. Consider laws about involuntary civil commitment. The deinstitutional movement remedied most of the abuses of the state-run and psychiatrist-guided coercion. It did so not by applying a narrow definition of mental illness but, instead, by laws limiting involuntary commitment to individuals who are both mentally ill *and* who pose a clear and present danger of serious harm, to themselves or to others. The new need is to help the large numbers of seriously ill people we have abandoned to the streets without proper care, but that problem, too, must be solved with better social policies, not definitions.

Alternative Definitions of Mental Disorders

Although I usually rely on the *DSM* definitions of mental disorders, I sometimes refer to alternative definitions as a reminder that there is no consensus about what mental disorders are. In a preliminary way, let us sample a few such definitions.

Organic Diseases

In opposition to Plato, Anthony Kenny recommends limiting mental disorders to organic malfunctions. They are "mental" disorders only because underlying biological malfunctions generate psychological symptoms—for example, irrational perception and disordered emotions and reasoning. Whereas brain disorders are real, "mental illness" in any other sense is a metaphor; literally, a myth. It amounts to "redescribing moral phenomena in medical terms." For example, sociopaths (or psychopaths) are not literally sick: "If a psychopath is given psychotherapy, we have a case in which neither the alleged causes of the condition (e.g. a broken home), nor its symptoms (e.g. petty theft), nor its cure (e.g. group discussions) has anything in common with the causes, symptoms, or cure of organic diseases."[29]

Earlier, the psychiatrist Thomas Szasz limited mental disorders to organic incapacitations. Everything beyond organic diseases, including most of the *DSM* categories, he said, are problems in living, such as difficulties in getting along with other people. "Mental illness is a myth," akin to witchcraft, "whose function it is to disguise and thus render more palatable the bitter pill of moral conflicts in human relations." For half a century, Szasz has vigorously campaigned against the abuses of psychiatric power that occur when we allow psychiatrists to redefine moral matters in health terms. In his view, we have created "a situation in which psychosocial, ethical, and/or legal deviations are claimed to be correctable by (so-called) medical action."[30]

Kenny and Szasz assert a morality-therapy dichotomy: health concerns organic incapacities, and organic incapacities lessen moral accountability; all other problematic behavior concerns problems in living which we are required to deal with responsibly. In my terms, they interpret the therapeutic trend as a replacement project, in which the domain of morality shrinks as the medical domain expands. But there is another possibility, the one I explore in this book: the therapeutic trend is primarily an integrative project. Plato did not replace morality by therapy but instead integrated them; so, for the most part, do Americans and psychiatrists.

In opposing medical tyranny, Szasz underscores the danger that superficial treatment of symptoms with pharmacology deflects attention from deeper problems, such as a troubled marriage or a dangerous work environment. But, to the contrary, using effective therapeutic approaches in helping people cope more effectively with problems is morally desirable. Restricting mental disorders to organic disorders limits the full potential for psychiatry to help people with a wide range of problems that have both moral and health dimensions. Problems with alcohol, drugs, low self-esteem, and myriad additional *DSM* matters can accurately be described as problems in living, but they remain mental health issues for which we need the resources of psychiatry.

Psychological Incapacity

Mental disorders are sometimes defined as the absence of normal psychological capacities, regardless of whether the absence is traceable to organic dysfunctions. Here "normal" is defined purely descriptively as capacities that are statistically typical. Thus, mental health consists in being able to perceive, feel, reason, and act in ways typical of humans at a given stage of development.

Mark Pestana adopts this conception of mental disorders and health in a book-length rejection of Plato's project. According to Pestana, mental health is a set of typical capacities or potentialities to act, feel, and reason. Whereas virtue is "activity which occurs in accord with the rules or principles of morality," "health not only does not entail a disposition to perform activities of a certain type [but] it, strictly speaking, does not entail *any* activities at all." Stated in another way, virtue consists in manifesting morally *good habits*, and vice consists in voluntary wrongdoing or culpable negligence. In contrast, mental health consists of *psychological capacities* that can be used for good or bad, and sickness is the absence of these capacities (in varying degrees). Moreover, the capacities have no impetus in moral directions, and a completely healthy person might be completely evil.[31]

Pestana's definition has some basis in common sense, for sometimes we do think of mental health as general psychological abilities.[32] But common sense has other, incompatible threads that are now more prominent. Usually we conceive of mental health as much more than simply *having* general capacities or potentialities to act and feel. Mental health includes *exercising* those capacities in healthy—and moral—ways, for example by maintaining self-esteem, coping effectively with stress, avoiding dangerous practices like drug abuse and reckless driving, and not engaging in repeated and egregious crime. In this connection, it is noteworthy that Pestana fails to offer a single example of an evil person who is mentally healthy. Hitler, Stalin, Saddam Hussein, and sociopaths are hardly paragons of psychological health.[33]

Severe Mental Incapacity

Another proposal is to restrict mental disorders to the most severe incapacitations, regardless of whether their origins are biological, psychological, or social. Rem Edwards offers such a proposal: "'Mental illness' means only those undesirable mental/behavioral deviations which involve primarily an extreme and prolonged inability to know and deal in a rational and autonomous way with oneself and one's social and physical environment. In other words, madness is extreme and prolonged practical irrationality and irresponsibility."[34]

One difficulty with Edwards's definition is the vagueness of "extreme inability." Is the mentally ill person physically unable to do otherwise, which would return us to Szasz's view? Or is the person unable without great effort, more than can reasonably be expected of a person, with values specifying what can "reasonably" be expected of an individual? Even if we could agree on a standard for "inability," however, it is clear that Edwards restricts mental disorders to full-blown madness, the moral equivalent of legal insanity. That definition is useful for some purposes, especially legal ones, but it is too narrow to guide our thinking about emotional and behavioral problems that do not involve madness, such as impulse control disorders and substance abuse problems.

Harmful Dysfunctions

Yet another suggestion is to make explicit the moral content of mental disorders while linking it to some notion of impairment. Thus, Jerome C. Wakefield defines mental disorders as harmful dysfunctions: "*Dysfunction* is a scientific and factual term based on evolutionary biology that refers to the failure of an internal mechanism to perform a natural function for which it was designed, and *harmful* is a value term referring to the consequences that occur to the person because of the dysfunction and are deemed negative by sociocultural standards."[35]

Wakefield's view of harm is relativistic—simply what social customs specify as objectionable. He would do better to replace it with a more objective notion of justified standards, such as the *DSM*'s tacit notion of rational desires to avoid unacceptable distress, disability, and danger. Such a shift permits us to say that until 1973 the American Psychiatric Association was mistaken in listing homosexuality as a mental disorder because unjustified moral standards were used. Even with this emendation, however, Wakefield's definition is still problematic in limiting mental disorders to biological dysfunctions. We have evolved with many additional psychological functions that can perform in healthy or unhealthy ways, and specifying these functions alludes to moral values.

Relativistic Definitions

A final approach is to define mental disorders as entirely relative to society's moral values. Mental health is simply whatever society approves as "normal," and disease and disorder are things it disapproves of. In Ruth Benedict's words, "the concept of the normal is properly a variant of the concept of the good. It is that which society has approved. A normal action is one which falls well within the limits of expected behavior for a particular society."[36] Relativistic definitions can be used to endorse expansionist proposals, but more often they are used to oppose expansionism by alerting us to abuses and by suggesting the ultimate arbitrariness of what counts as mental disorders. Again, relativistic definitions sometimes endorse psychiatrists' power, but more often they undermine psychiatrists' claim to have scientific authority for their definitions.

Social constructivism, a sophisticated version of relativism, claims that societies construct concepts of mental health and illness as subcategories of similarly constructed concepts of good and bad. Societies do so for many reasons, but primarily to assert the power of dominant groups. Psychiatrists, then, become agents of social control, as Michel Foucault illuminates. The problem with Foucault and social constructivists, indeed with all relativists, however, is that they leave little room for reasoned dialogue about when that control is morally justified or not—thereby reducing moral values themselves to expressions of social control.[37] Inspired by Foucault, Peter Conrad and Joseph W. Schneider reduce morality to "the product of certain people [with power] making claims based on their own particular interests, values, and views of the world." According to Conrad and Schneider, the therapeutic trend redefines social deviancy by medicalizing morality, and concealing morality as medicine fosters therapeutic tyranny: "Health standards and regulations can become little more than tools for political coercion and oppression."[38]

What do social constructionists have to offer as an alternative? Usually, they rest content with critiquing abuses of power, whether in the guise of morality or science. Precisely because they tend to undermine the validity of moral principles, they are left without a basis for engaging in moral reasoning aimed at showing what is and is not an abuse. Once they identify abuses, they have little further to contribute, and even their identification of abuses is without a firm basis in objectively defensible standards, which they believe do not exist. In opposition to social constructionists and other relativists, I proceed in the conviction that there are objective moral standards, including human rights and basic decency, in understanding mental health and in developing an integrated, moral-therapeutic perspective.

To conclude, there will always be controversy about the correct definitions of mental health and illness, if only because we disagree about the values that should shape the definitions. The important point is that moral values matter as we reflect on questions about mental health and mental disorders. Definitions serve different purposes. For the purposes of insurance payments for mental disorders, we might reasonably seek to limit the scope of mental disorders, congruent with financial resources. Even so, the emphasis in the *DSM* on mental disorders as significant and undesirable distress, disability, and danger of harm is for many purposes useful, and I make frequent reference to it. For other purposes, such as exploring personal growth and self-fulfillment, we might employ more positive definitions of mental health, such as those taken up in the next chapter.

2

MORAL HEALTH

Well-Being and the Virtues

Just as moral values shape conceptions of mental disorders, they structure positive conceptions of mental health. Positively conceived, mental health is the presence of psychological well-being and effective functioning, in addition to the absence of mental disorders. The most influential definition of positive health is set forth by the United Nations World Health Organization (WHO): "Health is a state of complete physical, mental and social well-being, not merely the absence of disease or infirmity."[1] The idea of *complete* well-being seems too ideal to be useful, and it also seems to encompass forms of well-being that go beyond health, for example financial success. Some thinkers recommend switching to *adequate* mental and physical well-being.[2] Yet, if "adequate" simply means the ability to function without being crippled by disorders, then positive and negative definitions coalesce, especially as the therapeutic trend expands the range of mental disorders. I find the distinction between positive and negative definitions worth preserving. To that end, I understand positive mental health as *ample* or *abundant* mental well-being, which falls somewhere between complete and adequate psychological well-being. In turn, mental health spans the range from ample to good, and from suboptimal to severe disorder. In any case, positive conceptions of health invariably embody or presuppose moral values.

In 1958, Marie Jahoda observed that "there is hardly a term in current psychological thought as vague, elusive, and ambiguous as the term 'mental health,'" and her observation remains true today.[3] It is a testament to her insight that the six (overlapping) criteria she identified for positive health remain the starting point for many contemporary discussions. With slight rewording, those criteria are (1) self-esteem, (2) psychological integration, (3) personal autonomy, (4) self-actualization, (5) social coping, and (6) realistic cognition.[4] I argue that these criteria are closely linked, respectively, to self-respect, integrity, moral autonomy, authenticity, responsibility, and truthfulness. They are not synonymous with these virtues, however, and each feature can be unfolded in

subjective or objective directions, thereby reflecting ambiguities in the therapeutic trend.

Self-Esteem and Self-Respect

Self-esteem is the cornerstone of most contemporary conceptions of positive
mental health, but what is it?[5] At one extreme, self-esteem is entirely subjective:
the tendency to have positive emotions and attitudes about oneself. The basis for
these emotions and attitudes might be driving a fancy car, being attractive,
succeeding as a thief, or any number of nonmoral things.[6] At the other extreme,
self-esteem includes self-respect—the virtue of properly valuing ourselves as
having moral worth. This ambiguity is present in the writings of both philosophers and health psychologists.

To begin with philosophers, John Rawls equates self-esteem with self-
respect, which "includes a person's sense of his own value, his secure conviction
that his conception of his good, his plan of life, is worth carrying out," together
with "a confidence in one's ability, so far as it is within one's power, to fulfill
one's intentions."[7] Rawls's definition fails to convey that self-respect, as a virtue,
implies a *justified* sense of one's worth based on engaging in *desirable* or *permissible* plans. Admittedly, the words "self-esteem" and "self-respect" are ambiguous in ordinary language. Sometimes they denote virtues of properly
appreciating one's worth; other times they merely denote positive self-regard
and self-confidence.[8] Some philosophers use "self-respect" to name a virtue, and
they think of self-esteem as mere feelings of self-affirmation. In contrast, Alan
Gewirth suggests that self-respect and self-esteem denote two different virtues.
Self-respect is the virtue of valuing "one's moral qualities, including one's
dignity as a moral person who is worthy of the respect of other persons"; self-
esteem (echoing Rawls) is the virtue of having "a secure sense of one's own
merits, and thus includes having the conviction that one's plans and purposes
are worthwhile and that one has the ability to carry them out."[9]

Turning to health psychologists, we again encounter a mélange of meanings
of "self-esteem," although most of them are linked to self-respect. For example,
Nathaniel Branden, a guru in the self-help literature, defines self-esteem as "the
integrated sum of self-confidence and self-respect," where self-respect is the
virtue of properly valuing oneself.[10] Brandon adds that the requisite self-
affirmation must be relatively stable and based on accurate beliefs. Likewise,
Richard Bednar and Scott Peterson tell us that "self-esteem is an enduring and
affective sense of personal value based on accurate self-perceptions."[11]

Despite these variations, there is a strong overlap between self-esteem, as used
in defining mental health, and self-respect. To see this, compare an ethicist's
example of lacking self-respect with a therapist's example of low self-esteem.
Ethicist Thomas E. Hill describes a "Deferential Wife" who is single-mindedly
devoted to her husband, organizes her life around him so as to meet his
needs, lives where he wants, entertains his friends, buys clothes for herself that

he likes, and has sex only when he initiates it. Rather than balanced give-and-take in trading sacrifices in one area for support in other areas, "she tends not to form her own interests, values, and ideals; and, when she does, she counts them as less important than her husband's." She does so, at least in part, because she loves her husband and "believes that the proper role for a woman is to serve her family."[12] The Deferential Wife lacks full self-respect, which Hill understands as the virtue of appreciating one's rights as a human being, together with authentically forming and living by personal standards. She manifests the vice of servility, unless her obeisance is required to secure a major benefit such as protection from an abusive husband.

Next consider psychotherapist Theodore Rubin's portrayal of his mother as "exasperating in her compliance" and "complete abandonment of herself" to her husband (Rubin's father). She had a "neurotic need to hate and efface herself" and a hidden rage that is transformed (via a reaction formation) into excessive devotion to others.[13] Rubin does not say whether he thinks his mother meets the *DSM* definition of a dependent personality disorder: "a pervasive and excessive need to be taken care of that leads to submissive and clinging behavior and fears of separation," as manifested in difficulty in initiating projects due to low self-confidence, needing constant reassurance from others, and excessive fears of being alone.[14] But he makes it clear that her self-esteem was distorted and improperly grounded.[15] As this example suggests, when health professionals use self-esteem as a criterion for mental health they typically mean valuing oneself in ways required by self-respect.

This strong overlap, if not strict identity, between self-respect and health-defining self-esteem is even clearer when we turn from low to inappropriately high self-esteem. The *DSM* characterizes narcissistic personality disorder as pervasive grandiosity, arrogance, snobbery, and admiration-seeking that involves excessively high self-evaluations and insensitive devaluations of the contributions of others.[16] Narcissists enter into personal relationships only when doing so brings recognition of their superiority. Whether we say narcissists have excessive self-esteem or the absence of proper self-esteem, their self-appraisals tend to be unstable in ways that render them especially vulnerable to perceived insults and defeats.

Narcissism is a failure of self-respect. Consider snobbery, which Hill understands as the failure to value persons in ways required by human dignity and respect for moral rights. A snob "lets assessments of merit become an exclusive and all-pervasive criterion for grouping people as honorable (insiders) and contemptible (outsiders)."[17] That is, snobs use rankings of social class, achievement, talent, or even virtue as a basis for dismissing entire groups of people as having lesser worth. Thereby, snobs fail to value persons as having moral dignity, and, ironically, they fail to properly value their own dignity. Snobbery distorts self-worth.

Finally, both self-respect and self-esteem take global and focused (feature-specific) forms. Regarding self-respect, *recognition self-respect* affirms our overall moral worth, whereas *appraisal self-respect* affirms our particular virtues and achievements.[18] We have recognition self-respect, Kant would say, when we appreciate our dignity as moral agents, which implies accepting our duties to ourselves, such as to develop our talents, keep our capacities for rational agency in good order, and take care of our health.[19] We have appraisal self-respect when we properly value ourselves for our particular virtues and achievements. In a parallel manner, psychologists distinguish global self-esteem (which is a broadly focused sense of one's general worth) and feature-specific self-esteem (which is focused on particular qualities or achievements).[20] When health professionals make self-esteem a mark of mental health, they usually have in mind justified, global, and stable self-esteem.[21] As such, health-defining self-esteem strongly overlaps with recognition self-respect.

Integration and Integrity

Psychological integration requires that the primary elements in our personalities are interrelated and expressed in ways that promote effective functioning.[22] This implies ongoing self-awareness and self-monitoring aimed at maintaining consistency.[23] Jahoda identifies several aspects of psychological integration, each of which alludes to moral values. One aspect is a "balance of psychic forces," which means that important parts of our personalities are expressed in acceptable and compatible ways. Another aspect is "resistance to stress," which is coping with problems without debilitating anxiety and depression. Still another aspect is "a unifying outlook on life," a perspective that gives meaning and purpose to life.[24] This requirement is prominent in the writings of humanistic psychologists such as Abraham Maslow, Erich Fromm, Victor Frankl, and Carl Rogers, who explicitly integrate mental health with moral values.

Words like "coherent," "important," "acceptable" "coping" and "meaning" allude to values. These words, however, can be construed objectively, in terms of justified moral values, or subjectively, in terms of attitudes that might or might not be justified. For example, does a meaning-giving outlook on life refer to a subjective sense of meaning, a sense of significance that might have little connection to justified values? Or does it allude to an outlook that bestows genuine worth on a life? Both senses enter into conceptions of mental health, often without clear demarcation.

Therapists routinely assume moral values in setting forth conceptions of psychological integration. In doing so, they establish links between moral integrity, understood as involving honesty and concern for others, and psychological integration. For example, Margaret Cohen argues that "the exercise of integrity rests fundamentally on the integration of the personality," and vice versa. Even infants develop "constructive, life-avowing impulses," and adults continue "trying to work out what is a reasonable way forward"—a therapist's way of alluding to moral values.[25] In contrast, ethicists typically drive a wedge between psychological integration and the virtue of integrity. Thus, in replying to Cohen, Amelie Oksenberg Rorty says that psychological integration merely requires coherence, lack of conflict, and reflective self-awareness. In contrast, integrity "conjoins honesty and fairness, sincerity and steadfast reliability."[26]

In adjudicating this dispute, we should distinguish isolated actions from general tendencies. Cohen and other therapists are concerned with general tendencies in which psychological integration and moral responsibility coalesce, but they allow isolated exceptions. Rorty is concerned with specific actions. Also, Rorty restricts integrity to honesty and authenticity, omitting basic decency, thereby departing from ordinary language.[27] Ask a person on the street whether a consistent, calm, self-aware evil tyrant has integrity, and the answer will probably be no. Integrity is soundness of moral character, built on a core of basic decency. Cohen captures this idea better than Rorty, as she plausibly connects psychological integration and basic integrity to mental health. Cohen's conception reflects ordinary beliefs in other ways. When parents seek to raise children to have integrity, as part of a healthy personality, they have in mind substantive moral values. Moral integrity and health-defining integration are not synonymous, but they significantly overlap.

Personal Autonomy and Moral Autonomy

Personal autonomy enters into most definitions of mental health, and strengthening personal autonomy is among the most frequently cited goals of psychotherapy, often under the heading of "empowerment."[28] Jahoda begins with a minimal definition emphasizing cognition: "Autonomy means a conscious discrimination by the individual of environmental factors he wishes to accept or reject." She then adds that "conscious discrimination" might involve different things: forming beliefs and desires by exercising reason, living according to one's values and beliefs, not being excessively passive or submissive in forming beliefs and desires, and maintaining an optimal degree of self-direction. In addition, autonomy implies self-control, which involves volition as much as cognition.[29]

For their part, ethicists distinguish personal and moral autonomy. Moral autonomy explicitly refers to moral values, as in Kant's idea of governing our conduct by universally applicable principles of duty. Moral autonomy is the virtue of forming a reasonable moral perspective and using it to guide conduct. In contrast, personal autonomy means self-governance, understood without reference to morality.

This contrast between moral and personal autonomy blurs, however, when autonomy functions as a criterion for mental health. Health-defining autonomy is typically understood to be exercised within the domain of what is morally permissible. When an individual's independent reflection leads to crime, difficulty in holding a job, and destructive personal relationships, it does not manifest health-defining autonomy. Even more obvious, self-control implicitly alludes to morally permissible forms of self-discipline. The compulsive gambler and drug abuser manifest an unhealthy loss of self-control.

Diana T. Meyers plausibly suggests that personal autonomy is best understood as a procedural matter in forming beliefs, desires, commitments, values, and decisions. The procedures consist in exercising certain skills of self-governance within the bounds of what is morally permissible. Autonomous persons are able to pose and answer the question, " 'What do I really want, need, care about, believe, value, etcetera?'; they must be able to act on the answer; and they must be able to correct themselves when they get the answer wrong."[30] Doing so requires exercising "coordinated skills that makes self-discovery, self-definition, and self-direction possible." Accordingly, threats to autonomy come from several directions: coercion and extreme social pressures, internalized social standards that are neither morally defensible nor supportive of human well-being—and psychopathology. As an illustration of psychopathology, Meyers describes a man whose commitments to his profession are neurotic. Sometimes he works with "fiery ambition," and other times he is utterly lackadaisical. His extreme swings in attitude, which arise from ambivalences and anxieties in his personality, undermine his personal and moral autonomy.[31] This is but one of many instances where moral autonomy overlaps with health-defining personal autonomy.

Self-Actualization and Authenticity

Most conceptions of positive mental health include the process variously called self-actualization, self-development, self-fulfillment, or personal growth. Here again we confront a subjective-objective ambiguity. Critics of the therapeutic trend tend to understand self-actualization as a subjective and selfish preoccupation with personal satisfactions. But many psychologists understand health-defining self-actualization by reference to moral values. In this connection, Jahoda highlights again the contributions of humanistic psychologists, who understand self-actualization as forming and pursuing meaningful commitments in love, work, and other valuable activities. As Abraham Maslow observes, "people who seek self-actualization directly, selfishly, personally, dichotomized away from mission in life, i.e., as a form of private and subjective salvation, don't, in fact, achieve it."[32] In this way, self-actualization is intimately connected to authenticity and meaning.

On the one hand, self-actualization is directly tied to the virtue of authenticity. Charles Taylor defines authenticity this way: "Being true to myself means being true to my own originality, and that is something only I can articulate and discover. In articulating it, I am also defining myself. I am realizing a potentiality that is properly my own."[33] Authenticity has become a fundamental virtue because it is an outgrowth of the moral worth of persons. Authenticity is not just any type of making up one's own mind; it implies an ongoing effort to unfold a reasonable conception of who we are and who we most want to be.

Establishing and maintaining an authentic self is difficult because so many forces fragment and diffuse identities. At the same time, we are suspicious of identities that are uniform at the expense of varied engagements and relationships. As the world becomes increasingly complex, our identities become increasingly multifaceted and protean.[34] Subjective tests for authenticity, such as "what feels right," are insufficient to provide guidance, and not only in situations where short-term pleasures overwhelm reason. Thus, an individual undergoing therapy or a major life transformation might initially "feel phony" in developing new modes of interaction.[35] Accordingly, feelings and reasoning must systematically interpenetrate. Despite this complexity, authenticity remains a fundamental moral value promoted by health-defining self-actualization.

On the other hand, health-defining self-actualization is linked to meaningful life. Each of us has multiple talents and moral capacities, only some of which can be fully developed. Self-actualization is personal growth in directions we choose autonomously and in ways we find meaningful. Both a subjective sense of meaning and objective meaning (intelligibility and value) are involved. Meaning is the intelligibility of a life in terms of values. Within therapeutic perspectives there is the tacit assumption that the requisite values are desirable, not just desired. Maslow, for example, begins his famous explorations of self-actualization by reflecting on his mentors whom he deeply admired for their remarkable creativity, openness to new experiences, and moral contributions.[36]

Alan Gewirth distinguishes between subjective and objective self-fulfillment. Subjective or "aspiration" fulfillment is developing one's strongest desires, where strength includes both motivational power and desires one most closely identifies with. In contrast, objective or "capacity" fulfillment brings to fruition one's best capacities, as identified by reference to the full range of (justified) values. In both modes, self-fulfillment is an important value, *if* it is limited by basic moral requirements of respect for human rights. Indeed, the justification of self-fulfillment and rights share a common root in the inherent moral dignity of human beings.[37] Gewirth also suggests that the lack of aspiration can be a sign of pathology, in that that it undermines self-fulfillment.[38] Gewirth's two types of self-fulfillment overlap considerably, and both enter into how health psychologists define mental health.

Coping and Responsibility

Successful coping, or what Jahoda calls environmental mastery, consists in normal functioning in work, interpersonal relationships, love, problem-solving, obeying the law, and other general aspects of social adaptation.[39] As a criterion for mental health, "normal functioning" is moral-laden, at least insofar as it implies meeting minimum standards of social adjustment. Kleptomaniacs and sociopathic murderers do not cope normally, regardless of how successfully they elude the law. At the same time, adequate coping leaves open a wide range of options, from morally minimally acceptable to morally ideal.

Psychologists often avoid explicit invocations of moral concepts in defining coping. For example, C. R. Snyder and Beth L. Dinoff define coping in terms of dealing with stress: "Coping is a response aimed at diminishing the physical, emotional, and psychological burden that is linked to stressful life events and daily hassles. The effectiveness of the coping strategy rests on its ability to reduce immediate distress, as well as to contribute to more long-term outcomes such as psychological well-being or disease status."[40] The reference to positive outcomes such as psychological well-being indirectly alludes to moral standards. Crippling guilt, shame, and self-hatred for betraying standards of decency and responsibility suggest failed coping. As a criterion for mental health, "effective" or "adequate" coping implies responses within the boundaries of morally responsible conduct.

Realistic Cognition and Truthfulness

Realistic cognition includes myriad ways of interpreting the world, but not all. Psychotics who hallucinate and paranoid individuals who see hostile forces everywhere have lost contact with reality. To a lesser degree, so have neurotics whose desires distort their perceptions. Thus, Freud built into mental health "the reality principle"—that is, the norm of living in accord with truth. (He also said the fundamental rule for psychoanalysis is that patients must make every effort to be and to speak truthfully.) The corresponding virtue governing realistic contact with reality is truthfulness—honesty as focused on truth, as distinct from honesty focused on trust (trustworthiness).

I postpone to chapter 13 a discussion of the connections between truthfulness and health-defining reality perception. There I discuss some psychological studies that challenge reality perception as a defining feature of mental health. Those studies portray self-deception and biased perception as healthy in maintaining optimism and hope, which are themselves taken to be health-making features. I argue that those studies overstate their case.

Subjectivity and Objective Values

Having linked Jahoda's criteria for mental health with the virtues, I can comment more fully on the tension between subjective conceptions of mental health and objective conceptions that allude to justified moral values. Self-esteem, as noted, might mean subjective self-affirmation (feeling good about oneself), but as a criterion of mental health it connects with the virtue of self-respect (proper valuing of oneself). Integration might be mere unity, but as a health-defining feature it typically overlaps with moral integrity (unity around a moral core). Autonomy can mean personal self-direction, but as a health-defining feature it connects with moral autonomy(self-direction within the bounds of moral decency). Self-actualization can mean "doing one's own thing," but as a health-defining feature it alludes to the virtue of authenticity in drawing forth one's higher potential, including moral potential. Coping, as a health-defining feature, implies functioning within the basic domain of moral responsibility, whether in work, love, or communities. And realistic cognition might imply the mere absence of severe disorders or it might be connected with truthfulness about the world and one's experience of it.

These subjective-objective ambiguities add complexity to the therapeutic trend. They should caution us against facile characterizations of the therapeutic trend as abandoning morality by unequivocally sliding toward subjectivism and self-centeredness.[41] The slide to subjectivism is a genuine danger, but it is a danger for both therapeutic and moral perspectives. It needs to be opposed with a sound conception of mental health that embodies *justified* moral values. There are widely shared moral values, defining minimum decency, that shape definitions of mental disorders such as antisocial personality disorder, pyromania, kleptomania, and so. Beyond minimum decency, definitions of positive health reflect the pluralism of morally permissible values in our society. In this way, reasonable moral differences signal moral complexity but not subjectivity.

Moreover, which moral values enter into positive definitions depends on the purposes for which the definitions are used. Employers, for example, might adopt thin specifications of mental health, aimed at assessing the satisfaction of workers with their jobs, and thereby rest content with basic moral responsibility at the workplace. In contrast, psychologists interested in helping individuals pursue meaningful lives might use thick conceptions that embody additional virtues. Thus, recent "positive psychologists" are returning to themes in value-rich humanistic psychology in exploring the full range of virtues.[42] This is a "return" because, as Michael E. McCullough and C. R. Snyder remind us, psychologists used to pay far greater attention to positive dimensions of health linked to the virtues. They cite the change that occurred during the 1920s as Gordon Allport urged replacing the language of *character* with a new language of *personality*, which sounded more scientific.[43] As a result, virtues receded into the background, but they never stopped influencing conceptions of mental health.

There is an obvious objection to using value-laden conceptions of mental health. Psychology and psychiatry are sciences. Insofar as the criteria for mental health embed moral values, how can mental health be studied scientifically? Aren't values themselves subjective, in ways that preclude scientific study? The brief answer is that the identification of sound values is a matter of moral reasoning, but once the values are identified they can be studied empirically.

Consider the research conducted by Carol D. Ryff and Burton Singer, who underscore the multitude of criteria used by leading researchers, including developmental psychologists, cognitive psychologists, and humanistic psychologists. In searching for an integrated, moral-therapeutic outlook, they examine what several leading ethicists say about morally good lives. This examination leads them to observe that "it is the chronic neglect of philosophical perspectives on 'the goods' in life that has handicapped efforts, including well-intentioned efforts, to understand positive health, and has produced instead deeply impoverished conceptions of human functioning."[44] Ryff and Singer's criteria for positive health slightly modify Jahoda's criteria: self-acceptance, environmental mastery, positive relationships with others (which Jahoda included under environmental mastery), autonomy, personal growth, and purpose/meaning in life (which Jahoda included under personal growth and integration).[45]

In operationalizing the criteria and testing them for reliability (i.e., consistency of application), Ryff and Singer rely on self-assessments using self-reporting psychological inventories. Quite simply, they ask people whether they believe their lives had certain features. Experimental subjects were then scored by how highly they ranked themselves using a 6-point scale with "strongly agree" at one end and "strongly disagree" at the other end. An individual would have "quality" or positive relationships with others, for example, if she strongly agreed that she had "warm, satisfying, trusting relationships with others; is concerned about the welfare of others; capable of strong empathy, affection, and intimacy; understands give and take of human relationships."[46]

Clearly, this self-assessment procedure risks a slide toward subjectivism. As Ryff and Singer admit, reliance on questionnaires yields only subjective self-assessments, which might be at odds with reality.[47] Nevertheless, their criteria can be morally examined for their justifiability beyond what individuals' report, even though there will never be complete consensus on the exact criteria and their precise meaning. That is true of moral values in general, and it is equally true of moral values as they enter into understanding positive mental health. Even more broadly, they should invite reasoning about the moral values whose implications are then investigated scientifically by psychologists.[48] And in formulating the "core criteria" defining positive mental health, they should engage wider moral debates in moral philosophy.

In short, empirical research that acknowledges the embeddedness of moral values in mental health is promising. Reliance of self-evaluations is in line with standard psychological approaches, although it might be augmented by other tools (such as interviews) if reliable assessments of individuals is needed. Most impressive, Ryff and Singer invite dialogue with philosophers and the public in discussing the values that shape conceptions of positive mental health.

This and the previous chapter outlined some ways in which moral values are embedded in conceptions of mental disorders and positive health, rendering "moral sickness" and "moral health" something beyond mere metaphors. The next chapter builds on this embeddedness theme while shifting to therapeutic critiques of morality. Typically, these critiques invoke positive conceptions of health in arguing that conventional morality is unhealthy. Because these conceptions of health embed selected moral values, however, we should be prepared to find that therapeutic critiques of conventional morality are also moral critiques. What initially appear to be replacements of morality by mental health turn out to be integrations of them. Whether particular integrations are successful is a further matter.

3

SICK MORALITY

Freud, Nietzsche, and Guilt

Freud ignited America's therapeutic trend and in doing so reshaped Western morality.[1] Many of his insights were anticipated by Nietzsche, who continues to influence ethics as the prophet of postmodernism. Both thinkers attack traditional morality as unhealthy and sick—as psychologically unrealistic in its demands to care about others, neglectful of human needs for self-affirmation, and the source of needless depression and anxiety. Both identify guilt as the culprit: society generates "the deep sickness" of guilt (bad conscience) and lessens happiness "through the heightening of the sense of guilt."[2]

At first glance, Freud and Nietzsche seem to appeal to morally neutral concepts of health in critiquing conventional morality. In fact, both thinkers embed selected moral values in their conceptions of health. Although the moral values they embed center on the self in ways that invite insular forms of egoism and neglect the positive role of guilt, they offer insightful therapeutic critiques of distorted forms of morality. They also interweave two of my themes: sound morality is healthy, and moral values are embedded in mental health.

Freud: Psychological Realism and Irrational Guilt

As common ground, let us agree that much guilt is irrational and pathological, as is much anger, hatred, and shame. Consider Irvin D. Yalom's depiction of a thirty-eight-year-old mother grieving over the death of her daughter four years earlier.[3] The extended bereavement destroys her marriage, alienates her two sons, and causes life-threatening blackouts. Early therapy sessions disclose guilt as the underlying problem. For several years her daughter suffered from leukemia and then died in her sleep on the day before her thirteenth birthday. The mother slept beside her daughter each night, but she has no memory of her final hours and fears she was not awake to comfort her. She also punishes herself for not summoning greater courage in helping her daughter cope with the illness, rather than pretending her condition was improving. At some level, she blames herself for not preventing her death. In addition, she has poor relationships with her two sons, one a drug addict and the other in prison, both of whom she resents for not keeping their agreements, which she forced on them, to share payments on an expensive family cemetery site. Frequently it occurs to her that one of her sons should have died instead of her daughter, but she immediately reproaches herself for that thought. From every direction she is consumed by guilt.

The word "guilt" is ambiguous. It can mean *being guilty* (culpability): the moral status of being responsible for wrongdoing. To ascribe guilt in this sense is to make a moral judgment. Alternatively, it can mean *feeling guilty* (an emotion and attitude)—the painful experience of feeling culpable for wrongdoing. And it can mean a *sense of guilt* (a sensibility): the general tendency to experience guilt for wrongdoing. When we say the mother's guilt is unjustified, we mean her emotions and sense of guilt are excessive in light of her actual culpability. She feels guilty for things she is not culpable for; she is less culpable than she thinks; the intensity and frequency of her guilt feelings are disproportionate to her actual offenses; and her responses to guilt feelings are unreasonable because they are based on unrealistic standards. Although some of her guilt is reasonable, in that she imposes unfair burdens on her sons (the gravesite payments) and fails to provide the support they need, she is unreasonable in how she copes with the guilt. She needs to stop torturing herself, make amends, and get on with her life. Therapy helps her do that.

As applied to guilt, terms like "excessive," "inappropriate," "unjustified," and "unreasonable" often suggest unhealthiness, as well as lack of moral warrant. The mother's guilt is unhealthy because it causes unnecessary suffering and impairs functioning. Regarding false beliefs, her pathology is manifested in obsessive ideas, distorted evidence, flawed reasoning, unreasonable demands, and hallucinations. Regarding emotion, her pathology is shown in the crippling intensity and debilitating recurrence of guilt feelings, shame, depression, and anxiety. And regarding coping, her pathology is shown in not making normal adjustments after a reasonable period of time. Not surprising, then, her therapy is a moral process that culminates in self-forgiveness and reconciliation with her sons, as well as a spiritual process in which her beliefs in reincarnation help her to accept her daughter's death.

Healthy guilt indicates a commitment to our obligations, expresses justified beliefs about wrongdoing, and manifests reasonable responses to culpability. Guilt is good insofar as it motivates responsible conduct and making amends for wrongdoing.[4] It provides a source of moral motivation by anticipating culpability, and it motivates prudentially by anticipating the pain of guilt feelings. In both regards, it is a supportive moral motive, subordinate to primary motives such as caring, conscientiousness, and self-respect. Morality also includes standards limiting guilt, by delineating obligations and grounds for excusing and forgiving.

Freud paints a bleaker picture. As a therapist, he encountered irrational guilt on a daily basis: "The patient represents his ego to us as worthless, incapable of any effort and morally despicable; he reproaches himself, vilifies himself and expects to be cast out and chastised."[5] According to Freud, guilt is rooted in aggressive and sexual instincts, together with unconscious defense against these instincts (as in the Oedipus complex of father-hatred and mother-love). Especially in *Civilization and Its Discontents*, he argues that guilt is far more destructive than commonly appreciated. It is one of the three main sources of human suffering, the other two being bodily dissolution and hostile environments. Nevertheless, he admits that guilt is a necessary evil, essential to civilization. Guilt arises when society instills a harsh judge within us, in the form of a partly unconscious superego, which is even more important in controlling aggression than establishing external authorities and punishment. The superego redirects aggressive instincts away from outer objects, including people we love, and toward ourselves with terrifying intensity. In this way, guilt amounts to fear of the superego's harsh demands.

By causing unmanageable anxiety, depression, and compulsions, guilt is the source of much psychopathology. The mother in Yalom's case study becomes sick because she internalizes (makes part of her identity) lost love objects (her daughter and sons) and then redirects her hostilities toward her children against herself. In response, Yalom and other therapists help patients accept and integrate their aggressive desires, transforming the irrational id into a rational ego. But guilt also routinely manifests itself in everyday unhappiness through depression, anxiety, and compulsions (which we misinterpret as having other sources).[6] This everyday discontent comes in many degrees and forms a continuum with neurosis. Therapy can help individuals, but the ultimate solution is to lower society's unrealistic moral demands, to soften the "cultural super-ego."[7] In particular, the Christian ideal of loving one's neighbor as oneself is an unrealistic ideal because it imposes impossible demands and dissipates our limited capacities for love.

Freud says the self-sacrifice Christianity enjoins is "wrong," something we "ought not" to do; it is "an injustice" to friends, family, and others who are "worthy" of our love.[8] Clearly, these words express moral (as well as therapeutic) judgments, and the moral judgments allude to moral values presupposed in his conception of mental health. What, then, is Freud's conception of mental health? Like most psychiatrists, he usually thinks of health negatively, as the absence of pathology. At the same time, he insists there is a continuum, not a sharp line, between normality and neurosis.[9] At key junctures he affirms a positive definition of mental health as the ability to work and love without excessive anxiety and depression. To this extent, he takes for granted conventional moral values about functioning responsibly in society, and he embeds those values in his conception of mental health. Yet he opposes relativistic definitions that reduce health to what society approves of, and he plausibly speculates that an entire society might be neurotic and promulgate unhealthy ideals.[10]

In light of this moral conception of mental health, I interpret Freud as undertaking an integrative project that interweaves therapeutic understanding with a modified version of conventional morality. He portrays himself as a scientist, and at most he admits that psychoanalysis is a practical therapy that uncovers morally relevant facts and encourages greater psychological realism.[11] But his therapeutic critique is clearly rooted in values that are both moral and therapeutic: compassion, honesty, self-respect, self-love, and the ability to love and work.

There is a complication, however, that leads critics of the therapeutic trend to charge Freud with eroding morality (as I discuss in chapter 5). Judeo-Christian ideals of altruism are central to traditional conceptions of morality, and in rejecting those ideals Freud largely assumes a self-interested value perspective. Indeed, he denies the very possibility of altruism, understood as concern for others for their sake, or at least he reduces altruism to "aim-inhibited" and sublimated expressions of egoistic instincts. Morality, he says, is a failed "therapeutic attempt" to use the super-ego to govern the self, but in controlling aggression it relies on the "narcissistic satisfaction" of thinking ourselves better than others.[12] And he says that other people deserve love only when they embody our own ideals and aspirations, so that in loving them we love ourselves.[13]

In effect, Freud's "pleasure principle" is a version of psychological egoism—the view that we are solely motivated by what we believe is beneficial to ourselves (pleasure-seeking, pain-avoiding). Within this framework, the only plausible value perspective is ethical egoism, which Freud includes in his "reality principle": we should adopt an enlightened view of our own good, controlling pleasure seeking in order to maximize our long-term well-being.[14] Now, if we define morality as requiring direct concern for others, then we might regard ethical egoism as skepticism about morality. In that case, we will interpret Freud as replacing morality with a self-interested therapeutic outlook—as pursuing a replacement rather than an integrative project. If instead we view ethical egoism as a (flawed) moral outlook, then Freud integrates a therapeutic outlook with a flawed moral perspective. I believe the latter interpretation is most plausible, but I grant there is room for disagreement. A similar disagreement arises concerning Nietzsche's health-oriented critique of morality.

Nietzsche: Vitality, Self-Mastery, Self-Love

Nietzsche says he awaits a "philosophical *physician*" who can diagnose the manifestations and distortions of health and power in philosophies and cultures.[15] In many ways he is that physician. Yet his therapeutic critique of morality is somewhat concealed by commingling it with his more contentious themes about the will to power and atheism. Nevertheless, his insights into guilt, aggression, and unrealistic ideals of altruism are illuminating and directly anticipate Freud.[16]

Far more radically than Freud, Nietzsche calls into question "the *value* of morality," voicing skepticism about "everything on earth that has until now been celebrated as morality." He dubs himself an immoralist who moves "beyond good and evil." His revaluation centers on rejecting altruism and guilt, where guilt is "cruelty turned backwards," toward oneself.[17] As such, he seems to replace morality with health. Certainly he rejects what many people consider morality: duty-oriented, altruism-emphasizing, guilt- and blame-oriented outlooks. Nevertheless, I believe he is better understood as undertaking an integrative project that embeds a virtue-oriented ethics in his conception of health. That is what he means when he writes that "many actions called immoral ought to be avoided and resisted" although for different reasons than conventional morality says.[18] Honesty, courage, self-control, and generosity are desirable when they are healthy expressions of the will to power, but their ultimate justification resides in how they express creativity and authenticity.[19]

Nietzsche explores a rich set of themes useful for integrative projects: health has inseparable physical and mental facets; it comes in many degrees; its requirements are relative to individual needs and capacities; it can be stimulated by episodic sickness; and occasionally it must be sacrificed to pursue even greater health.[20] Nietzsche also develops a robust conception of positive health—of well-being and well-functioning beyond the mere absence of disease. Yet, it is unclear exactly which virtues he uses to define health, as distinct from noting its typical manifestations and accompaniments. For example, he says the "standards" for health include "courage, and cheerfulness of the spirit."[21] Elsewhere he distinguishes health from the "strong, free, cheerful-hearted activity" that manifests and preserves health.Sometimes he portrays honesty as in tension with health, but other times he links deep truthfulness to "great health."[22]

According to some readers, vitality is the defining value in Nietzsche's conception of health.[23] Other readers believe self-mastery is central.[24] Still others note that self-love is the virtue prominent in most passages on health.[25] I suggest his conception of health combines these three values—vitality, self-mastery, and self-love—as overlapping and interdefined manifestations of the will to power.

Vitality consists in giving the instincts full creative expression in life-enhancing ways. Creativity comes from strong desires, powerfully mastered.[26] The desires are simultaneously physiological and psychological, reflecting the unity of body and mind. The most basic instinct, the will to power, includes aggression toward others, but its highest expression lies in creating the values that individuals and cultures live by.[27] Vitality is also manifested in expanding power by taking risks aimed at self-growth; in physical energy and vigor and the emotional dispositions of cheerfulness and joy; and in a plethora of pleasures that conventional morality renounces—for example, pleasure in seeing and inflicting suffering.[28] Sickness arises when the instincts are paralyzed and turned against ourselves.[29] An ethics of vitality transcends conventional morality, with its stock Do's and Do Not's, and calls instead for aspiration and authenticity.

Self-mastery, or self-command, consists in harmonizing diverse instincts, desires, and activities. It differs from conventional self-control, which suppresses the instincts and afflicts us with irritability and illness. Self-mastery concentrates the will to power, thereby increasing vigor, strength, and a sense of well-being.[30] In most creative lives, there is one "dominating passion" that serves to coordinate the personality.[31]

Self-love is self-acceptance, self-reverence, and authentic self-assertion. It is a tendency inherent in the will to power and, as a virtue, it is an achievement— something one must learn.[32] Genuine self-love requires effort and skill, much like learning to love music.[33] We must learn and continually relearn how to accept, trust, and risk ourselves in self-overcoming. In its highest stages, self-love becomes the love of life in its entirety (*amor fati*). Psychopathology caused by the absence of self-love is the source of the greatest cruelties against ourselves and others.[34]

In a way, Nietzsche's three-faceted conception of health refocuses Jahoda's six criteria. Vitality includes but goes beyond coping. Self-mastery includes psychological integration and autonomy. And self-love includes but deepens self-esteem and self-actualization. In each instance, standards of mental health are elevated. The healthy self is much like the fully authentic individual, although in some passages Nietzsche portrays health as the basis for pursuing authenticity, rather than its complete realization. Either way, it is clear that ethical values permeate his conception of health.[35]

In developing this conception of health, Nietzsche scatters his therapeutic critique of morality throughout his writings, but its fullest expression is *On the Genealogy of Morality*. "Genealogy" means uncovering the historical and psychological origins of moral values, which leads to showing how they function as pathological distortions of instincts. Each of the three essays composing *On the Genealogy of Morality* diagnoses pathologies rooted in the conventional distinction between good and evil, but there is a discernible shift in emphasis as the essays progress—from self-love, to self-mastery, to vitality.

Thus, the first essay links health to self-love. The origin of noble, aristocratic morality is "a triumphant yes-saying to oneself." Ancient aristocrats celebrated honor, honesty, and dominance that emerged from an "overflowing health" manifested in "strong, free, cheerful-hearted activity." In contrast, the slavish morality of Judaism and Christianity, and their legacy in humanitarian ideals of equality and selfless love, are ruses. They constrain the powerful by lowering their status and simultaneously elevating the status of the poor; they prop up the fragile self by denigrating others. Egalitarian values arise from *ressentiment*, a sick form of hatred and envy. As illustrations, he reminds us of Tertullian contemplating Judgment Day when Christians will enjoy watching the sinners "blaze together" in hell, and Aquinas pronouncing that we enjoy our virtue more when we see its absence in the sinners God punishes. In contrast, self-affirming individuals celebrate their own power and quickly express or shrug off their hatred and shame.[36]

The second essay accents self-mastery. Historically, guilt arose within debtor relationships. It functioned as a psychological surrogate for payments on a debt to a stronger person, who enjoys seeing the guilty person suffer. Over time, punishment acquired multiple rationales, including deterrence of crime and preventative detention, but punishment still embodies power in the form of blame and punishment. Guilt is the sickness caused when instincts turn against the self, in response to societal demands for self-control. This sickness, however, is like pregnancy; it can lead to good or bad. The bad is "psychic cruelty" in which we torture ourselves with excessive demands for self-control, sapping vitality and joy. The good is self-mastery that deepens self-love and vitality.[37]

The third essay celebrates vitality, while linking it to self-love and self-mastery. Religious ideals of humility, chastity, poverty, and self-sacrifice are disguised forms of cruelty toward oneself. Camouflaged as altruism, they express self-hatred, waste energy, and stifle creativity. Priests and other religious authorities exploit guilt feelings, using sin as a weapon. Like *ressentiment* and guilt, however, ascetic ideals have a creative potential to foster honesty with oneself, ultimately an "honest atheism" that overthrows morality and religion.[38]

Although Nietzsche's conception of health is a rich resource for integrative projects, it is flawed in several respects. For one thing, Nietzsche is an elitist who in valuing creative individuals denigrates common humanity—the "herd" whose only value is to make possible the few great individuals.[39] As Jonathan Glover reminds us, Nietzsche's outlook "contains much that is terrible. It includes intermittent racism, contempt for women, and a belief in the ruthless struggle for power. He rejected sympathy for the weak in favour of a willingness to trample on them."[40] With this in mind, we might think of Freud as democratizing Nietzsche's insights, integrating them within a humanistic framework and extending healing techniques to them.

For another thing, although Nietzsche celebrates selected virtues, his perspectivism leads him to claim that no values are objectively justified. Values are expressions of the will to power, and that will is expressed in different perspectives, none of which is privileged. In my view, Nietzsche's therapeutic critique of morality is strengthened by rejecting his subjectivism. In some form, self-love, self-mastery, and vital functioning are all defensible moral-therapeutic values. Moreover, in rejecting his radical perspectivism, we can embrace a pluralistic outlook that tolerates moral perspectives which unfold self-love, self-mastery, and vitality in different directions.

Finally, like Freud, Nietzsche is a psychological egoist who believes we are only motivated by self-seeking; altruism is a distorted manifestation of the will to power. He construes self-love and authenticity in egoistic terms, claiming that the will to power is "*essentially* appropriation, injury, overpowering of what is alien and weaker."[41] Indeed, his celebration of the self to the neglect of community is itself a pathological (narcissistic) exaggeration. These aspects of his thought can be renounced while retaining his moral insights into positive health and healthy morality, or so I will next suggest.

Love, Shame, and Forgiveness

We can accept Freud and Nietzsche's insights in critiquing traditional morality while retaining a positive role for guilt and rejecting their psychological and ethical egoism. In contrast with Nietzsche, we should attend to the health-promoting dimensions of altruism. Needs for love and community are as fundamental as any other "instincts" and as essential to vital functioning. Granting the importance of self-assertion (the will to power), we can affirm its expression through community and caring relationships. Nietzsche diagnoses the distortions of love, but he fails to appreciate authentic forms of love and morality as creative expressions.[42] These forms include religious love that expresses strength, self-mastery, and inner abundance. Tertullian's outlook was sick, and Aquinas's outlook was not entirely healthy, but it is absurd to say that Albert Schweitzer, Martin Luther King Jr., and Mother Teresa lacked vitality, self-mastery, and self-love.

Similarly, we can embrace Nietzsche's insights into how power enters into ideals of justice, fairness, and reciprocity.[43] Sometimes power distorts these ideals into sheer vengeance and hatred, but other times the ideals express a healthy will to power. Again, unhealthy forms of guilt manifest cruelty toward us, but healthy guilt plays a positive role in strengthening respect for other persons.

Turning to Freud, we can insist that any plausible conception of mental health will leave room for altruism. In this connection, psychoanalyst Michael Friedman rejects Freud's psychological egoism because it is based on an implausible drive theory: "According to [Freud's] drive theory an individual's deepest motivation is by definition egoistic, having as its goal the discharge of his own accumulated tensions. Any benefit that may accrue to others must be derivative, a result either of sublimations of or defenses against egoistic motivation."[44] Yet, as Friedman rightly insists, we have evolved as creatures with altruistic, pro-social instincts, including love, loyalty, and justice. Furthermore, Friedman identifies a positive role for guilt. Guilt is not merely a fear of the superego or merely a necessary evil. It is an emotion based on the belief that we have wronged people we care about. At some minimal level, care is owed to humanity at large, and falling below standards of minimum decency warrants guilt. As with virtually any emotion, guilt can become pathological, as in Yalom's example. In discussing pathological guilt, Friedman cites studies of the "separation guilt" experienced in growing apart from parents and other people we love, and the "survivor guilt" experienced by Holocaust survivors (and perhaps the mother in Yalom's example). In pathological forms of survivor guilt, individuals are unable to accept the role of chance and tragedy in shaping their fate and, instead, torture themselves for failing to prevent the death of people they love.

Earlier than Friedman, Erich Fromm showed how a therapeutic critique of conventional morality need not abandon all guilt. Fromm explicitly embeds moral values in his conception of the healthy self: the mature, integrated, productive self.[45] He views us as self-actualizing creatures pulled by ideals of authentic humanitarian love—responsible caring that expresses power, joy, and vitality—and the same is true of self-love, which is the opposite of selfishly cutting ourselves off from fulfilling caring relationships.[46] Against this background, he distinguishes between healthy guilt arising from a "humanistic conscience" and unhealthy guilt generated by an "authoritarian conscience"— Freud's super-ego.[47] The humanistic conscience is the positive voice of a moral self, the social being that aspires to unfold its highest nature. That nature includes social needs for reciprocal caring relationships, self-transcendence through creative expression, being at home in the world by participating in communities, identity as a unique and authentic self, and personal meaning grounded in an understanding the world.[48] Healthy guilt signals the failure to meet responsibilities to others.

Consider an objection. Bernard Williams believes we should accept more of Nietzsche's and Freud's critique of guilt than I have done. He draws a technical distinction between ethics and morality. Ethics includes all meaning-giving value perspectives, whereas morality is a specific ethics which he believes we should reject because of its guilt-and-blame orientation: "Blame is the characteristic reaction of the morality system. The remorse or self-reproach or guilt . . . is the characteristic first-personal reaction within the system."[49] Like Nietzsche and Freud, Williams thinks most guilt arises from excessive demands for impartiality of the sort embedded in Christianity, utilitarianism, and Kantian duty-ethics. Guilt-and blame-oriented morality is a "peculiar" ethical outlook that "we would be better off without."[50] In its place, he recommends a virtue-oriented ethics that replaces impartial duties with more personal commitments and replaces guilt with shame.

Like guilt, shame is a painful emotion generated by perceived failures, but the types of failures differ. With guilt, the failures are violations of duties to others; with shame, the failures are not becoming who we aspire to be. Williams believes that guilt is more prone to excess in self-punishing because it is tied to general rules and duties, whereas shame is focused on our own good. Shame functions as a self-protective emotion that tends to unify us, rather than turn us against ourselves: "By giving through the emotions a sense of who one is and of what one hopes to be, it [shame] mediates between act, character, and consequence, and also between ethical demands and the rest of life."[51]

In reply, there is no reason to think a shame-oriented ethics can avoid the excesses of guilt-oriented morality. Shame is equally liable to irrational excesses, and those excesses cut to the core of the self in exceptionally painful ways.[52] Just as much as guilt, shame is woven into social demands, and when those demands are unrealistic they generate a level of self-cruelty that rivals irrational guilt. And as with guilt, the self-diminishment can be manifested through depression, anxiety, and self-hatred, and toward others in the forms of humiliated fury and revenge.[53] So intimate are these connections that we can feel shame for the weaknesses of people we love—for example. a parent—or otherwise identify ourselves with.[54]

Finally, forgiveness—of self and others—deserves special mention within an integrated, moral-therapeutic perspective on guilt. Recently, therapists have explored the health aspects of forgiving others and are using it "as a cognitive and emotive psychotherapeutic technique to diminish excessive anger in a number of clinical disorders."[55] They have studied how self-forgiveness can heal the suffering caused by guilt and other forms of self-blame. Some therapists recommend forgiveness as a knee-jerk response, rather than a discriminating and voluntary choice, thereby debasing it with an excessive emphasis on self-interest.[56] Just as an integrated perspective brings therapeutic understanding of forgiveness, it will bring a moral understanding of therapeutic excesses.

To sum up, in calling for a healthy value perspective, Freud and Nietzsche caution about the excesses of guilt and blame conventional morality, yet they underestimate the positive role of guilt. As a forward-looking, guardian motive, guilt turns us away from wrongdoing and motivates reform and making amends when we harm others. Justified guilt and blame, as well as approbation and praise, contribute to positive growth.[57] Again, Freud and Nietzsche rightly call for greater psychological realism in acknowledging predominant needs for self-love and self-assertion, but they fail to acknowledge that psychological realism also implies appreciating human capacities of caring for others.[58] Their one-sided focus on the self, to the neglect of altruism and obligations, illustrates a danger in many therapeutic perspectives. As we see next, critics of the therapeutic trend highlight, though also exaggerate, that danger.

Part II
RESPONSIBILITY FOR HEALTH

Our duties towards ourselves constitute the supreme condition and the principle of all morality.

Immanuel Kant, *Lectures on Ethics*

For *most* people in reasonably affluent, middle-class circumstances in Western societies, personal responsibility for health is possible, and thus a reasonable social demand.... At best, we can argue mitigating circumstances, diminished responsibility, and mild victimization—but only a small minority can claim they lack responsibility altogether.

Daniel Callahan, *False Hopes*

4

RESPONSIBILITY IN THERAPY

Part I introduced the themes of healthy morality and the moral-ladenness of health, and I turn now to my third theme: responsibility for health. This responsibility provides an obvious bridge between morality and health, but its meaning, extent, and foundation are less clear. The unclarity renders the notion especially liable to abuse in the form of blaming victims for their misfortune. This chapter discusses responsibility for health in the context of client-therapist relationships, chapter 5 explores broader social contexts, and chapter 6 responds to concerns about blaming victims.

I begin with Samuel Butler's *Erewhon*, a novel that adumbrates our current uncertainty about responsibilities for health and provokes us to clarify the meaning and foundation of those responsibilities. Next I critique two ideologies about therapy that distort our understanding of responsibilities for health. One ideology concerns the sick role: to be sick is to be an innocent victim, and nonjudgmental therapy implies not holding patients responsible for their sickness. The other ideology concerns science and causation: sick people (as well as healthy ones) are completely determined by biological and environmental forces in ways that remove moral responsibility. These ideologies, I argue, are as inimical to effective therapy as to sound morality.

Erewhon's Inverted Ethic

In *Erewhon*, Butler imagines a society that inverts conventional morality: physical sickness is wrongdoing, and wrongdoing is mental illness. On the one hand, physically ill Erewhonians are charged with the "crime" of poor health. They are brought to trial, publicly ridiculed, and punished according to the severity of their offense. A mild cold is dealt with leniently, but a terminal case of tuberculosis warrants a life sentence in prison. More generally, victims of misfortune of all kinds, not only sickness, are held in contempt and ostracized. On the other hand, wrongdoers are regarded as mentally ill. Forgers, thieves, arsonists, and other violent criminals are sent to the hospital at public expense or, if they are wealthy, their "fit of immorality" is treated at home.[1] The same is true of addicts, whose compulsions are believed to be caused by or "part of" the mental disease constituting their addictions.[2] Therapy for such "moral ailments" is administered by a "straightener" who diagnoses the specific mental disorder and writes a prescription which the patient is expected to heed rigorously.[3] Often the cure is not pleasant. In fact, it looks much like what we call punishment, reconceptualized as therapy.

A case in point is Mr. Nosnibor, a wealthy stockbroker who suddenly begins to augment his earnings illegally. At first he dismisses his criminal inclinations as minor "symptoms," but he knows he is seriously ill when circumstances lead him to commit fraud on a massive scale. A straightener raises concerns that he might be permanently impaired, but subsequent investigations reveal grounds for hope in light of the sound "moral health" of his parents and grandparents. The straightener writes a prescription for monthly floggings during the next year. He also prescribes paying double the amount of his fraudulent earnings to the government. In light of her despicable misfortune, the woman whose money Mr. Nosnibor embezzled is repaid nothing.

The Erewhonians' reversal of conventional morality emerges from both empirical beliefs and moral standards. As for empirical beliefs, the Erewhonians are convinced that individuals have greater control over their physical health than is usually appreciated, such that all physical illness indicates culpable failure to take care of their health. They also believe that immoral activities are beyond control and due entirely to "pre-natal or post-natal misfortune." As for moral standards, the Erewhonians embrace an ethic of luck: good luck warrants veneration, and bad luck warrants contempt.[4] This inverted ethic parodies the utilitarian ideal of maximizing social well-being. Thus, good fortune is revered because it inspires joy; ill fortune is reviled because it makes other people uncomfortable and tends to be contagious. Punishing sickness motivates people to take better care of their health, and even therapy for crime, such as the lashes given to Mr. Nosnibor, is sufficiently unpleasant to deter future wrongdoing.

Butler's satire is effective because we are closer to the Erewhonians than we like to think. We too admire (and envy) people for their talents, beauty, physical vitality, privileged upbringing, wealth, fame, and other good fortune, whether earned or unearned. In principle, our admiration is nonmoral; in practice, it shades into something like moral esteem. Furthermore, often we turn away in pity from victims of misfortune, rather than offering help, even lapsing into "blaming the victim." Like the Erewhonians, we regard addictions as mental disorders requiring therapy. At the same time, we hold people responsible for their excessive drinking, smoking, alcohol abuse, and overeating.[5] Sometimes we are ambivalent, torn between punitive and therapeutic responses to criminal offenses. Just as Mr. Nosnibor is given psychotherapy for his crime, we believe prisoners should be offered counseling and therapy, if only to reduce recidivism when they return to society. Again, we mix penalties with therapy, as in drug courts where judges coerce drug abusers into therapy programs. Yet we are aware that scientists continue to uncover genetic and environmental influences that make crime and mental disorders seem more like misfortunes. Typically, these discoveries are expressed as statistics about groups, leaving us unsure what to conclude about specific individuals. In charging the Erewhonians with confusion, we must acknowledge our own uncertainties about responsibility for health.

Dimensions of Responsibility for Health

What is responsibility for health?[6] In its core meaning, it comprises responsibilities—*obligations*—to take care of our health. The extent of these obligations needs to be explored contextually, but it is clear they require avoiding destructive habits such as alcohol abuse, drug dependence, crime, and obsessive hatred and envy. Numerous influences contribute to habit formation, but typically they are risk factors rather than complete causal determinants. We retain the ability, in varying degrees, to prevent bad habits from taking over our lives, to seek help when they do, and to stop them from harming others.

Although obligations form the core of responsibility, responsibility has additional dimensions that cluster under the heading of *moral accountability* for meeting obligations. Accountability refers to capacities and answerability. In its capacity sense, moral accountability means having general abilities such as moral reflection, caring, and self-control, which are required for meeting obligations. In its answerability sense, moral accountability means susceptibility to being held to account for specific actions in light of obligations and standards for meeting those obligations.

Moral accountability is complex. It includes (1) having obligations; (2) accepting obligations as justified and binding; (3) being willing, on appropriate occasions, to give an account of failures to meet obligations, whether in the form of explanations, excuses, or justifications (all of which are subject to appraisal); (4) engaging in appropriate forms of apologizing, compensating, repenting of wrongdoing, and responding to others' wrongdoing with forgiveness; (5) assessing who has the requisite capacities for having obligations and being answerable for them; (6) reacting on appropriate occasions with attitudes such as praise, gratitude, resentment, indignation, guilt, and shame; and (7) punishing and rewarding in accord with reasonable standards of enforcement.

What is the justification of responsibilities for health? At one extreme, libertarians tend to reduce responsibilities for health to responsibilities to pay for one's own health care, which is required by not imposing on others' resources. They believe we have a right to smoke and to pursue other unhealthy practices, as long as we do not impose burdens on others to pay for our health care.[7] In a similar vein, but within a utilitarian framework, John Stuart Mill said we are not accountable to others for our drunkenness, but only for violations of duties caused by our drunkenness.[8] At another extreme, the communitarian John Knowles grounds health obligations in national well-being: "I believe the idea of a 'right' to health should be replaced by the idea of an individual moral obligation to preserve one's own health—a public duty if you will."[9] If we acknowledged a responsibility to be prudent in matters of health, "our country would be strengthened immeasurably, and we could divert our energies— human and financial—to other pressing issues of national and international concern."[10]

In contrast to all these approaches, Kant identified a twofold foundation, which I find compelling. Responsibilities for health are grounded in self-respect and also in the general requirement that we maintain our capacities to meet other responsibilities. On the one hand, responsibilities to maintain our health are part of what it means to respect ourselves. In the absence of special circumstances, ruining our health manifests a lack of respect for our rational autonomy—our ability to govern our lives responsibly. Kant primarily thought in terms of duties, but self-respect is also a virtue—a mandatory virtue, whose absence signals a moral failing.[11] On the other hand, duties to maintain our health are prerequisites for meeting all other duties: "The supreme rule is that in all the actions which affect himself a man should so conduct himself that every exercise of his power is compatible with the fullest employment of them."[12] Conscientious, responsible human interactions require self-control; maintaining contact with reality; summoning the requisite commitment and energy; and avoiding pathologies of irrational fear, hatred, self-contempt, and impulsiveness.

I am not endorsing all aspects of Kant's account. In particular, the virtue of self-respect is more care-oriented, emotionally resonant, and intimately linked to our happiness than he recognized.[13] To respect ourselves is to care about ourselves, or, as Nietzsche said, to love and revere ourselves, which implies caring about our health. Furthermore, we should reject Kant's absolutism— that is, his condemnation of all suicide and each instance of getting drunk. A plausible approach affirms prima facie duties of health—duties that have exceptions when other duties outweigh them in particular circumstances. A plausible approach also allows considerable flexibility in how health responsibilities are interpreted and balanced with other duties.

In balancing conflicting duties, we need to distinguish medical good and total good.[14] Our medical good is health, but health is only one dimension of our overall good, however important. Again, maintaining our health tends to contribute to our overall well-being, but not always. Sometimes well-being requires risking our health, or even sacrificing our lives for more important values. To complicate matters, some risks to health contribute to health in other ways, as when smoking reduces stress and controls weight. Again, competent adults have the right to pursue their overall well-being, but how they exercise that right is open to appraisal within a wider set of values.

Acknowledging responsibilities for health does not, of course, imply coercing individuals into meeting them. In practice, coercion largely concerns paternalism: When is it permissible to interfere with people's liberty to promote their good, by pressuring them to accept greater responsibility for their health? No doubt some paternalism is fully justified in light of major health benefits of relatively minor inconveniences, such as mandatory use of seat belts and motorcycle helmets, and avoiding dangerous drugs.[15] But the present point is that accountability should not be confused with paternalism and coercion. In many instances, accepting accountability is best promoted by encouragement and positive incentives to accept responsibilities regarding health.

The Sick Role Ideology

The classical medical model of the sick role, as articulated by Talcott Parsons, drives a wedge between (a) responsibility for causing sickness and (b) responsibility for contributing to its cure.[16] The model assumes that we are not responsible for causing the sickness, thereby treating us as victims of forces beyond our control. Furthermore, depending on its severity, sickness excuses us from work and certain other social requirements. We are responsible for our sickness only in the sense of being expected to try to get well, which often means seeking and cooperating with medical help provided by nonjudgmental physicians. We are also responsible for taking reasonable precautions to prevent further illness.

Even today, psychiatrists who write for the general public reinforce this sick role ideology. Consider *Am I Okay?: A Layman's Guide to the Psychiatrist's Bible*, written by Allen Frances, who is the chairperson of the task force on *DSM-IV*, and Michael B. First, who is the editor of the *DSM-IV* text and diagnostic criteria. Frances and First claim we are never responsible for causing or contributing to mental disorders. In response to the question, "Is having a psychiatric disorder my fault?," they write: "The answer is a resounding no. . . . No one holds anyone responsible for having diabetes or hypertension or heart disease or cancer, but there is a tendency to look down on someone for being depressed, anxious, or addicted to a substance. . . . This is illogical, unfair, unhelpful, and counterproductive."[17]

Is it illogical to hold people accountable for some physical ailments? Smokers are at least partly responsible for heart and lung diseases caused by their habit, and a "logical" approach to combating those ailments demands responsibility about smoking. It is also fair to hold individuals responsible for alcohol abuse, drug dependency, compulsive gambling, kleptomania, and myriad other mental disorders listed in the *DSM*. Frances and First vastly overgeneralize when they lump together genetically caused brain disorders, over which we lack control, with bad habits, over which we have significant control. Furthermore, the claim that it is unhelpful and counterproductive to hold people responsible for their mental maladies is ambiguous. Holding responsible might mean (1) blaming or (2) acknowledging obligations to take care of one's mental health. True enough, within the context of a patient-therapist relationship, it is unhelpful and counterproductive for therapists to blame individuals for their past errors. But it can be helpful and productive to encourage individuals to accept responsibility for their health—for example, by avoiding harmful addictions.

Recall that the *DSM* has a strong Cautionary Statement, which says that diagnosing a mental disorder does not by itself answer questions about "individual responsibility, disability determination, and competency."[18] The *DSM* defines mental disorders by patterns of behavior, emotion, and desire. It does not claim, for example, that the "dysfunctions" and "impairments" of pedophiles, pathological gamblers, and alcoholics constitute forces beyond their control or provide automatic excuses. As editors of the *DSM*, Frances and First endorse the Cautionary Statement.[19] However, they seek to drive a wedge between responsibilities for causing disorders, which they deny patients have, and responsibility for causing harm, which they admit patients usually have. This wedge is problematic, both conceptually and morally.

The wedge is conceptually problematic because the *DSM* defines many mental disorders by reference to illegal and socially objectionable conduct—and implicitly by reference to moral values and harm caused. For example, the discussions of kleptomania, pyromania, drug abuse and dependency, and antisocial personality disorder (sociopathy) all refer to morally objectionable behaviors. It is contradictory to say that we are never at fault for having a "maladaptive behavior," which is defined in terms of objectionable behavior, and then to say we are responsible for the harm inherent in that objectionable behavior.

The wedge is morally problematic because the *DSM* defines mental disorders in terms of patterns of behavior, desire, mood, and emotion—not in terms of incapacities that make it impossible to act otherwise. That is why the Cautionary Statement is so important. Whether individuals are morally responsible for causing or contributing to habits of drug abuse, excessive gambling, kleptomania, and so on is a moral judgment, not a purely scientific one. Psychiatrists do great damage when, in writing for the public, they encourage a sweeping inference from "sick" to "not responsible."

Nonjudgmental Therapists and Responsible Patients

If we have responsibilities to take care of our health, what is the basis for requiring psychiatrists and other psychotherapists to be nonjudgmental? Does encouraging patients to accept responsibility for contributing to their problems imply blaming them, in ways inimical to healing? And do nonjudgmental attitudes undermine moral accountability?

Therapy is a special moral context in which some aspects of moral accountability are suspended or modified. Professional ethics requires therapists to adopt attitudes that promote healing, which typically includes suspending blame and moral judgment about wrongdoing. It does not follow that patient responsibility has no role in therapy. As we have seen, even the sick role ideology requires patients to accept responsibility for contributing to the healing process.

But encouraging patients to accept responsibility for solving their problems does not mean blaming them, and even in everyday contexts blameworthiness does not mean we must actually blame (as opposed, say, to ignoring or forgiving an offense).[20]

Another question is whether, in opposition to the sick role ideology, we should remove the wedge between responsibility for healing and responsibility for (sometimes) contributing to sickness. We should, and successful therapy often requires us to. As Irvin Yalom writes:

> We must encourage our patients to assume responsibility—that is, to apprehend how they themselves contribute to their distress.... The therapist may have to say, in effect, "Even if ninety-nine percent of the bad things that happen to you is someone else's fault, I want to look at the other one percent—the part that is your responsibility. We have to look at your role, even if it's very limited, because that's where I can be of most help."[21]

Thus, patients' responsibility for contributing to the healing process is linked to responsibility for contributing to the problem in the first place. Yalom is not saying that victims of childhood traumas share responsibility for causing their problems. Instead, he is asserting that they must accept responsibility for how they deal with the effects of those traumas in their adult lives. And in most other instances, accepting responsibility for present solutions requires acknowledging some role in causing the problems in the first place.

Nonjudgmental therapy means avoiding or suspending blame and other negative attitudes toward clients, while conveying positive attitudes of hope and encouragement. Therapists often know their clients have engaged in wrongdoing, but they are trained not to blame them and instead to adopt a supportive and future-oriented stance. Even the examination of past behavior is aimed at understanding habits and attitudes that need to be modified or abandoned. The same stance is familiar in helping a friend or someone we love. But suspending blame is one thing; asserting complete innocence is something else.

More fully, there are two main reasons why therapists suspend blame and seek to maintain positive attitudes of support. One reason is to promote healing and problem solving. Positive support creates a context of trust that enables clients to explore problems, including difficulties about guilt and self-blame, without fear of condemnation that would only worsen their depression, hopelessness, fear, and self-loathing. Clients need to be able to speak freely, explore dreams and fantasies, and "open up" emotionally in ways that render them vulnerable. The other reason is to respect clients as persons, which means respecting their autonomy and values, even when the therapist disagrees with them. This is a fundamental professional norm, justified by the therapists' role in helping. It is also justified, as a procedural norm, by respect for persons' autonomy. Therapists fail to respect client autonomy when they lapse into a paternalistic stance that interferes with clients' autonomy, albeit for the client's own good.

The autonomy respected and promoted in psychotherapy is not social and political liberty—that is, freedom from coercion, oppression, and poverty. Instead, as Edwin Erwin points out, therapists are interested in promoting (and respecting) "inner autonomy," which has three aspects: "(1) the capacity for rational reflection; (2) the tendency to eliminate defective desires; and (3) the capacity for self-control."[22] The capacity for rational reflection is the ability to reflect on desires and preferences, along with the ability to change desires in light of higher-order (more important) values. In particular, it is the ability to change defective desires, including irrational desires based on false information or logic, inconsistent desires, futile desires that can never be satisfied (such as the desire for everyone to love us), and neurotic desires rooted in unconscious and infantile desires. Self-control consists in the ability to bring one's desires into line with reasonable value judgments. All these ideas—"rational reflection," "defective desires," and "self-control"—have moral dimensions, whether or not therapists explicitly discuss them as such.

To be sure, promoting autonomy is not universally endorsed as the primary goal of therapy. Aims of therapy depend substantially on the specific types of psychotherapy, which Erwin estimates to be over 400. Thus, some therapists adopt the goal of promoting mental health, understood according to their specific criteria for defining mental health. Other therapists focus exclusively on the "presenting problem," the symptoms or difficulties that prompt a client to seek therapy. Even therapists who adopt autonomy as a primary goal might define it in different ways: perhaps narrowly in terms of resolving clients' presenting problems and aims, or perhaps broadly in terms of wider values. Nevertheless, respecting and supporting autonomy is both a means and a primary goal in most psychotherapy.

To sum up, nonjudgmental therapy does not mean nonmoral therapy, if only because there are moral reasons for therapists to be nonjudgmental. Nor does it mean encouraging patients to view themselves as helpless victims, for that would undermine their agency in reshaping their lives. Much less does it imply hostility to morality. Moral values permeate therapy, especially the values of compassion, caring, respect for autonomy—and accepting responsibility. In addition, therapists generally want their clients to be more active than passive in their work and pleasure seeking, more involved in relationships than socially isolated, and more sexually fulfilled than celibate.[23]

Determinism and Autonomy

Hard determinism is the second ideology associated with therapeutic outlooks, specifically with the scientific worldview underlying them. Hard determinism is the view that because all actions (like all other events) are caused by biological and environmental forces beyond our control, we are not morally responsible for anything. Whereas the sick role ideology focused on pathology, hard determinism applies to all behavior. Hard determinism was endorsed by early psychotherapists as otherwise different as Freud and B. F. Skinner, and it still influences many therapeutic perspectives. Yet, hard determinism is inimical to therapy, as well as to morality in general, for in undermining morality it undermines responsibility for health.

Hard determinism is overthrown by finding a way to reconcile universal causation with moral responsibility. The current name for that reconciliation is *compatibilism*: even if all events and actions are caused, we are still responsible for (many) actions. I believe that compatibilism is correct, in some version.[24] Defending that belief here, however, would immerse us in the enormously complex issue of free will versus determinism. Instead, I will simply outline how compatibilism enters into an integrated, moral-therapeutic perspective.

A moral-therapeutic perspective takes science seriously. It accepts that all events, including human actions, have causes that can be investigated empirically. If there are areas of noncausation, they occur at the level of subatomic particles described by quantum physics, a level that has no direct relevance to understanding moral responsibility. All actions are caused, then, but it does not follow that we are complete victims of biology and environment. Instead, we contribute to the causal nexus through our conduct. Our desires, beliefs, values, and capacities for agency are causally influenced *and* (sometimes) causally efficacious in ways that render us morally accountable.

All the freedoms we cherish—moral freedom to choose, freedom to reason and think, self-control, freedom to change and improve, and political freedom— are compatible with the view that every event has a cause.[25] In Owen Flanagan's words, universal causation is compatible with "self-control, self-expression, individuality, reasons-sensitivity, rational deliberation, rational accountability, moral accountability, and the capacity to do otherwise, unpredictability, and political freedom."[26] We do not cherish free choice that severs our actions from our past, our character, and our present reason-guided engagement in the world. Without the link between past character formation and present actions, it would be unreasonable to hold a person accountable. A wholly uncaused "free will" would undermine responsibility by severing the link between a person (as presently constituted) and her actions. We exempt or excuse individuals not because their actions are caused, but because they are caused in particular ways—for example, by external forces beyond their control or by exceptional burdens and obstacles. Individuals are accountable when they have these capacities, or would have if they had acted responsibly in developing them, and when they can reasonably be expected to exercise them in particular situations.

Unfortunately, some leading compatibilists have encouraged the view that mental disorders automatically excuse or exempt from responsibility. In particular, Peter Strawson insightfully argues that metaphysical debates about free will and determinism are irrelevant to ordinary practices of holding individuals responsible. What matters is whether individuals have normal capacities to participate in moral practices, such as moral reasoning, guilt and shame when we fail to meet moral standards, gratitude for acts of kindness, mutual love among adults, resentment toward people who wrong us, indignation toward people who unjustly harm others, and forgiveness when others repent and make amends. In defending compatibilism, however, he assumes that psychopathology undermines normal capacities, such that to be sick is to be exempt from responsibility. Moreover, he is generous in his list of responsibility-exempting pathologies: schizophrenia, insanity, neurosis, compulsion, sociopathy, and "warped" and "unrealistic acting out of unconscious purposes." Insofar as a person is sick, we adopt "objective attitudes" toward them, viewing them as objects for therapy rather than as participants in personal relationships. Although he admits he is working with a "crude opposition of phrase where we have a great intricacy of phenomena," he leaves the impression that mental disorders automatically exempt from moral responsibility.[27] Here I briefly comment on several of Strawson's examples, leaving fuller discussion to Part III.

Consider neurotics, who act in unrealistic ways because of unconscious purposes. Suppose the unconscious purposes lead to sexual exploitation of the sort Judge Lanier engaged in, or to compulsive behavior involving violence, as with serial killers and rapists; or suppose that the unconscious purposes produce alcoholism that leads to drunk driving and manslaughter, or kleptomania that leads to significant theft of property. In these cases, sickness does not exempt from responsibility, morally or legally. People with serious addictions, compulsions, and impulse control disorders face special obstacles, and our moral responses should take them into account. But they are not exempt from accountability. Most compulsions and impulse-control disorders are not completely debilitating, rendering the person literally unable to resist impulses to engage in harmful conduct. And even if persons are impaired at the moment of acting, they remain responsible for allowing the compulsion to gain control over them, and that responsibility extends to responsibility for actions. They are also responsible for seeking and cooperating with help.

Next consider sociopaths—"moral idiots," as Strawson calls them, or persons with antisocial personality disorders, as psychiatrists now call them. Bearing in mind that only a small percentage of sociopaths are violent, are we "uncivilized" to react with deep resentment and outrage when they kill someone we care about? Sociopaths do not *care* about moral values in the way most of us do. Because of this, they have a major moral impairment—a disorder that makes them unfit for many moral aspects of interpersonal relationships. Nevertheless, sociopaths are not legally insane, and they are routinely held accountable before the law. They are also morally accountable for adhering to society's basic norms. For, although they do not care about moral reasons, they are able to discern what society sets forth as legal and moral standards. We hold people accountable primarily for their actions, not their motives (although motives have additional moral significance). Hence, in holding sociopaths accountable, we are demanding that they do not murder, cheat, or steal, and self-interest provides reasons for them to adhere to these moral reasons. Of course, sociopaths are not always motivated by enlightened self-interest, but neither are most of us.

With these examples in mind, we can ask why Strawson assumes that the "civilized" view is that psychopathology automatically exempts from responsibility. One reason is that he is preoccupied with "reactive attitudes," such as indignation and blame, and pays too little attention to obligations. In one passage he virtually reduces obligations to attitudes: "The making of the [moral] demand *is* the proneness to such [reactive] attitudes."[28] Essentially, he assumes that accountability and moral community are entirely about reciprocal attitudes within relationships based on mutual good will.[29] Since sociopaths generally fail to reciprocate our good will, they are excluded from the moral community. If we focus on obligations rather than emotions, however, there is every reason to hold sociopaths accountable. They have the same obligations as all of us—not to murder, rape, steal—and their disorders do not exempt them from accountability for meeting those obligations. In any case, moral attitudes need to be justified by reference to obligations. When we express justified resentment or indignation, we are not merely expressing feelings. We are asserting that individuals have violated their obligations, and we are manifesting our commitment to standards of decency as essential to social life.[30]

Another reason Strawson thinks psychopathology exempts from responsibility is that he assumes responsibility implies the capacity to act morally at a given moment. Because compulsives are out of control in a given moment, they are not responsible.[31] This view overlooks responsibilities for acquiring and maintaining sound moral habits of self-control in the first place. Failure to develop sound moral habits often amounts to culpable *moral negligence*. Drunk drivers might well be completely unable at a given moment to avoid killing a pedestrian, but they are culpable for getting into the situation. Similarly, many moral failures are traceable to longer-term negligence in failing to form habits and even traits of character necessary in meeting the minimal obligations incumbent on us all as members of a moral community. As Jonathan Jacobs observes, agents might become "ethically disabled" by forming powerful habits and attitudes that make it far more difficult or unlikely they will act responsibly in some situations, but they remain morally accountable.[32]

To conclude, we have laid the foundation for blocking any automatic inference from "sick" to "not responsible." Within limits, which should be explored contextually, we are responsible for our health, and even within the therapist-client relationship this responsibility plays a key role. We are also accountable for the negligence that leads to morally objectionable and unhealthy habits. Although this chapter focused on the relationship of therapists to clients, we have already broached the topic of the next topic: the transfer of therapeutic attitudes from the clinic to the wider community.

5

RESPONSIBILITY IN COMMUNITY

When he published *The Triumph of the Therapeutic* in 1966, Philip Rieff was mourning a loss, not celebrating a victory. The loss was traditional morality as embedded in religious communities. The triumph was psychotherapy, at the time dominated by psychoanalysis, which he claimed replaces moral agents with "psychological man." Each decade since, Rieff's themes have been reworked, most notably by Christopher Lasch in *The Culture of Narcissism* (1979), Robert Bellah and his coauthors in *Habits of the Heart* (1985), and James D. Hunter in *The Death of Character* (2000).[1] Hunter's opening lines convey the dire tone of most of these books: "Character is dead. Attempts to revive it will yield little. Its time has passed."[2]

These critics interpret the therapeutic trend as a replacement of community-oriented morality with self-oriented therapeutic values such as self-esteem, self-fulfillment, and authenticity. They charge that exporting therapeutic attitudes from the clinic to the community erodes moral responsibility by fostering moral subjectivity and shallowness, lowering moral aspiration, and encouraging selfishness and a victim mentality. In responding to these charges, including their application to self-help groups and moral education, I argue that the critics identify genuine dangers but exaggerate them. For the most part, the therapeutic trend integrates morality with therapy, albeit with varying degrees of success, rather than abandoning it.

A Soprano's Overture

The Sopranos is a dark but illuminating TV drama structured around a mobster's visits to a psychiatrist for help in coping with his problems. In the opening episode, Tony Soprano faints during his son's birthday party, and, when no physical cause is found, he is referred to psychiatrist Jennifer Melfi. Together they explore his "job" dissatisfaction, depression, anxieties about death, fears of losing his family, and ambivalence toward his mother, who has borderline-personality disorder and colludes in an attempt to kill him. From the outset, the therapy sessions are emotionally charged with more than usual eroticized attractions of patient to therapist (transference) and therapist to patient (countertransference). Like us, Dr. Melfi is fascinated by Tony's world of power and violence, at least when it does not physically injure innocent bystanders, and she is intrigued by his ability to compartmentalize love for his family and brutality in crime. For his part, Tony knows that psychotherapy places his life at risk from other mobsters who fear he will divulge secrets about them.

Widely praised for its honest portrayal of therapy, *The Sopranos* also dramatizes criticisms of the therapeutic trend. One criticism is that therapists' nonjudgmental stance fosters relativism and subjectivism by reducing morality to individual preferences. Thus, Dr. Melfi is criticized, by her husband and others, for participating in a "moral never-never land" and for assuming a "cheery moral relativism" that colludes with evil rather than confronts it. The criticism is implicit in the premise for the series: a nonjudgmental psychotherapist helps an emotionally distressed mobster cope with a life of extortion, racketeering, and violence.[3] At the same time, it is clear that a full confrontation by Dr. Melfi would end the therapy and prevent Tony from obtaining help. Melfi occasionally does help Tony morally—for example, when she encourages him to notify the police about a pedophile soccer coach rather than take the law into his own hands. The event reflects how traditional conceptions of complete neutrality are under scrutiny within the therapeutic community.[4] It also reminds us that a thoroughgoing nonjudgmental stance shades into amorality.

Another criticism is that the therapeutic trend fosters a victim mentality in which sickness is used to excuse immorality. With wonderful irony, Tony, the mobster, complains that psychiatry undermines personal responsibility: "Nowadays everybody's got to go to shrinks and counselors and go on Sally Jesse Raphael and talk about their problems.... It's dysfunction this, dysfunction that."[5] Excuses are used to deflect blame: "I am sick, hence a victim, hence not at fault." They are used to gain exemption from onerous duties: "I am sick, hence unable to meet responsibilities, hence excused." And they are used to gain benefits: "I am sick, hence deserving of compassion and help."

Yet another criticism concerns the tyranny of health professionals in guiding moral education. When his thirteen-year-old son is called before the school authorities for getting drunk on stolen communion wine, Tony assumes he should be punished. Instead, the principal sends him to the school psychologist who diagnoses him with borderline attention deficit disorder, nearly forcing him to take medication and transfer into a "special needs" classroom. The psychologist says the boy should be "consequenced" for his wrongdoing, an awkward euphemism for punishment that blurs what is at stake morally. Likewise, the critics of the therapeutic trend charge that therapeutic attitudes are systematically blurring our understanding of morality.

Autonomy versus Subjectivism

The critics charge, first, that the therapeutic trend reduces moral values to subjective preferences. It encourages individuals to choose their values autonomously, rather than to accept religion-based morality, society's authority, and objectively defensible obligations. In the words of Bellah and his coauthors, the therapist seeks "to teach the therapeutic client to be independent of anyone else's standards" and "to rely on his own judgment without deferring to others." As therapeutic attitudes spread to the wider society, they encourage "'finding oneself' in autonomous self-reliance."[6]

This criticism fails to distinguish several ideas: moral self-governance; ethical subjectivism; authenticity in developing and expressing one's deepest commitments; and economic independence and self-reliance. In particular, both Bellah et al. and their interviewees fail to distinguish between moral self-governance and ethical subjectivism. In its classical, Kantian meaning, moral self-governance means exercising independent reasoning in making reasonable moral judgments rather than passively relying on others to make them for us. As such, it is the opposite of ethical subjectivism, the view that values are mere personal preferences unsupported by reasons. Bellah's group and other social critics generally assume that sound morality is rooted in religion, so that independent moral thinking is suspect when it strays from mainstream religious beliefs. But with or without religion, moral self-determination based on independent moral reasoning should not be confused with ethical subjectivism.

Second, the critics object that the therapeutic outlook is morally shallow or vacuous because its nonjudgmental stance discourages moral judgments. Spread to the wider culture through self-help books and the media, therapists' nonjudgmental stance places all moral judgments on a par, with none more justified than others.[7] As Rieff says, "because the clinical attitude aspires to moral neutrality, its therapeutic effect is culturally dubious."[8]

In reply, it is indeed disastrous to slide from nonjudgmental attitudes in therapeutic contexts to abandoning moral judgment in everyday life. We need to remain attuned to the contextual nature of moral judgments—therapy is a special context of helping, and there are many others. In fact, good therapists help us make nuanced, contextualized moral judgments. They remind us that "insight and self-understanding do not flourish in an atmosphere of self-depreciation or blame" and that when we want to help others we often do best to reign in our passion for blaming.[9] Furthermore, therapeutic outlooks are not morally neutral; as we have seen, they embody moral values. Even a therapist's suspension of blame is required by professional distance, which fosters a secure environment in which individuals can explore their inner conflicts as part of therapy. Therapeutic neutrality is embedded in a wider network of moral values that include respect for clients' autonomy, care for their well-being, obtaining informed consent, maintaining confidentiality, and minimizing harm to third parties.

Third, critics charge that the therapeutic trend lowers moral aspiration. According to Rieff, it teaches us to "survive, resign yourself to living within your moral means, suffer no gratuitous failures in a futile search for ethical heights that no longer exist—if they ever did."[10] According to Bellah et al., it encourages narrow "instrumental" thinking about means to self-interested goals, rather than broader reflection on valuable goals in a good life.[11] Obligations to the wider community are replaced by "honest communication among self-actualized individuals."[12] Honesty, loyalty, and commitment are embraced, but they are distorted when pressed into the service of self-interest, as with Tony Soprano.

Interestingly, this criticism acknowledges that therapeutic outlooks are not morally neutral after all. Instead, they embed selected moral values: honesty with oneself aimed at self-understanding, tolerance and effective communication with others, prudence and realism in forming and pursuing goals, kindness toward oneself and caring for significant others. The problem, according to the critics, is that these values are weighted toward self-seeking at the expense of others. I agree that therapeutic emphases often slide toward subjectivism. Nevertheless, therapeutic attitudes are not inherently at odds with community-oriented values. Self-respect, honesty, compassion, and other therapeutic values are integral to morality, and the criteria for mental health embody standards of minimally acceptable behavior. To think otherwise is to stereotype morality as exclusively concerned with other-oriented obligations, thereby forgetting duties of self-respect, and to stereotype therapy as exclusively about self-seeking.

Obligations versus Selfishness

A fourth criticism is that the therapeutic trend fosters immorality by encouraging self-absorption and selfishness, discouraging civic and religious involvements, eroding moral commitments at work, and threatening obligations of family and love. Within the therapeutic worldview, says Rieff, "nothing [is] at stake beyond a manipulatable sense of well-being" and skills to "manage the strains of living as a communally detached individual."[13] In Lasch's words, the "therapeutic sensibility" has at its core "the feeling, the momentary illusion, of personal well-being, health, and psychic security," but no sense of obligation.[14]

In reply, there is no such thing as "the" therapeutic outlook; there are hundreds of different ones. Some disregard community and obligations, but many others pay heed to how caring relationships and community involvements contribute to mental health. They acknowledge responsibilities to others, as well as to oneself. The critics neglect the community-oriented aspects of therapy, whether within counseling or in the public attitudes it fosters, just as they downplay the self-oriented aspects of morality. Thus, humanistic psychologists, such as Erich Fromm and Abraham Maslow, insist that caring relationships promote both moral meaning and mental health. Indeed, reciprocal caring relationships enter into definitions of the healthy and responsible "self." Again, contemporary marriage and family counselors generally focus on entire families and other meaningful personal relationships. Good counselors, whether in helping their clients or writing a self-help book, appreciate the importance of reciprocal caring to self-fulfillment. Moreover, today many psychotherapists are attuned to the religious beliefs of their patients, and public health experts heed the values of caring and justice.[15]

More cautiously, Bellah and his coauthors accuse Americans of confusion rather than selfishness, as they oscillate between moral language and "the language of individualism."[16] Part of this self-oriented language is linked to "expressive individualism": when Americans talk about the values structuring their families, love, work, and communities, they speak primarily of satisfying their preferences. Another part is "utilitarian individualism," the means-to-ends instrumentalism concerned with meeting self-interested goals of success and wealth. (Bellah's use of "utilitarian" is the exact opposite of Bentham and Mill's meaning of promoting the general good.) As for the therapeutic attitude, "the very language of therapeutic relationship seems to undercut the possibility of other than self-interested relationships." Again, "the therapeutic view not only refuses to take a moral stand, it actively distrusts 'morality.' . . . The question 'Is this right' becomes 'Is this going to work for me now?'"[17]

In reply, I agree that the critics identify tensions in Americans' value perspectives. Americans are pulling back from some traditional loyalties to large organizations such as government and corporations, as well as showing gradual decreases in community involvements in organized religion, local civic organizations, and other forms of community. We are developing what Bellah et al. call "lifestyle enclaves" centered on personal relationships within groups of our choosing (including virtual communities on the internet). But the therapeutic trend is not the source of our "endemic individualism," and the recent erosion of community involvement is due to broader political and economic forces. These forces include increased competition from global capitalism, mobility of managers and labor which severs ties to local communities, increasing respect for pluralism and diversity rather than uniform values, the dominance of large bureaucracies of all kinds, and value distortions promulgated by mass advertising and marketing.[18]

Why, then, don't the critics target these deeper forces? And why don't they celebrate the positive contributions of the therapeutic trend in helping people cope with the dislocation caused by economic turmoil and eroding political structures?[19] I suspect the answer lies in their tacit support of traditional, organized religion. Traditional religion differs from popular forms of spirituality, which are more individualistic and upbeat, and less blame-oriented, than much traditional religion. These new forms are flourishing in America, and they are attuned to therapeutic themes about healthy morality and self-fulfillment.[20]

Responsibility for Health versus Victimism

A fifth criticism, made by Charles Sykes in *A Nation of Victims*, is that the therapeutic trend fosters a self-serving victim mentality. Sykes begins with an

FBI agent who embezzles government money and loses it gambling in Atlantic City. After being fired, the agent gets his job back by arguing that his pathological gambling is a handicap protected under federal law. Sykes assembles dozens of additional illustrations from lawsuits, criminal defense proceedings, talk shows, and self-help books, to support his contention that "victimism" has become "a generalized cultural impulse to deny personal responsibility and to obsess on the grievances of the insatiable self." He interprets the therapeutic trend as replacing personal responsibility with pathology: "Almost by definition, disease is caused by agents or forces largely beyond the control of an individual—by viruses, microbes, genetic deficiencies, or environmental factors. If someone who drinks excessively is sick, then the notion of personal or moral responsibility becomes highly problematic."[21]

The "almost by definition" is a considerable exaggeration, one that Sykes shares with the Americans he criticizes. The mental disorders specified in the *DSM* have multiple causes that might include morally bad habits. Although mental disorders can seriously impede moral agency, most do not make it impossible. Sykes is right, however, that pathologizing undesirable conduct creates a *temptation* to regard ourselves as hapless victims. In addition to natural self-favoritism, responsibility can be an onerous burden we eagerly seek to escape.[22]

With regard to both physical and psychological disorders, we eagerly equivocate on the word "victim": I am a victim of sickness, in the sense of suffering from it; therefore I am an innocent victim, in the sense of a hapless object of forces beyond my control. Moreover, the extent to which illness is caused by factors beyond our control is often ambiguous, making it easy to appeal to disorders as excuses. Sykes and others exaggerate when they condemn the *DSM* as a recipe book for "making us crazy" and for "manufacturing victims" by turning us into wounded, abused, sick individuals.[23] But they are partly correct. Influential ideologies of the sick role do portray patients as blameless, as we saw in chapter 4. The *DSM* Cautionary Statement, which disavows that mental disorders are automatic excuses, cannot by itself remove this danger.

My claims about what therapeutic outlooks can accommodate might seem irrelevant because the critics' concern is with what is actually happening, on a societal scale, not what would happen if we were all thinking clearly. But I believe we should be wary of what these critics "discern" in our society, especially when they are nostalgic for religious-based ethics and societies. The dire warnings of Rieff and other critics should be opposed by the report by sociologist Alan Wolfe, who documents some of the creative moral-therapeutic integrations taking place: "Many of our respondents find themselves more comfortable with the language of psychology than they do with the language of sin. But this hardly means that character is dead. . . . Our respondents are not so much rejecting character as they are asking for new ways to form it that are compatible with a generally positive view of human potential."[24]

Self-Help Groups: Communities
or Forums for Evasion?

Therapy-oriented self-help/mutual-aid groups, which operate in the social space between the clinic and the broader community, are a favorite target of critics of the therapeutic trend. In particular, Wendy Kaminer derides these groups: "Today's popular programs on recovery from various (and questionable) addictions actively discourage people from actually helping themselves."[25] The self-help sector includes books, videos, audiotapes, and Internet ("virtual") communities, but Kaminer singles out Alcoholics Anonymous (AA) and its progeny of twelve-step recovery groups, including Al-Anon (for spouses of alcoholics), Narcotics Anonymous, Overeaters Anonymous, Workaholics Anonymous, Debtors Anonymous, Gamblers Anonymous, Sex and Love Addicts Anonymous, Procrastinators Anonymous, Clutterers Anonymous, Fundamentalists Anonymous (for those withdrawing from overzealous religious groups), and Codependents Anonymous (where codependents are covictims and facilitators within destructive families). She attacks these groups for their moral shallowness, victim mentality, psychobabble, and naïve faith that there is a "spiritual" solution to everything. Contrary to their professed goals of self-empowerment, the groups portray individuals as victims of diseases beyond their control. The first of the twelve steps is to acknowledge one's helplessness and inability to manage one's life, without the help of a "higher power."[26] This medicalizing of bad habits invites passivity ("I'm a victim"), self-absorption ("I'm sick and suffering"), pitiful pleas ("I need help"), and greed ("I deserve compensation").

We can grant that self-help/mutual-aid groups provide forums for moral evasion, self-indulgence, and bathos. But so do religion, family, politics, work, and every other area of human activity. The point is that self-help/mutual-aid groups are also forums for honesty, courage, and commitment. Preoccupied with excesses and abuses, Kaminer seems blind to this good. To admit that we are seriously addicted or otherwise sick, that we have lost control, and that we need help in coping with our difficulties is a profoundly responsible act, not mere whining. So is accepting needed help from others. Kaminer says twelve-step groups are a sad substitute for community; in fact, sometimes they offer the most supportive community available for individuals confronting overwhelming problems.[27]

Fair-minded critics offer more balanced assessments of recovery groups. After drawing attention to the enormous diversity and varied quality of the groups, Robert Wuthnow argues that twelve-step groups have the potential for both good and bad. At their worst, the groups reinforce narcissism and self-indulgence. At their best, they provide healing communities. Their proliferation in recent years manifests Americans' enduring search for the sacred, even though the sacred is redefined as more inward-looking and less oriented to religious authority and organizations. Wuthnow worries that such groups "encourage many members to regard biblical wisdom as truth only if it somehow helps them to get along better in their daily lives," thereby robbing "the sacred of its awe-inspiring mystery and depth."[28] Yet, he sees no reason to denigrate their therapeutic emphasis, and neither should we.[29]

Another balanced assessment is offered by Thomasina Jo Borkman, who characterizes self-help/mutual aid groups as forms of community in which "people work together to emphasize one another's strengths and capacities," whether or not the emphasis is on healing per se. In "viable self-help groups, the committed participants face their shared problem and, in telling their stories, relive the pain, stigma, and other negative aspects of their situation in order to work through it with dignity.... Some examine what it means to be a human being."[30] As Borkman points out, self-help/mutual-aid groups offer occasions for experiential learning and self-development. They provide structures for moral transformation. And they do not endorse a monolithic ideology and set of values. For example, groups dealing with problems of being overweight cover the spectrum from those that accept social norms of slimness (TOPS: Take Off Pounds Sensibly) to those that reject them (Fat Is Beautiful). The groups generally adopt nonjudgmental approaches, asking participants to restrain their tendencies to indulge in blaming themselves and others. This nonjudgmental stance, however, is very much a moral stance. It serves the moral goals of evoking empathy and compassion, fostering self-acceptance and self-respect, and ultimately enabling individuals to accept responsibility for their conduct.

Taken as a group, Americans' self-help/mutual-aid groups are like a Rorschach test: what we see reveals much about our values and biases. Kaminer's religious skepticism, Wuthnow's religious concerns, and Borkman's pragmatism highlights what they find valuable or worrisome about such groups. Although some individuals use therapy-oriented groups to evade personal responsibility, others use them to accept moral responsibility. These "self-chosen communities" make important contributions by combining, in Robert Jay Lifton's words, "highly fluid arrangements with some of the supportive elements of the traditional community."[31] Instead of signaling the death of morality, they contribute to community and help us cope with social fragmentation.

Self-Esteem and Moral Education

Moral education is another favorite target of the critics. In particular, James Hunter studies moral education as a prism through which to view an entire society in which "the self—its appetites, preferences, and interests—is not alone on stage, but it is at center stage—and without serious rival or competition."[32] He argues that self-esteem, rather than obligations to others, is emphasized in moral education in schools, including sex education and drug-prevention programs, as well as in self-help books for parents. He concludes that Americans are experiencing a "death of character." A closer look at his data suggests a less bleak picture.

Halfway through his book, Hunter makes a remarkable admission: most programs in moral education do integrate values such as justice, tolerance, reciprocity, and compassion. The programs teach caring for other people and for community, typically using the theme that proper self-esteem empowers us to care for others. His real objection is that the programs give the wrong *reasons* for caring for others—namely, benefits to oneself. For example, one typical self-help book tells parents that when children ask why they should be kind to others, the answer should highlight benefits for the child: because being kind makes you feel good about yourself, gives you a strong sense of self, helps you function better in society, makes your world happier, and helps you make friends.[33] Such an approach corrupts morality by reducing it to ethical egoism, the view that reduces morality to self-interest.

Most often, however, Hunter discovers programs mixing appeals to self-esteem and caring for others. This impurity alarms him. Consider, for example, what he says about the Character Counts! Coalition, founded by Michael Josephson, which blends appeals to self-interest with moral reasoning. Josephson teaches children to feel good about themselves when they do the right thing: "We have to make them [the children] committed to doing right, meaning it feels good to do right. Teach them that it feels good to do right." Such teachings, Hunter complains, send a mixed message by blending self-interest and morality. So do religious books that conjoin self-esteem with benevolence: "There is considerable ambivalence in the mix of both traditional biblical teaching and psychological assumptions, concepts, and methods."[34]

Hunter's call for purity manifests a lack of psychological realism. There is nothing objectionable about teaching morality by mixing appeals to self-interest and the well-being of others—as long as both appeals are taken seriously. Parents, clergy, and educators have always done that. They know that human beings are most strongly motivated by self-interest and have only limited capacities for altruism, and they know that morality and self-interest are both valid and mutually reinforcing. As for feeling good about doing the right thing, that can be a mark of genuine moral commitment, not impurity. And when Hunter objects to grounding morality in the rights of autonomous individuals, he is dismissing the human-rights ethics that has guided Americans throughout their history—an ethics that includes respect for others' rights, as well as asserting one's own.[35]

Like Hunter, William Damon claims that self-esteem oriented curricula foster selfishness by elevating self-interest over respect for others. In bolstering positive attitudes toward oneself independently of moral standards, educators fail to teach caring about others' feelings and needs. The "inflated sense of self-importance that is fed by our culture's overemphasis on self-esteem" is part and parcel of "failing to give children firm rules and guidelines," which "is a sure way to breed arrogance and disrespect." Damon insists that building self-esteem should not be a direct goal in moral education, whether self-esteem is understood as self-acceptance or positive feelings about oneself. Instead, "we would do better to help children acquire the skills, values, and virtues on which a positive sense of self is properly built."[36]

In reply, health-defining self-esteem, the kind that largely overlaps with the virtue of self-respect, is one of the primary virtues that should be taught. Damon, like the other critics, overreacts to the one-sided emphasis on self-esteem by dropping it altogether. But proper self-esteem is one important value among others. To be sure, excessive preoccupation with self-esteem eclipses moral motivation and obligations to others. Self-esteem is not a sufficient foundation for moral education, and vastly exaggerated claims have been made on behalf of self-esteem. For example, the California Task Force to Promote Self-Esteem and Personal Responsibility conceived of self-esteem as an all-purpose vaccine for social ills: "Self-esteem is the likeliest candidate for a social vaccine, something that empowers us to live responsibly and that inoculates us against the lures of crime, violence, substance abuse, teen pregnancy, child abuse, chronic welfare dependency, and educational failure."[37] Such claims provoked massive research which, overall, failed to substantiate them.[38] A distinguished set of researchers, initially hoping to document the claims of the California Task Force, concluded that "the associations between self-esteem and its expected consequences are mixed, insignificant, or absent."[39]

I should add that self-esteem research and debates about the importance of self-esteem are handicapped by the absence of a shared definition of self-esteem. If self-esteem is simply feeling good about oneself, then of course it is not correlated with good character. What is more commonplace than the self-affirming, narcissistic criminal?[40] Yet, as noted in chapter 2, health-defining self-esteem embeds additional values, such as reasonable beliefs about oneself, warranted degrees of self-confidence, and appropriate ways of valuing oneself. As such, it interweaves with the virtue of self-respect: properly valuing oneself as deserving the same recognition as other moral beings, as opposed to both having an inferiority complex or a narcissistic personality disorder. Educators are supposed to support and teach appropriate self-esteem, not just any kind of self-elevation.[41]

The Authentic Self in Community

I have suggested that critics of the therapeutic trend identify but exaggerate genuine abuses and dangers. I conclude with an overview (to be developed in Part IV) of how an integrated, moral-therapeutic perspective links self-fulfillment with responsibilities to others, as well as to oneself. I take my bearings from Charles Taylor. Taylor shares the critics' concerns about how the therapeutic trend encourages moral subjectivism rather than the recognition of values independent of us, but he understands the threats to values in Western culture as having far deeper roots than Bellah and the other critics discern.[42] He also insists that the critics' attacks on ideals of autonomy and self-fulfillment are wrongheaded. These ideals are themselves objectively defensible aspects of authenticity—a profoundly important moral value that must not be confused with sheer egoism.[43] Popular culture tends to debase authenticity by sliding from moral autonomy to subjectivism and selfishness. The remedy is to rethink, not reject, authenticity and autonomy.

Authenticity is a distinctively modern value and a product of Romanticism, but its contemporary implementation comes through the "affirmation of the ordinary"—of love and work, of everyday life. Authenticity is the idea that "each of us has an original way of being human" and there is a moral imperative to be "true to my own originality," which "is something only I can articulate and discover."[44] Authenticity, as well as autonomy and self-fulfillment, cannot stand alone as isolated values. They need to be "part of a 'package,' to be sought within a life which is also aimed at other goods."[45] To fulfill ourselves requires identifying our deepest desires and aspirations, but doing so within "the horizon" of moral values. These values place limits on conduct, but they also enlarge possibilities for meaningful life.

As social creatures, our identities are "narrative constructions" in which we tell a story about who we are, where we have been, and where we are going. Postmodernists tend to construe the self as an arbitrary creation, the product of a "story" told to ourselves any way we choose. They illuminate the fragility and contingency of the self, and this meaning explains why we tend to defend them so fiercely when they are threatened. They help explain why self-esteem is so unstable and at risk in contemporary society.[46] Yet, their skepticism about objective values leads to nihilism and the loss of meaningful lives. Defensible narratives connect the self to wider horizons of objective values and meaning. Authenticity is debased by the slide to subjectivism, whereby feelings and choices become self-certifying, rather than making them subject to appraisal in light of values whose validity is independent of our own will. Subjectivism undermines meaning-giving resources for achieving authenticity, especially personal relationships and community involvements.

The idea of narratives also enters into many therapeutic outlooks. Nearly all "talk therapies" rely on dialogue aimed at telling a life and retelling it to make it more intelligible and estimable.[47] This dialogue might be permeated with bias, illusion, contingency, variability, and multiple interpretations. But it can also be built on truth and justified values.[48] Indeed, "self-fulfillment" and "community" are value-laden concepts. Rather than a mere grouping of individuals, communities are societies linked by shared identities, mutual concerns, and overlapping values that contribute to personal meaning.[49] The critics of the therapeutic trend often assert commitments to traditional religion-based communities and, offended by Freud's aggressively antireligious stance, view the therapeutic trend as opposed to community. Yet, even Freud was not hostile to community per se—whatever that might involve. He understood the healthy self as able to work and love, two types of relationship that invite wider social involvements. Sound therapeutic outlooks affirm a plurality of views about community, including many options lying between traditional forms of religion and superficial forms of "lifestyle enclaves."

To conclude, the critics insightfully alert us to the self-oriented excesses in the therapeutic trend. In doing so, they interpret the therapeutic trend as replacing morality with therapy; hence, "the death of character." In philosophical terms, they identify a social movement toward increasing ethical egoism, and, hence, at most toward flawed integrative projects of the sort found in Nietzsche and Freud. Recasting their criticisms, and dropping pejorative stereotypes of therapy, we can draw on the critics' insights in developing a sound integration of morality and therapy. Our next concern is whether a sound integration of morality and therapy leaves some room for blame. I argue it does.

6

BLAMING VICTIMS

D on't blame the victim, we say, but what if victims of mental disorders or physical diseases largely create their own problems by smoking, abusing alcohol, using illegal drugs, overeating, or gambling compulsively?[1] Is blame then appropriate because they are no longer victims (hapless objects) of forces beyond their control, even though they remain victims of (sufferers from) the malady itself? Or, somewhat paradoxically, are they blameworthy as agents who cause their sickness, but not blameworthy as victims who suffer? In general, how can we take seriously responsibilities for health while avoiding destructive forms of blame?

Blame tends to be counterproductive, therapeutically and morally, in helping contexts. Even when individuals are blameworthy for engaging in dangerous acts, the helper's role requires suspending or greatly limiting blame while encouraging them to accept responsibility for their health. Nevertheless, not all blame is destructive, and sometimes it motivates individuals to accept responsibility for their health. I explore how an integrated, moral-therapeutic perspective encourages acceptance of responsibility for health without unfair and destructive forms of blame. The discussion is structured around four health-related contexts: (1) preventing sickness, (2) assigning financial liabilities for health care costs, (3) giving meaning to suffering, and (4) interacting with health care professionals. What we say about blame in one of these contexts is relevant to but does not dictate what we say in other contexts.

Preventing Sickness: Justice and Compassion

Audre Lorde, the distinguished African-American poet, was diagnosed with breast cancer in 1978 and underwent a mastectomy. While reading a medical magazine, she came across a letter from a physician who claimed that "no truly happy person ever gets cancer." The letter endorsed the idea that positive attitudes suffice to prevent cancer, a superstition that physicians should dispel rather than disseminate. Lorde reports that in her vulnerable state the letter momentarily "hit my guilt button," but indignation quickly followed. Making victims feel guilty "is a monstrous distortion of the idea that we can use our psychic strengths to help heal ourselves," and it "is an extension of the blame-the-victim syndrome."[2]

Lorde accurately identifies a "monstrous distortion," but when we turn from breast cancer to, say, smoking-caused cancers and nicotine-use disorders, the ethics of blaming becomes more complex. Ample and readily available evidence establishes causal connections between smoking and lung cancer, emphysema, and heart disease. It can be enormously difficult to stop smoking—for most people, harder than overcoming heroin addiction. It can also be difficult not to start smoking, given peer pressure, advertising, and the influence of movies. Nevertheless, smokers are not mere victims of forces beyond their control. The same is true of many individuals who are overweight, abuse alcohol, fail to exercise, and take foolish risks. We have responsibilities to take care of our health. Anticipating blame can be a supportive motive for meeting those responsibilities. At the same time, we do best to emphasize the positive ideal of taking due care to meet our responsibilities concerning health.[3]

In its primary meaning, blame is a negative moral response to persons rather than to actions, but the response takes various forms.[4] *Judgment blame* is the simple judgment that individuals are culpable for specific wrongs. Paradigmatic blame, however, involves this judgment plus additional elements. Thus, *attitude blame* consists of negative attitudes and emotions: resentment, indignation, anger, contempt, or hatred (in blaming others); and guilt, shame, depression, or self-hatred (in blaming oneself). These attitudes and emotions have varying degrees of intensity, from mild to vehement, and they can be episodic or recurring.[5] *Censure blame* consists of public criticism, including formal condemnation and reprimand (the strict sense of "censure") and informal criticism such as snide remarks, angry denunciations, and shunning. Finally, *liability blame* consists of assigning liabilities (costs, penalties, punishment) for harmful consequences, whether or not attitude and censure blame are involved.

The imperative "Don't blame the victim" is used to protest all these forms of blame toward individuals who are not responsible for specific harms. The forms of blame are distinct, however, and some are less appropriate than others. For example, even if we believe that individuals ought not to smoke (judgment blame), we can avoid negative attitudes toward them (attitude blame), whether out of friendship or indifference. And if for public policy reasons, smokers are assigned financial penalties in the form of higher insurance premiums (liability blame), it does not follow we should shun them (censure blame). Assigning liability can be done with the professional detachment of a judge or an insurance agent.

With these distinctions in mind, we can clarify why it is immoral, as well as a confusion, to blame innocent victims who have done nothing wrong. Two key values are violated: justice (including fairness) and compassion. In most instances, the primary objection is *justice based*: it is unjust to blame persons for harms they are not responsible for. Blaming the innocent inverts justice, creating the topsy-turvy world of *Erewhon*. Usually, compassion is also violated, and in some situations the primary objection to blaming victims is *compassion based*. Suppose that victims are ordinary mortals (not tyrants) who do foolish things which primarily hurt themselves. For example, a promising young athlete is left physically disabled and mentally impaired because she drove recklessly and without a seat belt. She caused her own suffering, but to adopt punitive attitudes toward her would be callous. "Don't blame the victim," we say, even though (and partly because) she is the victim of her own mistakes; she has suffered enough. Similarly, regardless of whether individuals partly cause their coronary disease or injuries, adopting harshly negative attitudes toward them is usually uncompassionate.

In using the compassion-based objection to blaming victims, we highlight suffering and set aside questions about its causes. We view individuals as victims of (suffering from) the sickness or injury, regardless of their role in producing it. This compassion-based objection to blaming generates confusion, however, when it blurs the protest against injustice. In what follows, I take account of the compassion-based objection, but I emphasize the justice-based objection.

As Kant emphasized, responsibilities for our health are rooted in self-respect and in the general obligation to maintain our ability to meet all other responsibilities. These responsibilities do not by themselves justify blaming people for causing their sickness. For one thing, the exact requirements of self-respect are unclear. It is doubtful, for example, that self-respect entails an absolute prohibition of smoking, even though it establishes a strong presumption against it. Perhaps an individual judges that smoking is the best compromise in dealing with a stressful life. If we disagree with that judgment, we should still avoid assuming there is only one reasonable view of what self-respect requires. For another thing, failing to meet a responsibility does not by itself justify blame, at least not in all its forms. And when we do blame, usually we should target specific behaviors and flaws, rather than a person's entire character.[6]

Additional ambiguities remain. The extent to which individuals cause their maladies is often unclear. Cause and effect relations might be in doubt. Singling out one causal factor over many others might be based on contested value judgments. Often it is uncertain which precautions can reasonably be expected of an individual, given their resources, obstacles, and additional responsibilities. Thus, specifying responsibilities for health is a moral matter, not a purely scientific one. It involves selecting and weighing particular causal factors as relevant to accountability and discounting others. Even saying that a drunk driver is responsible for causing an injury presupposes a moral standard of what can reasonably be expected of drivers.[7] Of course, poor health habits do not always cause sickness, but responsibilities for health require acting in light of probabilities rather than certainties. Taken together, these ambiguities often create a presumption against blaming, but they do not remove blameworthiness for failing to take obvious precautions.

In short, an integrated, moral-therapeutic perspective urges great caution in blaming. Nevertheless, abandoning all blame would undermine moral convictions and motivation in deterring wrongdoing and prompting reform. That is obviously true of judgment blame, but it is equally true of attitude, censure, and liability blame. Blame can strengthen moral motivation through public outrage at cruelty, resentment when rights are trampled, and maintaining self-respect through a healthy sense of shame and guilt.[8] Reasonable blame is based on humane attitudes, wide sympathy, sensitivity to valid excuses, generosity in forgiving offenses, and an overall positive aim in making the world better. Except regarding extreme wrongdoing, blame should be moderate and expressed in what Joseph Butler called a "settled and deliberate" calm manner.[9]

Financial Consequences: Liability versus Culpability

In a frequently cited letter to the *New England Journal of Medicine*, written at the beginning of Ronald Reagan's presidency, two professors warned of "a potentially dark side to a policy that might emphasize only individual responsibility in health." Acknowledging that we have responsibilities for our health, they nevertheless criticized political conservatives who were withdrawing health care funding for economically disadvantaged groups, in disregard of environmental and economic causes of poor health. Any one-sided emphasis on personal responsibility has "the effect of blaming the victim of poor health and social conditions."[10]

The "and" in the last quotation conjoins two things: being a victim of sickness (suffering from it) and being a victim of forces that led to the sickness. In doing so, it juxtaposes two different matters: compassion-based concerns about blaming people for their poor health, and justice-based concerns about blaming people for causes of poor health not under their control. The authors were primarily making a justice-based protest against blaming the poor for unfair social conditions and lack of resources to promote health—resources such as money, education, and time. "Elite moralism about health," they charged, ignores the complex economic, environmental, and genetic factors that influence who will suffer severe illness. Yet, by blending justice-based and compassion-based pleas, the authors blurred their primary focus on injustice.

Policy issues are complicated because they involve both prevention and liability. On the surface, prevention of sickness requires compassionate effort to get individuals not to harm themselves, whereas liability for health care costs concerns economic justice for such payment. In fact, prevention and liability coalesce at key junctures. Insofar as policies assigning financial liabilities motivate us to take better care of ourselves, assigning personal liability is integral to a compassionate approach to preventive medicine. Thus, compassionate prevention sometimes favors a tough stance in motivating individuals to avoid sickness. Furthermore, assigning financial costs for sickness involves weighing a host of factors such as individuals' ability to pay, their difficulties in finding affordable health care, and general questions about how to fairly distribute costs while being compassionate toward human suffering. In this way, both compassion and justice enter into prevention and liability.

John Knowles urges individuals to accept responsibility voluntarily. In contrast, Leon Kass recommends building in sanctions to national health insurance, even "refusing or reducing benefits for chronic respiratory disease care to persons who continue to smoke," when formulating insurance plans for health coverage. Smoking should carry financial penalties, even if that means denying life-supporting therapy for smokers. He insists that we confront the hard realities of health care and accept the need to ration health care toward irresponsible individuals.[11]

Critics of Knowles and Kass charge that they are blaming victims and that the lines of causality of sickness are too blurry to support a tough stance. Some smokers, especially young ones, might be partly the victims of massive advertising campaigns by tobacco companies, Hollywood images, and peer pressure; others might actually contribute to their health by using smoking to manage stress and control weight. Even after we affirm that individuals have responsibilities for their health, the exact extent to which they cause their health problems remains ambiguous, and we do well to focus on creating supportive social environments rather than blaming victims of sickness.[12] Furthermore, focusing primarily on individual responsibility deflects attention from deeper problems, such as poverty and societal enticements to engage in dangerous activities. Robert Crawford says the emphasis on individual responsibility is an "ideology" that serves to "avert any serious discussion of social or environmental factors" while unfairly blaming victims of these factors.[13] Lorde agrees, warning us that blaming the cancer victim neglects larger social issues about environmental pollution that causes cancer.[14] In addition, there are ethnic, class, and gender issues concerning the smug affluent who preach lifestyle correctness to the disadvantaged.[15]

I believe we should explore the middle-ground position staked out by Daniel Callahan in *False Hopes*. Callahan emphasizes that the ideals of humane medicine require that "the sick are to be treated regardless of the cause of the sickness or the culpability of the afflicted person." Neither physicians nor health care agencies should become moral judges. Nevertheless, most middle-class Americans deserve blame for their laxity in health matters: "We *ought* to be blamed. We are our own worst enemies and the victims of our own choices." We also harm others by our foolishness, given the financial interdependencies established within insurance and government programs. Callahan recommends a strong set of incentives and penalties, including higher insurance premiums, increased taxation on alcohol and cigarettes, and mandatory participation in health education programs.[16]

Many questions remain. Concerning money and motivation, what about individuals who do not pay medical insurance, either because they cannot afford it or because they have other priorities? Will acknowledging an obligation to care for them provide an incentive for widespread laxity? Compassion is best preserved by distinguishing financial liability from moral culpability. Financial liability concerns who should pay the costs, not guilt and resentment. As Gerald Dworkin points out, fundamental consideration in assessing liability is fairness: "People ought to bear the costs of their activities." But the enormous complexity of causal relationships should lead us, in setting public policy, to downplay attitude-blame and concentrate on reasonable distributions of liability costs.[17] Moreover, equally important considerations are utilitarian: effective incentives and accountability for dangerous practices might be cost-effective. In any case, the best combination of individual accountability and sharing of costs within the community is an empirical matter that must be investigated with regard to specific problems.

Coping with Illness: Meaning and Identity

Public policy concerning financial liability is widely discussed in medical ethics, but until recently ethicists said little about coping with illness. Here the issue concerns not only future-oriented acceptance of responsibility but also interpreting the meaning of illness.

A Hindu woman is terminally ill and suffering horribly. Her family asks her to recall any unrepented sins. She remembers having once eaten improperly prepared food and also inadvertently causing the death of a (sacred) cow by failing to attend to its care. After confessing these sins, she dies peacefully. The woman believes in the "natural law" of karma, that wrongdoing begets eventual suffering for the wrongdoer and requires ritualistic confession. Within this religious context, blame plays a positive, therapeutic role insofar as it alleviates suffering through repentance, forgiveness, and self-acceptance. Her judgment of fault promotes self-transcendence, not self-denigration. In this way, accepting blameworthiness can be a sign of caring for oneself and others—when it occurs within moral practices or religious rituals that contribute to human well-being and self-affirmation.[18]

Richard Shweder and his coauthors use this example to illustrate how religious meanings can render suffering more manageable. They suggest that religious doctrines about responsibility for health can be reasonable when applied to foolish habits such as unhealthy eating and engaging in unprotected sex: "In many cases, blaming yourself when you get sick can be the rational thing to do." They add, however, that "of course, there are illnesses and other conditions of suffering for which the sufferer is not 'at fault'" because the disease is entirely caused by forces outside one's control.[19] This "of course" blankets a number of complexities about scientific and religious views of causation. Many people believe that God works through natural (and social) processes.[20] Even when a natural cause is well-established, religious faith can interpret it as linked by divine law to other "sins," as illustrated by Jerry Falwell's former view that AIDS is a divine punishment. We can only hope that religious believers exercise the humane pragmatism recommended by Shweder's group: "a casuistic flexibility in applying the appropriate moral discourse and theodicy to particular cases or situations."[21]

Coping with illness requires making sense of it, for "what actually arouses indignation against suffering is not suffering in itself, but rather the senselessness of suffering."[22] Religious or not, most people do assign personal meanings to illness, transcending scientific explanations. As Lorde suggests, cancer is survived partly "by scrutinizing its meaning within our lives, and by attempting to integrate this crisis into useful strengths for change."[23] Given the enormous variety of moral and spiritual responses, this integration will always have a highly personal dimension. Often there are ambiguities about when sickness results from violating responsibilities for health and about when it illustrates another troubling truth: the causes of much terrible suffering are random and chaotic. Either way, acknowledging moral and religious meanings of sickness easily degenerates into blaming victims. Far more than in the context of public policy, questions about blaming victims must be confronted piecemeal and contextually.

Susan Sontag opposes this piecemeal approach. In *Illness as Metaphor*, she challenges all attempts to give meaning to sickness. Although her primary concern is cancer, she generalizes: "Nothing is more punitive than to give a disease a meaning—that meaning being invariably a moralistic one." Because meanings are typically expressed with metaphors, "the most truthful way of regarding illness—and the healthiest way of being ill—is one most purified of, most resistant to, metaphoric thinking." Attaching symbols and stereotypes to diseases introduces superstition, blocks understanding, places undue burdens of guilt on innocent sufferers, and stigmatizes the vulnerable. The prototypical stigma is that illness is a punishment, thereby blaming victims for bringing about their own suffering. Another stigma is that the sick are morally weak in failing to conquer their illness, thereby exaggerating mind-over-body attitudes and assigns "to the luckless ill the ultimate responsibility both for falling ill and for getting well."[24]

Sontag's demythologizing of disease is one-sided because she does not confront responsibilities for health. In my terms, she raises compassion-based objections to blaming victims without discussing justice-based issues about causes of sickness. She also conflates moral and moralistic meanings. "Moralistic" is a pejorative term. It suggests, as Linda Gordon reminds us, "preaching about the practices of others; being improperly rigid, lacking in the flexibility that acknowledges human variation and imperfection; being uncontextualized, offering judgments not based on a full examination of the actual universe of choice available to the one who is criticized."[25] Moral meanings need not be punitive, parochial, and pompous. They can be rooted in compassion and fairness.

Metaphors are abused by the insensitive, but Sontag's generalizations extend well beyond criticizing the insensitive. Consider two of her specific criticisms. First, she renounces military metaphors such as "battling" diseases as foreign "invaders." She claims that military metaphors support violence, state-sponsored oppression, and dominance by the medical profession. But metaphors, including military metaphors, are malleable and can serve more positive aims. For example, Lorde found military metaphors therapeutic. Like Amazon women who underwent breast amputations as part of their culture, "women with breast cancer are warriors, too. I have been to war, and still am."[26] When a nurse urged her to wear a prosthesis so as not to damage other patients' morale, Lorde saw the nurse trivializing a wound that symbolized a warrior's courage.

Second, Sontag warns that assigning meanings to disease invariably leads to punitive attitudes that undermine healing. Yet, moral and religious meanings can be therapeutic, as with the Hindu woman. Many persons interpret illness as a trial, a test of faith for themselves and others, or a call to accept mystery (as in the Book of Job). Even when sickness is interpreted as a punishment, the tone need not be punitive. We reap what we sow; old sins cast long shadows; what goes around comes around. These sayings can be used to offer encouragement to change rather than hostility, or resignation rather than resentment.

Finally, Arthur Frank goes too far in the opposite direction from Sontag when he suggests that patients have a responsibility "to witness their own suffering and to express this experience so that the rest of us can learn from it."[27] This view places additional demands on sick and vulnerable individuals.[28] I believe Frank confuses responsibilities with rights. Obviously we have a right to give meaning to our illness, but I doubt there is an obligation to do so.[29] With their illness narratives, which speak to human vulnerability and courage, the sick offer us gifts rather than duties fulfilled.[30]

Patients: Cooperation and Double Binds

Because the interactions between patients and health care professionals are structured by authority and power, they give rise to special dangers of blaming victims. Consider Kat Duff, who at age thirty-six was diagnosed with chronic fatigue and immune dysfunction syndrome (CFIDS). She was unable to climb stairs or even get out of a chair, and she needed twelve hours of sleep a day. Her concentration and memory were impaired, she would occasionally blank out altogether, and she suffered from recurring bouts of depression. Compounding these difficulties, she confronted a medical community which viewed CFIDS as a psychosomatic illness. Subsequently, in reflecting on the experience, she expressed resentment that sick people are blamed for not adopting positive attitudes of faith, hope, and courage: "Many sick people are shamed by friends, family, or even their healers into thinking they are sick because they lack these 'healthy' attitudes, even though illnesses often accompany critical turning points in our lives, when it is necessary to withdraw, reflect, sorrow, and surrender, in order to make needed changes."[31]

Whereas Lorde objected to the notion that positive attitudes suffice to prevent disease, Duff objects to demanding positive attitudes from the sick.[32]

Duff's attitude is more controversial and elusive, for the moralistic "healthism" to which she objects should not lead us to overlook patients' self-indulgence that places unfair burdens on caregivers. But Duff is right that patients are often put in a double bind: they are to actively participate in their care but passively accept the recommendations of medical authorities, with failure either way rendering them blameworthy. The double bind is especially troublesome in treating chronic illnesses because of characteristic patterns of improvement, relapse, and numerous in-between states of uncertainty. Also expressing this concern, Arthur Kleinman quotes the frustrated words of a man needing renal dialysis for kidney disease caused by diabetes: "The signals are constantly switching. . . . Do I leave it up to them, or do I take part? When I'm well, they're constantly pushing me to do more and be responsible for the care. When I get sick, they tell me I brought it on myself by doing too much. You can't win."[33]

Kleinman suggests the problem is inevitable in high-tech settings where time pressures lead health professionals to dictate when patients should be actively involved (primarily in outpatient services) or passively compliant (emergency and inpatient services). But the problem arises in other settings as well, including psychotherapy, and it can be traced in part to the traditional sick-role model discussed in chapter 4. That model ascribes several responsibilities to the sick: The sick are not responsible for overcoming their illness by themselves; they are exempted (in varying degrees) from usual social obligations; they are obligated to try to get well; and, to that end, they are obligated to seek and cooperate with medical help, and to take reasonable precautions to prevent a threatened illness.[34] The dual obligations placed on patients—try to get well, and cooperate with medical professionals—generates a double bind.

Healers are human. They have natural inclinations to respond more positively to the cooperative patient and less supportively to the patient who fails to meet expectations. Unless those inclinations are restrained, they add to the plight of patients who already experience feelings of confusion, shame, and guilt that work against recovery from acute illness and management of chronic illness. For example, one study of why patients abandon renal dialysis programs noted the tendency of the medical staff to see some patients as obnoxious and to respond accordingly. In addition, "throughout the course of treatment, if the patient gained too much weight or failed to function up to staff expectations, the staff's exhortations, if not heeded by the patient, would be followed by anger, withdrawal, and explicitly expressed disinterest in the patient."[35]

Double binds arise in part because of uncertainties about how much can reasonably be expected of a given patient. Good clinical judgment usually finds a suitable combination of sympathy and firmness. It remains focused on providing support in the form of education, reassurance, helpful suggestions, and encouragement to change bad habits—without becoming moralistic. Nevertheless, even though it is generally disrespectful, uncompassionate, and therapeutically self-defeating to censure patients, encouraging patients to accept their responsibilities remains essential to therapy.

Several times during his public television series *Healing and the Mind*, Bill Moyers asked physicians about blaming victims of sickness. David Felten, a physician-researcher studying how attitudes affect the immune system, acknowledged the need for caution to avoid making patients feel guilty when there is little they can do about their condition. At the same time, he insisted that "we can't let a patient totally reject all responsibility for getting in there and fighting." Dean Ornish, a researcher on coronary diseases, elaborated on the same theme. It is harmful "to say [to a patient] that you have nothing to do with it at all, and that you're just a victim of fate, or bad genes, or bad luck. If you're just a helpless victim, there's not much you can do about your condition. But to the degree that your behaviors and attitudes are contributing to the problem, you can do something about it—and that is empowering."[36]

This theme echoes Irvin Yalom's emphasis during psychotherapy on the area of control that patients have. Therapists should also help clients distinguish two targets of blame: specific behaviors (often an appropriate target) and overall character (probably never an appropriate target in medical settings). Then they should encourage clients to see the positive aspects of their character even when specific behaviors may have contributed to the harm from which they suffer.[37] But Sharon Lamb identifies further complexities. She reports that victimizers tend to blame themselves too little, but victims of abuse tend to blame themselves too much, both for the harm that befalls them and for not quickly overcoming anger, depression, and other psychological effects of the harm. Ironically, unwarranted self-blame can generate a sense of control. If we can say, "I did it, so I deserve it," we can manage the anxiety of a threatening and chaotic world. This occurs even when the sense of control is illusory, as it often is, and Lamb documents that we tend to exaggerate the control we have in many areas of our lives.[38]

To conclude, I have argued that moral and therapeutic reasons combine to encourage personal acceptance of responsibility while fostering positive attitudes of compassion, hope, and self-respect. Rather than banishing blame altogether, moral judgments should take account of how justice and compassion interact in different contexts. Prudence and moral responsibility are essential in maintaining our physical and mental health; fairness and social utility enter into assigning liability for health care costs; authentic personal meanings are salient in coping with illness; and compassion and respect for autonomy are crucial when patients interact with health professionals.

Part III
WRONGDOING AS SICKNESS

It is no coincidence that the picture of psychological health maps so well onto the ordinary conception of moral character or virtue, while psychopathology has correlates in vice.

Lawrence C. Becker, *A New Stoicism*

The great thing, then, in all education, is to make our nervous system our ally instead of our enemy.... For this we must make automatic and habitual, as early as possible, as many useful actions as we can, and guard against the growing into ways that are likely to be disadvantageous to us, as we should guard against the plague.

William James, *The Principles of Psychology*

7

ALCOHOLISM

In Part III I develop an integrated, moral-therapeutic approach to a wide range of undesirable behaviors: alcoholism, pathological gambling, crime, violence, and bigotry. In each instance, I argue that the same pattern of conduct can be wrongdoing for which we are responsible and sickness for which therapeutic responses are appropriate. I begin with alcoholism because of its historical importance. Beginning in the mid-1930s, Alcoholics Anonymous (AA) invigorated the therapeutic trend by convincing health professionals and the American public that alcoholism is a disease rather than a morally bad habit. In contrast, I argue that alcoholism is both a sickness and a morally bad habit. It is a disorder of agency that has physical, psychological, and moral dimensions. Much of what I say applies to other, cross-functional addictions—that is, addictions interchangeable with alcoholism's psychological functions.[1]

Alcoholism as Ailment and Activity

Typically we regard occasional alcohol abusers as *irresponsible* agents, but as their dependence on alcohol progresses, we are encouraged by the health care industry to think of them as *nonresponsible* victims of the disease of alcoholism, or, in terms of the *DSM*, substance dependency disorder. We continue to hold them responsible, however, when their drinking results in drunk driving, spouse abuse, rape, and other serious harm. Hamstrung by a morality-therapy dichotomy, we seem to lack a coherent conceptual framework for saying alcoholism is both immorality and sickness.

Although alcoholism takes too many forms to be encapsulated in any one example, Caroline Knapp's remarkable memoir, *Drinking: A Love Story*, identifies key issues. As her title suggests, Knapp compares the passions and yearnings in drinking to romantic love. During twenty years of abusive drinking, she cherished alcohol as a source of pleasure to accent life's joys, a coping device to deal with problems, and a reliable source of comfort and self-assurance. All the while, she viewed alcoholism as a moral matter, but she never thought of herself as an alcoholic. Then, after attending AA meetings, she became convinced that alcoholism is a physical disease for which she was not morally responsible. AA also taught her that "not drinking is a choice one makes every day." The tension between these two claims—alcoholism is a disease, yet not drinking is a choice—is unresolved in her memoir, as it is in our society.[2]

Is Knapp responsible for her drinking? The question prompts two polarized responses. Yes, she and other alcoholics are responsible for choosing to drink in ways that cause harm. No, she and other alcoholics suffer from a disease for which they are not responsible. The affirmative answer is grounded in a moral perspective: a network of beliefs and attitudes about responsible agents that employs concepts such as integrity and dishonesty, right and wrong, guilt and blame. The negative answer is grounded in a therapeutic perspective: a web of beliefs and attitudes about healthy organisms that employs concepts such as disease and symptoms, wellness and suffering, treatment and therapy.

These simple yes-and-no answers, rooted in a morality-therapy dichotomy, frame debates about alcoholism among experts, as well as in popular culture. As an illustration, consider Harvard Medical School's *Mental Health Review* on alcohol abuse and dependence, which contains opposing essays by psychiatrist George E. Vaillant and philosopher Herbert Fingarette.[3] Vaillant, a distinguished alcohol researcher, insists that anyone who has worked in an alcohol clinic knows that alcoholism is a disease. Fingarette, author of *Heavy Drinking* and other writings that influenced legal rulings, argues that the notion of alcoholism as a disease is a sheer myth. Whereas Vaillant confidently speaks for the medical establishment, Fingarette criticizes the establishment in ways that have provoked enormous controversy.[4] He defends the traditional view, held by thinkers from Aristotle to Dewey, that abusing alcohol is a moral matter.[5]

Fingarette's and Vaillant's views can be reconciled by applying my three themes. First, a sound moral perspective on alcoholism will be healthy. It will be psychologically realistic in its demands and take account of ongoing scientific inquiry into alcoholism, while keeping visible the *agent* whose conduct is made in response to these influences. Second, we are responsible for our health, mental as well as physical, which requires taking prudent measures in taking care of ourselves, within limits set by our opportunities and other obligations. Specifically, we have obligations to avoid harmful addictions and, should they arise, to seek and cooperate with available help in overcoming them. Holding people accountable for meeting their obligations should not be equated with blaming.[6] Third, moral values permeate mental health and psychotherapy. Alcoholism was labeled a "disease" in part because the modern, industrialized world required a disciplined work ethic. Moral values also structure the goals and procedures of therapy for alcoholism. Whether the specific goal is to stop drinking altogether or to provide skills for controlled drinking, the overall aim is to restore responsible control over alcohol.

In applying these themes, I structure my discussion around four aspects of alcoholism: the condition itself (its defining features and symptoms); its causes (and prevention strategies); its cures (treatment, coping, and management); and its consequences (especially harm, but also benefits). Moral and therapeutic perspectives apply to all four aspects.

Condition: Self-Control and Impaired Agency

What is alcoholism, the condition itself? Numerous definitions have been offered, tailored to the contexts of law, public policy, psychiatry, clinical experimentation, and self-help therapy groups.[7] As an intuitive definition, we might think of alcoholism as long-term heavy involvement with alcohol in ways that lead to systematic loss of control and to significant problems—for example, by threatening goods such as health, safety, family, jobs, and financial stability. The expression "loss of control" will raise flags, but I intend something visible in conduct: failing to exercise responsible control over drinking. I do not mean a complete incapacity to exercise responsible control, and in fact most alcoholics do retain significant degrees of control over drinking. This reference to responsible agency seems to slant matters in favor of moral perspectives, but even therapeutic perspectives refer to moral values in defining alcohol disorders.

In particular, the *DSM* defines *alcohol abuse* as a long-term pattern of maladaptive use of alcohol that results in repeated failures to "fulfill major role obligations at work, school, or home," recurrent physical hazards, repeated legal problems, or persistent interpersonal problems.[8] And the *DSM* defines *alcohol dependence* as "a maladaptive pattern of substance use" that leads to impairment or distress shown in three (or more) of the following features: tolerance (the diminished effect of a given amount of the substance, or the need for increasing amounts to achieve a desired effect); withdrawal symptoms (significantly distressful symptoms from ceasing or reducing use of the substance); heavy use of the substance beyond what was initially intended; unsuccessful effort to reduce usage; large amounts of time spent in obtaining the substance or recovering from its effects; giving up many other activities because of the substance use; and continued use despite knowledge of the recurrent problems it causes.[9] Words like "obligations," "maladaptive," and "causing problems," allude to moral values. Furthermore, the *DSM* defines alcohol dependency in terms of overt behavior, without specifying any particular etiology. And in referring to failed intentions and efforts to change, the *DSM* says nothing about the extent to which individuals have the ability to change by exercising greater self-restraint, altering their life style, and seeking help. In these ways, the *DSM* definition clarifies what it means to lose responsible control over drinking.

Returning to Knapp: Was her drinking voluntarily chosen and under her control? Yes, in some respects; no, in others. On the one hand, she had considerable choice during the early formation of her drinking habits. Even after years of heavy drinking she had some control over when, where, how much, and for what purposes to drink. For example, she carefully maintained a two-drink limit whenever she was around her mother, whom she had promised to stop abusing alcohol. Most striking, she imposed strict rules on herself never to drink at work. She was a "high-functioning alcoholic" who succeeded in her profession despite abusing alcohol, and perhaps partly because of it. At the height of her heavy drinking she wrote a book and several award-winning articles. She reports deliberately using alcohol to shape her personality away from fear and self-doubt and toward confidence and discipline in her work.[10]

On the other hand, at some point she lost overall control, as well as some episodic control, manifesting the "maladaptive behavior" specified in the *DSM*. She experienced intense cravings (desires) for alcohol, and whether alone at night or in restaurants with friends, she felt unable to stop after a few drinks. Her attempts to shape her identity backfired, and self-deception about the drinking eroded her self-confidence. She managed to stop drinking only after entering a drug-rehab clinic, followed by three months of daily AA meetings.[11]

Knapp was sick. Her long-term abusive drinking manifested a disordered and impaired agency that had physical, psychological, social, and moral dimensions. Perhaps she also suffered from suboptimal cognitive and emotional functioning, shown in the self-deception, emotional turmoil, and unsteady self-esteem. But the sickness of alcoholism is the disordered agency itself, as defined in terms of overt behavior and failed intentions. The *efficacy* of her will was impaired: she had great difficulty carrying out her resolve to drink responsibly. In addition, the rational *deliberateness* of her will was impaired: many of her choices and reflections were guided by impulse rather than reasoned choice.[12]

I emphasize again that the sickness, the impairment of agency, is defined by the overt behavior patterns and experiences specified in the *DSM* criteria, not by what she was capable of choosing. Of course, we can speculate about her capabilities. Short of having extensive clinical studies of her, her testimony concerning the degree of control is relevant but not decisive in settling her abilities. After all, her beliefs about losing self-control might be rooted in the same rationalization and denial that she confesses regarding her drinking. What could be more comforting than to excuse twenty years of abusive drinking as something she was incapable of controlling and hence cannot be faulted for? Even if she honestly reported her experiences, she might have had more actual control than she believed. Perhaps she could have made a greater effort, not so much through brute exertions of will but primarily through intelligent, skilled resistance to temptation by planning ahead.[13] At some point, however, it is futile to speculate about the possible control she might have exercised in different circumstances, and such speculation is irrelevant to whether she was sick. She was sick simply because she systematically lacked responsible self-control in ways that caused substantial harm.

Alcoholism is a disorder, but is it a disease? Vaillant insists it is, but all he means is that the individual "has lost the capacity consistently to control how much and how often he drinks."[14] He does not mean complete loss of the possibility of exercising control; indeed, that meaning is incompatible with his therapeutic optimism about restoring control. As long as we are clear that "disease" has this nontechnical meaning, we can call alcoholism a disease. But doing so is misleading insofar as it suggests there are specific bodily abnormalities always present.[15]

Fingarette points out that "disease" has no clear meaning or application regarding alcoholism, and he also avoids talk of sickness, impairment, disorder, and dysfunction. Nevertheless, his limited aim is to debunk the myth of alcoholism as a physical disease, not to argue against all ways in which it might be a sickness.[16] In fact, he conveys much the same idea of impairment when he draws attention to the debilitating effects of deeply entrenched habits of heavy drinking. In his view, alcoholics make drinking a "central activity" in their lives, fundamental habits that they come to rely on as much as work, religion, family, and other basic roles defining who they are.[17] Drinking becomes a preoccupation, influencing every area of their lives, from how they spend their time to their choice of friends. Like other central activities, drinking expresses their choices and also acquires a powerful momentum that greatly adds to their difficulty in exercising responsible self-control. Hence, outside help is often needed to restore control. Yet, alcoholics rarely lose all capacity for self-control—witness Knapp's ability to set rules for her drinking.

In short, with regard to defining the condition of alcoholism, Fingarette and Vaillant differ in emphasis but not substance. Both agree that (a) alcoholism is a severe disruption of self-control over alcohol; (b) the disruption is identified by overt conduct and as such is a behavioral impairment and disorder of agency; (c) the lessened self-control and impaired agency take effect through physiological mechanisms involving a drug (alcohol) that one chooses to ingest in response to a multitude of influences; and (d) the drinking poses a threat to physical health, mental well-being, and responsible conduct. Both think of alcoholism as an activity and an ailment—an activity involving an ailment (impaired self-control), and an ailment defined by an activity (abusive drinking).

Causes: Choices and Influences

Disagreement about calling alcoholism a disease might dissipate if we could pinpoint genetic, congenital, or environmental factors that predestine individuals to become alcoholics (in the absence of preventative measures). The scientific search for these factors began at least two hundred years ago, and research continues unabated.[18] Much has been discovered about the physiological mechanisms that impair judgment and control, and research has uncovered an array of biological indicators, such as characteristic metabolic patterns and brain chemistry. Numerous additional factors within families, peer groups, and cultures have also been identified.

After canvassing the relevant literatures and conducting his own long-term studies, Vaillant recommends a biopsychosocial explanation that integrates multiple contributing factors: genetic predispositions, biochemical processes, psychological elements, and social and cultural factors. In this regard, he compares alcoholism to hypertension and coronary disease, for which there are also predisposing factors. Just as light can be conceived as a particle and as a wave, he writes, alcoholism is "both a conditioned habit and a disease."[19] "Conditioned habit" refers to social influences rather than personal choices.

Predisposition, however, is not predestination. Most predisposing factors are *influences*, which individuals have some ability to resist, not complete determinants. Even a genetic predisposition is only a risk factor that interacts with environmental influences and personal decisions in complex and nondeterministic ways.[20] Moreover, unlike cancer and heart disease, the risk factors can be controlled completely by choosing not to drink. Here Vaillant waffles. In a few passages he admits that individuals are partly the source of their drinking problems by choosing to drink in irresponsible ways. He immediately downplays this admission, however, insisting that choice diminishes as individuals become alcoholics. Later, in discussing ways to prevent alcoholism, he urges that individuals must learn to form healthy drinking habits and to drink in moderation.[21] Yet he fails to pursue the implications of this recommendation concerning responsibility for choices.

Not surprisingly, Fingarette devotes considerably more attention to the early choices that shape drinking habits. Any number of influences lead individuals to form habits of drinking in the course of responding to anxieties and problems, but persons have choices about how to respond to these influences. Alcoholics tend to use alcohol as a blanket solution to difficulties. The vast majority of people do not intentionally choose to become addicts, and only in a rare case does that occur.[22] Like most habits, drinking patterns are typically formed unreflectively, as drinkers drift into abusing alcohol, influenced for example by stress, peer pressure, and ample self-deception.[23] We are responsible for our habits, even when we form them carelessly.

Additional support for Fingarette's view concerns preventive measures. Alcohol abuse can be modified by changing the environment to which individuals respond on the basis of reasons. The changes include increasing the cost of alcohol, reducing its availability, and restricting advertising. They include adopting strong social attitudes against abusive drinking, tough penalties against drunk driving, and policies of refusing to serve additional drinks to intoxicated individuals. They also include improving how youth are socialized into drinking through education, family and cultural practices, and designated-driver programs.

Does Vaillant's or Fingarette's account explain why Knapp became an alcoholic? Both do, with different emphases. Vaillant would stress that Knapp's father was an alcoholic, as was his first wife, and one of their children suffered from fetal alcohol syndrome. Regardless of whether these facts suggest a genetic link or an environmental influence, or both, Vaillant's integrated biopsychosocial model applies. Additional environmental influences are suggested when Knapp complains about the aloofness of her father, who was a psychiatrist who was more intellectually intrusive than emotionally intimate, and when she recalls that as a child she felt more comfortable with him after he had imbibed a couple of cocktails. Knapp also reports strong peer expectations to drink at high school parties and in college dorms, where alcohol was readily available. Fingarette, like Vaillant, would interpret all these contributing factors as influences, not determinants. Knapp is responsible for the cumulative and uncritical choices she made in response to the influences. Over many years she gradually made drinking a central activity in her life as a way of dealing with fear, insecurity, anger, and a host of everyday problems. Far from being coerced, she chose to drink in response to problems and influences, and she gradually drifted into a habit that gradually became central in her life.

With regard to causes, then, no fundamental disagreement between Fingarette and Vaillant emerges, only a difference in emphasis. Vaillant's future-oriented preoccupation with altering drinking patterns leads him to acknowledge but downplay the role of voluntary choices in causing those patterns, while acknowledging that no one is fated to become an alcoholic. Fingarette's moral perspective leads him to highlight the cumulative choices that generate habits of heavy drinking, but like Vaillant he acknowledges the myriad cultural, family, peer, and biological influences that we are free to respond to in alternative ways.

Cure: Therapy and Recovery

Vaillant's primary argument for viewing alcoholism as a disease is that doing so promotes healing. Getting alcoholics to believe they suffer from a disease encourages them to seek and receive help—if not a permanent cure, then improved skills for coping during a lengthy (sometimes lifelong) recovery. Typically the help begins with medical supervision as the patient undergoes withdrawal symptoms and then continues through some form of therapy, although some drinkers change with the help of family and friends or even by themselves.[24] Ironically, merely believing that alcoholism is a disease provides hope by relieving alcoholics of the guilt and shame that fuels their abusive drinking. In addition, the disease model encourages them to enter the health care system where they can benefit from medical research and clinical expertise, and it prompts them to participate in AA and other self-help/mutual-aid programs conducted by laypersons. Moral perspectives, by contrast, intensify guilt and blame in ways inimical to therapy.

Nevertheless, the therapeutic effects of believing that alcoholism is a disease do not establish that it actually is a disease. If it could, similar heuristic appeals could justify virtually any belief, rational or irrational, whenever placebo effects contribute to healing. Perhaps, however, the therapeutic implications of beliefs about alcoholism can serve as a buttressing consideration rather than a primary argument. By Vaillant's own admission, the main reason for viewing alcoholism as a sickness centers on systematic loss of self-control. In addition, we can affirm the importance of nonjudgmental attitudes in therapeutic contexts. Can these concerns be met without making alcoholism a physical disease?

I believe that viewing alcoholism as a *sickness*, in a loose colloquial sense, can be equally effective in encouraging people to seek therapy. After all, most people do not carefully distinguish "disease," "disorder," and "sickness," and all three terms are commonly used without scientific precision. What is essential is to (a) firmly convey the attitude that alcoholics are sick and need help (including self-help/mutual-aid), (b) create a supportive framework in which clinicians suspend blame and other negative attitudes as part of maintaining "professional distance," and (c) offer genuine hope to clients that they can regain responsible control. These elements suffice to make sense of how Knapp and many others find renewed hope and strength at AA.

Indeed, in a few places Vaillant suggests that therapeutic perspectives tend to increase a sense of responsibility for taking care of oneself. He emphasizes that alcoholics must accept responsibility, and he even admits that alcoholics recover by exercising their own powers to "heal themselves." Alcoholics, he adds, need social support in the form of finding more positive "substitute dependencies" rooted in a fresh "source of inspiration, hope, and enhanced self-esteem."[25] The implication is that therapy has moral aspects and is itself a (special) moral context. Therapy is nonjudgmental, not nonmoral.

All this is in tune with Fingarette's view, which encourages drinkers to accept moral responsibility in changing their habits. Alcoholics must re-configure the central activities in their lives—not all at once by a fiat of will but by gradually transforming their daily activities.[26] This reconfiguring is exactly what Knapp does at AA, helped by camaraderie and mutual support.[27] Al-though Fingarette does not say so explicitly, he is not rejecting all aspects of therapeutic perspectives. The language of therapy permeates his penultimate chapter entitled "Helping the Heavy Drinker." There he recommends the kind of counseling or therapy that one might seek in dealing with any problem, but he is well aware that modifying heavy drinking requires significantly more help than is needed in changing most habits. Like Vaillant, he insists it is naive and destructive to believe that brute willpower suffices to overthrow deeply en-trenched dispositions to drink. Heavy drinkers usually need help in developing "appropriate tools and strategies for reshaping their lives."[28] Far from dis-mantling health care services for alcoholics, Fingarette calls for rethinking their rationale, approaches, and aims.

When Vaillant opposes moral perspectives he primarily has in mind re-sponsibility-as-blameworthiness.[29] Fingarette, in contrast, is mainly concerned with the need for drinkers to accept responsibilities (obligations), and he agrees that blaming is self-defeating in therapeutic contexts. Fingarette's perspective does not imply blaming during therapy. He is well aware that self-berating and harshly condemning attitudes from other people are self-defeating within contexts of helping.[30] Blame is best focused on specific actions rather than global (and usually self-righteous) condemnations of a person's entire character. Even outside therapeutic contexts, there are alternative responses to wrongdoing, including excusing when there are extenuating circumstances that excuse or mitigate blame, and forgiveness, which is the recognition of wrongdoing combined with a voluntary refusal to blame.

In response to Vaillant's claim that the disease model is needed to draw people into therapy, Fingarette notes that disease-talk actually turns some people away, either because they are offended by the stigma they attach to "disease" and "mental disorder," or because they believe they are the primary source of their problem.[31] We might add that moral concern motivates people to seek help. A sense of moral responsibility played a very large part of Knapp's motivation for seeking and cooperating with help. After her parents died, she began to realize that if she continued to destroy her life there would be no one to help her. She reports that on one occasion she drove recklessly, and in a precipitating event that led her to therapy, she nearly harmed her friend's two children, with whom she was playing when she was completely intoxicated.

Consequences: Responsibility for Harm

Alcoholism causes enormous harm to drinkers, their families, and innocent bystanders. The harm includes financial waste, property damage, loss of jobs, car fatalities, and violent crimes such as rape, spouse abuse, and child abuse. It also includes coronary disease, cirrhosis of the liver, fetal alcohol syndrome, mental illness, and a loss of autonomy and authenticity (as Knapp emphasizes). Alcohol causes more health-related damage than all illegal drugs combined.[32] Hence, as a major public health concern, alcoholism undeniably invites therapeutic perspectives. It also invites moral perspectives. Premature deaths, unnecessary injuries, destroyed careers, and broken relationships are both moral and medical matters.

Fingarette holds drinkers accountable for the harm they cause, but what about Vaillant? He agrees that alcoholism is not an excuse for harming others. Yet, by neglecting public policy issues, he fails to confront the objection that his one-sided therapeutic perspective excuses irresponsible conduct and reinforces alcoholics' rationalizations. The difficulty is to see how to reconcile the idea of alcoholism as a sickness with holding people accountable for the harm it causes.

Inspired by the morality-therapy dichotomy, Vaillant and the wider therapeutic community adopt a *two-topic approach*: they sharply distinguish between (1) the condition of alcoholism—that is, the drinking problem that includes heavy alcohol consumption, alcohol dependency, impaired agency, and the need for help—and (2) the harm caused by alcoholism. The disease model is applied to the first topic (one is a victim of sickness) and a moral model to the second topic (one is responsible for wrongdoing caused by the sickness). This two-topic approach is tidy but untenable. Alcoholism and its harmful effects are intimately connected. As we have seen, the very definition of alcoholism makes reference to the loss of control that causes harm. And if we hold persons accountable for drunk driving, we must also hold them accountable for drinking in situations where they know or should know it is likely to cause harm.

I develop this criticism of the two-topic approach within three contexts: therapeutic practice, public policy and law, and everyday assessments of character. To begin with therapeutic practice, AA is only one of many therapies, but it remains the most widely recognized and influential one. Adopting a two-topic approach, AA separates alcoholism itself, which is a disease for which alcoholics are not responsible, and harm caused, for which alcoholics are accountable and must make amends as part of the therapeutic process.[33] Regarding the condition itself, AA says alcoholics are "powerless over alcohol" without the help of "a Power greater than ourselves." Regarding harm caused, AA calls for making "a searching and fearless moral inventory of ourselves" and for making amends to persons one has harmed. In this way, both the goal and the means of therapy center on accepting responsibility—for the harm caused and for coping with the disease (with the help of the higher power). Succinctly stated: "One is not morally responsible for one's alcoholism, but one has responsibility for doing something about it."[34]

Contrary to AA, I do not understand how we can reasonably hold individuals responsible for harm caused directly by a disease over which they are entirely powerless, whether entirely or episodically. If I kill someone because I have an unforeseeable heart attack while driving, I am not responsible for murder. Similarly, if alcoholics are wholly powerless over their drinking, then they are not responsible for the harm it causes when their powerlessness results in drunk driving. And prospectively, if alcoholics are responsible only after (and while) they receive the help they need, whether from a higher power or from the group's support, then they are given a standing invitation to avoid accountability by evading help. Moreover, if alcoholism is a "disease of denial," whose symptoms include rationalization and self-deception, individuals are accountable for their dishonesty.

AA has a spiritual foundation. Historically, it derives from a quite familiar religious view of human frailty and the need for God's grace, a view embedded in the evangelical Christianity of the founders of AA and in many other religions. These religious views are not inherently opposed to moral perspectives, assuming they acknowledge a role for moral effort, for obligations to seek help, and accountability for wrongdoing. In fact, AA acknowledges these things, even including restitution for harm as one of the twelve steps. Fingarette says AA is "a new way of life, rather than a treatment program."[35] Surely it is both.

Turning next to public policy and law, they, too, are often based on a two-topic approach: alcoholics are responsible when they break the law, but they need therapy to overcome the disease of alcoholism over which they lack control. In an important discussion, Ferdinand Schoeman attacks polarized positions but ultimately accepts much of the two-topic approach: "It is not unusual now for alcohol abusers to be deemed responsible by a court and then sentenced to participate in programs [like AA] that tell the abuser that he/she is not accountable for continuing patterns of drinking. However incoherent this compound picture strikes one as being, we don't have available a more satisfactory picture."[36] In fact, we can make better sense of public policy by abandoning the morality-therapy dichotomy and adopting an integrated approach. There is no inconsistency when judges and legislators hold alcoholics accountable before the law and then send them to therapists who, to achieve their purposes, suspend moral judgment and focus on alleviating the sickness involved. Nor is there inconsistency, as Schoeman notes, in attending to differences in context. Thus, we are justified in feeling resentment and blame when alcoholics cause harm by failing to exercise good judgment and self-restraint, for example by driving while intoxicated, but "the alcoholic, the abused spouse, the disadvantaged, all deserve our support, sympathy, and constructive endeavors on their behalf."[37] Indeed, we reasonably hold all drivers fully accountable and blameworthy when they drive under the influence of alcohol.[38]

Finally, we cannot avoid making assessments of character when individuals cause enormous harm to us or to people we care about. The assessments, however, must be contextually nuanced and target specific aspects of character, in order to avoid wholesale denigration. An integrated, moral-therapeutic approach invites sensitivity to an array of variables regarding causes, degrees of impairment, types of resulting harms, and available help. Here again, our moral reactions are not neatly separated in the way the two-topic approach suggests. Justifiably, wefeel resentment when individuals shun help and continue to drink in ways that place others at risk, even if, like Knapp, they are lucky enough to avoid causing great harm. But we also admire persons for their courage in acknowledging their problems and seeking help. When we suspend moral judgments (outside of therapeutic contexts), it is often because individuals face exceptional difficulties. Sometimes we forgive, partially forgive, excuse, or simply ignore drinking because it seems integral to highly creative lives.[39] If justice is contextualized, as Schoeman emphasizes, so is compassion. Some alcoholics are more deserving of our sympathy than others, and sometimes "tough love" reveals deeper caring than an indulgent sympathy for irresponsible individuals.

We also assess our own character. We do so as responsible agents seeking moral integrity, and we do so as vulnerable beings who sometimes struggle to maintain self-esteem.[40] Self-assessments should show the same caring, firmness, and balance that are used to judge others. In passages where Knapp questions what alcoholism reveals about her character, she casts matters in extreme terms: either she is a worthless sinner or an innocent victim.[41] She is neither. She is a generally good person who is bad at managing her drinking.

To conclude, when we look beneath the disagreements about alcoholism, we uncover agreement on many key points: alcoholism raises major medical and moral issues; alcoholism is not dictated by a simple biochemical abnormality; most alcoholics retain significant episodic control; most have difficulty (in varying degrees) in controlling their overall patterns of drinking and need help;

drinkers have responsibility to avoid causing harm, to cooperate in solving their drinking problems, and to make amends for the harm they cause; and self-righteous blaming and destructive self-blaming are objectionable on both moral and therapeutic grounds. These conclusions provide a partial roadmap for thinking about additional forms of wrongdoing as sickness.

8

PATHOLOGICAL GAMBLING

In 2003 the *Washington Monthly* reported that William Bennett lost $8 million in gambling during the previous decade, mostly during lavish trips to Atlantic City and Las Vegas where he enjoyed $500 slot machines and video games. During a two-month period his losses were $1.4 million, and on one weekend alone he lost $500,000. The report drew national attention because Bennett was a prominent politician who for years had called for a higher moral tone in American life and who had served as Secretary of Education, chair of the National Endowment for the Humanities, and America's first "drug czar" in the war on drugs. Because much of his gambling money came from his best-selling anthology, *The Book of Virtues*, the article exposing his gambling was titled "The Bookie of Virtue."[1]

Bennett insisted that nothing is wrong with gambling on any scale, if one can afford it, which is why he omitted it from his catalog of vices. Nevertheless, he had written of the "need to set definite boundaries on our own appetites," and he emphasized "that too much of anything, even a good thing, may prove to be our undoing."[2] He was also closely associated with conservative organizations that campaigned against gambling. James C. Dobson, the head of one of those organizations, released this statement: "We were disappointed to learn that our long-time friend, Dr. Bill Bennett, is dealing with what appears to be a gambling addiction" of the sort that is "a cancer on the soul of the nation" and which "has the power to ensnare and wound not only its victims, but also those closest to them."[3] Dobson inferred that Bennett was addicted because of the scale of his gambling, thereby conflating morally excessive gambling with gambling addiction.[4] Much of the public concluded that Bennett was a hypocrite who wrote politicized jeremiads while indulging his favored vices, and the furor forced Bennett to publicly renounce gambling.

Traditionally, gambling that causes significant harm to oneself and others was a moral matter; today, "pathological gambling" is a mental disorder.[5] An integrated, moral-therapeutic perspective makes sense of how it can be both.

Except for the absence of ingested substances, my account parallels what was said about alcoholism, for pathological gambling also has physiological and psychological underpinnings such as irrational beliefs and cycles of longing, excitement, depression, and shame. In this way, pathological gambling exemplifies the wider range of addictions involving resilient, intense, and pleasurable activities such as excesses of consumer spending and pornography.[6]

Alexei's Moral Affliction

Like alcoholism, problem gambling takes many forms, and a single case can only identify some key issues. Dostoevsky's *The Gambler* is the most famous case in the clinical literature, as well as in fiction.[7] The novel combines Dostoevsky's psychological insight with a fictionalized version of his own problem gambling that began four years before the novel's publication in 1866 and continued five years afterward. The protagonist, Alexei Ivanovich, chooses to gamble based on an initial curiosity, then excited fascination, and soon a well-entrenched habit. Alexei's choices reflect his life circumstances and connect with his other interests. He is a university-educated but financially insecure tutor for the children of a retired general. The general, too, is a compulsive gambler who awaits the death of an elderly aunt in order to gamble with the money he inherits. Alexei is in love with the general's stepdaughter, Paulina, but Paulina treats him with alternating aloofness and restrained affection. Only after gambling ruins his life does he discover she reciprocates his love. Thus, when Alexei first tries his hand at roulette he is frustrated in love, lacks a stable sense of self-worth, and urgently needs money to change his humble circumstances and win Paulina's love. He is also confident that his studied approach to roulette will ensure success. An initial small loss followed by a large win transforms his confidence into a cycle of depression and exhilaration. He is hooked, and the remainder of the novel chronicles his self-destructive decisions.

Alexei is not alienated from his gambling; he does not experience it as unwanted or forced on him. Although he painfully regrets his losses, his enjoyment of the pastime never diminishes. Indeed, his gambling expresses his basic beliefs, desires, and values. Money is one value (48).[8] Obtaining money through gambling is not only acceptable but romantic, and he contemptuously dismisses his society's hypocrisy in celebrating aristocratic gambling for entertainment while denigrating plebian gambling for monetary gain. Social recognition is an equally important value, and he revels in the admiration from observers at the casino during his winning streaks. He immensely enjoys the activity of gambling itself, down to the clinking of coins as he approaches the gaming rooms and the thrill in tossing the dice. Above all, he values risk taking. In a prospectus for his book, Dostoevsky described a character whose "need to risk something ennobles him in his own eyes" (5). For Alexei, taking risks at roulette is an exhilarating, existential wager of his current identity for a new one (28). Momentous risk taking is courageous and heroic (172); it expresses his cultural identity as an adventurous Russian; it elicits cosmic pleasures of challenging fate (40); and episodes of winning bring joy and power (148). Does Alexei have other moral values that could counterbalance his enthusiasm for taking risks? Apparently not. He is averse to judging himself when he gambles (31). In addition, he expresses contempt for moralists who praise the prudent and disciplined accumulation of wealth through hard work, noting how quickly they are silenced when individuals win (170). He also rejects the advice offered by his friend Mr. Astley, who warns him that he has lost contact with responsibilities and reality (174).

Alexei is sick, in the colloquial sense that refers to an abnormal state involving harm to the self. The abnormal state consists of entrenched patterns of lacking self-control over gambling. We would not call him sick if he lost control once or twice, perhaps as a novice roulette player. He is sick because he continues to gamble despite obvious and substantial harm, and in ways manifesting a patent lack of good sense, even though he is highly intelligent. "Good sense" alludes to standards of prudence and morality, and hence "self-control" is a normative expression referring to values defining responsible conduct. Unlike infants and the insane, Alexei does not lack capacities for autonomy. Instead, his loss of self-control refers to his actual patterns of conduct in gambling, together with related patterns of desire, emotion, and irrational reasoning. And if his agency has become impaired, the impairment is defined in terms of his overt behavior.

In short, Alexei is sick, but he also chooses to gamble based on his beliefs, desires, and values. If we think in terms of a morality-therapy dichotomy, it is contradictory to say that he is both an agent and sick, at the same time and with regard to the same activities. According to that dichotomy, behavioral problems are either moral matters concerning choice, responsibility, and character; or they are therapeutic matters concerning health. But pathological gambling is both wrongdoing and sickness, and hence the morality-therapy dichotomy should be renounced.

Responsibility for Health and Sickness

As I proceed in this discussion, I respond to the opposing view set forth by Sheila Blume in her essay, "Compulsive Gambling and the Medical Model." Blume leaves some room for moral responsibility in accepting medical help, in tune with the sick role ideology, and to that extent she rejects an absolute morality-therapy dichotomy. Her main thesis, however, is that compulsive gambling is a disease rather than wrongdoing, and hence she seeks to replace moral perspectives with therapeutic ones. This replacement is needed, she claims, in "lifting a large burden of irrational guilt from both patient and family" in order to facilitate healing.[9] In contrast, I argue that pathological gamblers have moral obligations, and are accountable for meeting them, with respect to all four aspects of pathological gambling: (1) the condition itself, (2) its causes, (3) its cure (alleviation, coping), and (4) its consequences.

Condition

What is pathological gambling, the condition itself, understood as a psychological disorder? It is a systematic loss of self-control over gambling as manifested in the harmful patterns of conduct, desire, and emotion spelled out in the *DSM*. The *DSM* defines pathological gambling in terms of overt patterns of behavior, not in terms of dubious claims that individuals are literally unable to choose differently. As such, the *DSM* provides a more precise specification of what it means to systematically lose responsible self-control, all the while presupposing moral values about the responsible use of money. Pathological gambling is "persistent and recurrent maladaptive gambling behavior" that meets at least five of the following criteria.[10] Dostoevsky's novel suggests that Alexei meets criteria 1, 2, 4, 5, 6, and 9:

1. Preoccupation: has repeated thoughts about gambling, including past experiences, future plans, and present ways to find money to gamble with.
2. Tolerance: in order to achieve the same degree of excitement, gambles with increasing sums of money.
3. Failed intentions: repeatedly tries and fails to limit or stop gambling.
4. Withdrawal: irritable when trying to limit or stop gambling.
5. Escape: gambles to escape from personal problems and negative moods such as depression or anxiety.
6. Chasing: after losing, often gambles to regain losses.
7. Deception: lies to family and others to conceal the extent of gambling.
8. Illegal acts: finances gambling by illegal activities.
9. Jeopardy: the gambling jeopardizes or ruins significant relationships, jobs, or other important opportunities.
10. Bail out: uses others to provide money to alleviate problems caused by loss of money by gambling.

Blume accepts the *DSM* definition, but she suggests Alexei's loss of control exempts him from responsibility.[11] Adopting this medical model liberates him (and others) from self-destructive guilt and paves the way for cooperating with medical professionals to bring about change. I agree that therapists should largely set aside questions of guilt and blame in order to help gamblers accept responsibility for changing. It does not follow that gamblers are exempt from responsibilities concerning money, whether before, during, or after their addiction.

We are responsible for our habits. As a habit, gambling gains power over individuals in two ways. First, all strong habits have a momentum, as Herbert Fingarette said, once they become a central activity in our lives. They acquire a projective force, as Dewey called it: "The nature of habit is to be assertive, insistent, self-perpetuating." Second, habits interact with each other, reconfiguring our identities by penetrating all areas of life. As Dewey writes, "We are the habit"; "when we are honest with ourselves we acknowledge that a habit has this power because it is so intimately a part of ourselves."[12] Alexei doesn't merely gamble; he *is* a gambler. His gambling expresses his beliefs, desires, and values—his identity. For that reason, changing his self-destructive behavior requires reconfiguring his self-conception and sense of self-worth. He needs to modify his values, in particular his contempt for patiently earning rewards through work.

Unlike Alexei, some pathological gamblers are alienated from their gambling. They disapprove of it and desire to end it, even as they feel strong urges to continue. By the time they voluntarily seek help, they are seriously conflicted, which largely explains why they seek help—although some accept help only reluctantly or by court order. Self-alienated gamblers are not exempt from moral and legal accountability, however. In varying degrees, they understand, or should understand, that they have obligations they are undermining. They would not experience conflict in the first place unless the gambling expressed at least part of their identity.

Causes

Most current explanations of compulsive gambling rely on eclectic models that cite multiple and interacting influences at the levels of biology, psychology, and society. Blume, too, adopts a biopsychosocial perspective. But after beginning with the promising suggestion that the medical model used in the *DSM* does not specify any particular causes, she insists the disease model rules out personal agency as part of the etiology: "Involuntariness is part of the general idea of disease; it 'happens to' one." This leads her to say that pathological gamblers are not responsible for causing their addiction.[13]

Yet surely individuals do contribute to the genesis of pathological gambling. Indeed, the *DSM* definition wisely refrains from stating any specific etiology and instead defines pathological gambling in terms of overt behavior and psychological states. The *DSM* leaves open for investigation the extent to which individuals have a role in generating and failing to prevent their gambling problems. Furthermore, Blume's claim of complete passivity in the genesis of pathology is inaccurate even with regard to many physical diseases like hypertension and cigarette-caused lung cancer. Early in her essay she points out that medical problems like ulcers and asthma arise from the interaction of individuals and their environment, but even there she seems to think of persons as passive victims of inner and outer forces, denying any significant role to their own agency.

Many explanations of Alexei's compulsion have been offered in the clinical literature. Psychoanalysts explore Alexei's neurotic defense mechanisms, including denial, projection, and splitting or compartmentalizing.[14] They also take note of Alexei's family-like involvements in the general's family, linking them to pre-Oedipal—oral and anal—instincts manifested in his obsession-compulsions.[15] Self-esteem theorists attend to the unstable levels of self-worth that plunge Alexei from self-hatred, depression, anxiety, or boredom to excessive confidence and manic mood elevations, underlying Alexei's gambling patterns.[16] Biological perspectives focus on the physiological basis of the patterns of low and high moods, as well on genetic predisposition to addictions in general.[17] Most convincing, to my mind, social learning theorists and cognitive psychologists highlight the extent to which Alexei irrationally perceives matters of sheer chance as subject to skill and to rational comprehension in discerning "a certain pattern" in winning numbers (40).[18]

For example, cognitive psychologist Michael B. Walker would emphasize the dramatic extent to which Alexei instantiates three "core beliefs" of the regular gambler:

1. That through persistence, knowledge and skill it is possible for a person to make money through gambling.
2. While many will fail in the attempt, the gambler believes that he or she, unlike those others, has the resources needed to win.
3. That persistence in applying oneself to the task will ultimately be rewarded."[19]

Alexei's irrational thinking includes illusions of excessive control and skill, biased evaluations of outcomes (such as interpreting wins as signs of skill or magical good fortune), rationalizing or downplaying losses, and becoming entrapped in failed strategies (such as chasing losses). Walker's explanation is also tailored to particular forms of gambling characterized by particular kinds of irrational beliefs. For example, because horse racing and poker involve greater elements of skill, they invite irrational beliefs connected with these skills. In contrast, lotteries and slot machines involve pure chance and tend to generate irrational beliefs that some numbers in a lottery are "more lucky" than others.

A moral perspective can accept insights from all these explanatory approaches, assuming that the causes are understood as *influences* rather than fully determining forces entirely beyond the agent's control. All human conduct—healthy and unhealthy alike—is a product of multiple psychological, social, and biological influences. These influences restrict and shape conduct without reducing people to robots.

Cure and Coping

An integrated, moral-therapeutic perspective sees morality partly through a therapeutic lens, emphasizing caring and helping aimed at restoring responsible self-control, rather than punitiveness, especially when individuals harm primarily themselves. A punitive response, and especially a self-righteous moralistic one, tends to compound already-present feelings of shame and guilt, thereby generating resentment, depression, and anxiety—all of which can reinforce compulsive gambling and other self-destructive activities.[20] Thus, in many situations harsh blame is incompatible with helping, whether as a friend, family member, compassionate observer, or therapist. Even when blame is deserved, it can elicit reciprocal anger rather than contrition.

Compassionate helping, however, does not preclude "tough love" and accountability for wrongdoing. It is compatible with firm social policies designed to minimize social damage, such as placing limits on the amount of credit available to problem gamblers and limiting temptations to gamble.[21] These policies are integral to a public health approach to preventing and controlling pathological gambling. Pragmatic adjustments in moral and therapeutic perspectives that hold gamblers accountable while recognizing the need for help are now being developed.[22]

Difficulty in directly controlling impulses is a feature of all strong and problematic habits.[23] Changing bad habits is usually accomplished indirectly, by developing other habits and skills, rather than by brute force in the form of will power over troublesome impulses.[24] Usually, but not always, some form of help is needed, whether from professional counselors or from lay groups like Gamblers Anonymous.

Like most adherents of the moral-health dichotomy, Blume's central argument is that therapeutic approaches work.[25] But working is not the same as being based on truth. Belief in the chemical efficacy of a placebo might help an individual get better, but it does not follow that the placebo is chemically effective. Moreover, therapy does not require telling gamblers they are utterly helpless and lack moral responsibilities concerning their gambling. Pathological gamblers do need to be told that they are sick: they have lost control, their agency has become impaired, and they should seek and cooperate with help. But telling compulsive gamblers that they are not responsible (accountable) is harmful. In fact, Gamblers Anonymous, like Alcoholics Anonymous, says that gamblers' have responsibilities to change. "De-moralizing" gambling can be demoralizing: it undermines efforts to regain control.

Directly or indirectly, the aims of therapy are to help individuals be more prudent, accept their obligations, and deal responsibly with gambling—either by abandoning it or by dramatically modifying gambling habits. Although gamblers tend to exaggerate the extent to which they have power over the results of their gambling, part of the excitement of gambling, as Alexei illustrates, comes from placing one's fate outside oneself, in the roll of the dice. A sound therapeutic perspective challenges this idea: "The development of a more realistic internal orientation toward personal control and responsibility should always be made a major treatment goal for the pathological gambler."[26] Within a context of care, respect, and hope, the therapist should not reinforce clients' denial but instead to get them to confront their evasions and change their views and values—what is sometimes called "cognitive restructuring"—as part of accepting personal responsibility.[27]

Neither professional counselors nor support groups were available to help Alexei. Perhaps support from a religious commitment and community might have helped. Could a friend have helped? Evidently not, at least his friend

Mr. Astley was unable to do much. Astley confronts Alexei with moral judgments, even calling him unfortunate and lost, someone who has ruined his life by his failure to understand the importance of hard work. Although he makes these comments without anger or hostility, he does not adopt a therapeutic stance toward Alexei (179). Although Astley's comments fall on deaf ears, however, perhaps his advice and concern might eventually have an effect.

To her credit, and consistent with the sick role ideology, Blume emphasizes that pathological gamblers are responsible for seeking, accepting, and co-operating with available help.[28] Presumably, "responsible" means that individuals have obligations and are accountable for participating in curing their destructive gambling. Here, then, Blume abandons a strict morality-therapy dichotomy.

Consequences

Finally, does impaired agency remove responsibility for the harm done by gambling? Does it excuse the destruction of a family's financial resources, suffering imposed one one's spouse and children, unpaid debts or stolen money to support the gambling? It does not. An effective therapeutic perspective will not deny all accountability for these harms. Certainly a coherent public policy must encourage all of us as citizens to discourage destructive forms of gambling as being irresponsible. The *DSM*, in its Cautionary Statement, states that mental disorders such as pathological gambling are not automatic exemptions from responsibility.

Gamblers Anonymous urges individuals to assume personal responsibility for repaying their debts. Indeed, doing so is integral to therapy. Reflecting a similar distinction in Alcoholics Anonymous, on which it is modeled, Gamblers Anonymous adopts a "two-topic approach" in sharply separating the sickness of the gambling itself and moral (and legal) accountability for the harm caused by the gambling. Blume also assumes this distinction and grants that gamblers are legally accountable for crimes related to their gambling. It is implausible to say that individuals are complete victims, entirely lacking in responsibility for the "disease" of gambling and yet fully responsibility for its harmful consequences.

To conclude, an integrated, moral-therapeutic perspective on pathological gambling emphasizes helping individuals to accept responsibility, where responsibility refers to obligations rather than to blame. Such a perspective understands therapy as a special moral context rather than as replacing morality. The perspective highlights how habits shape identity and conduct, how loss of self-control is both an impairment and morally objectionable, and how moral values partly define problem gambling. It makes sense of how addictions, whether or not they involve ingested substances, can be both wrongdoing and sickness. Let us now widen the range of topics beyond addictions, beginning with serious crime.

9

CRIME AND PUNISHMENT

On the surface, punishment and therapy are contradictory responses to crime. Punishment is inflicting a penalty for wrongdoing; therapy is bestowing a good to restore health. In fact, crime often involves both law breaking and pathology. An integrated, moral-therapeutic perspective views punishment and effective therapy as complementary responses to violence and habitual law-breaking, what I call (for convenience) *serious crime*.[1] An integrated view of serious crime applies to all our themes: healthy morality, responsibility for health, and moral values embedded in mental health and therapy. I begin by noting how the morality-therapy dichotomy constricted classical debates about punishment. Next, using as examples kleptomania (compare compulsive gambling) and drug abuse (compare alcoholism), I show how serious crime can be both wrongdoing and sickness. These examples are familiar in debates about therapeutic approaches to crime, and they provide continuity with the preceding discussions of addictions. I then discuss the possibility of extending a moral-therapeutic approach to other serious crime, although I postpone violent crime to chapter 10. I conclude by commenting on legal insanity.

Punishment and Rehabilitation

Plato taught that punishment heals the "diseased souls" of criminals and improves their character.[2] Only in the mid-twentieth century, however, were serious attempts made to "rehabilitate" criminals. In *The Crime of Punishment*, Karl Menninger portrays punishment as primitive, hate-motivated vengeance that should be replaced by love-motivated therapy. Punishment fosters horrific abuses within the criminal justice system: excessive penalties for minor crimes, prisons that breed violence, unforgiving hostility toward criminals that prevents their reintegration into society, and practices that allow most criminals to escape penalties because of limited jail space. At a deeper level, punishment is an irrational infliction of suffering: it is "absurd to invoke the question of justice in deciding what to do with a woman who cannot resist her propensity to shoplift, or with a man who cannot repress an impulse to assault somebody."[3] Ill or immature, criminals need therapeutic intervention, broadly understood to include psychotherapy for mental disorders, education for immature individuals, and crisis intervention for people overwhelmed with situational difficulties.[4] Psychotherapists, educators, and social workers should replace judges, juries, and attorneys.

Menninger embraces hard determinism, the view that all human actions are determined in ways that preclude moral responsibility. The causal chains identified by science make justice meaningless: "There is no 'justice' in chemical reactions, in illness, or in behavior disorder."[5] In fact, hard determinism also undermines his appeals to love and compassion, which are moral values that we freely choose to apply. Moreover, Menninger grants that some actions are voluntary and others coerced. In fact, he acknowledges that penalties, understood as preset costs individuals voluntarily incur in violating social rules, are essential to therapy. In addition, he fails to recognize that justice, as much as love, is essential to therapeutic outlooks—justice in protecting the rights of the public and criminals, in obtaining informed consent, and in allocating medical resources to criminals and noncriminals alike.[6]

The main problem, however, is that Menninger's proposals do not work.[7] For example, his attempt to deal with property crimes on an "outpatient" basis, without prisons, increases rather than lessens property theft. Again, his proposal to institutionalize violent offenders in medical-oriented facilities fosters psychiatric tyranny in imposing medical procedures without informed consent. In general, during the 1960s and 1970s, most attempts at "rehabilitation" (without punishment) failed. As one psychiatrist observed: "The mental health professions have never been able to document their ability to 'treat' criminal behavior, if by treatment we mean to reduce the incidence of recurrence."[8]

Herbert Morris offers a more principled opposition to therapeutic approaches. He argues that punishment respects criminals as free and accountable agents, whose dignity implies a "right to be punished."[9] Treating criminals as sick is degrading because it reduces their actions to mere "happenings," like a runny nose or an epileptic seizure. Likewise, Antony Flew attempts to block the expansion of the domain of psychopathology, in order to protect moral responsibility. He agrees with Menninger that psychopathology is defined in terms of incapacities to act or extreme difficulty in exercising normal agency, such that the person is unable to inhibit or control impulses to engage in crime.[10] Thus, if kleptomaniacs are sick, then their behavior is exempt from moral judgment, just as Menninger said.[11]

Morris, Flew, and Menninger all think of therapy and punishment as opposed. They assume that psychopathology incapacitates in ways that remove or mitigate guilt. A pragmatic American public, however, favors a mixture of punishment and therapy whenever it proves effective, including cost effective, in controlling crime.[12] In the same vein, an integrated, moral-therapeutic framework helps us rethink, not abandon, moral justifications of punishment. These justifications include deterring crime, expressing and controlling public outrage, compensating victims, repairing damaged communities, and changing or controlling criminals so they do not commit further crimes.[13] Some of these purposes are more important than others, and different ethical theories disagree about which are primary. It will suffice to indicate how therapeutic approaches can be integrated with three theories: rule-utilitarian, retributive, and restorative.

Rule-utilitarianism endorses a set of rules about crime and punishment that produce the most overall good by deterring crime, keeping dangerous individuals in jail, and changing criminals before they reenter society. As such, their approach is straightforwardly compatible with therapeutic approaches that prove to be effective. Serious crime warrants prison time, but in prison therapy should be available. In contrast, retributive theories justify punishment in terms of the justice in making criminals pay for wrongdoing. Retributionists tend to be harshly critical of therapeutic attitudes toward crime, but that is because they interpret sickness as an excuse for wrongdoing. Rather than opposing therapeutic approaches, however, they should reject the assumption that sickness is an automatic excuse for wrongdoing. Therapy can then be made available in prisons and during probation in order to lower recidivism. In this way, retributive theories are in principle compatible with therapeutic interventions.

In contrast to both rule-utilitarian and retributivist theories of punishment, restorative justice focuses on repairing the injuries caused to victims and communities.[14] For example, it requires criminals to compensate victims and calls for broader moral and spiritual reconciliations between victims and perpetrators.[15] In distinguishing restoration and rehabilitation, defenders of restorative justice have gone too far in renouncing therapeutic approaches.[16] Restorative justice theories can take into account the healing of the criminal as part the broader goal of healing the society disrupted by crime.

Kleptomania: Sick Agency

Let us move from these abstractions to illustrate how crime can be both wrongdoing and sickness, to which punishment and therapy both apply. Consider Beth, a forty-five-year-old mother of five who has few close personal relationships.[17] In her youth she rarely stole, but since her divorce she steals frequently. Her desires to shoplift come and go, and she could easily afford to purchase the magazines, books, and postcards she pilfers. She is baffled about why she steals, and she experiences excitement about successful thievery, fear of penalties for stealing, enjoyable fantasies of being caught, and shame and self-hatred about actions incompatible with her professed values. Sometimes her stealing seems to her to just happen; other times she makes an effort to restrain her impulses to steal, with occasional success. She also has rules about stealing, such as not robbing people she knows and stores she likes.

Is Beth sick or a criminal who is legally and morally accountable? Forensic psychiatrist Marcus J. Goldman says she illustrates why kleptomania lies "somewhere between criminality (because of the theft) and mental illness (because of the bizarre nature of the act)."[18] His point is that kleptomania is unlike major mental illnesses such as schizophrenia that destroy agency, and it is also unlike theft motivated by greed. In fact, I suggest, far from showing kleptomania lies "between" criminality and a mental disorder, Goldman makes a case for saying it falls squarely into both categories.

On the one hand, kleptomania is a mental disorder, listed in the *DSM* as an impulse-control disorder. Like other mental disorders, it is defined in terms of patterns of behavior, desire, intention, and emotion that involve significant distress, risk of harm, or disability (where "disability" does not mean complete incapacitation). Specifically, kleptomania is defined by repeated failures to resist impulses to steal things not needed, based on motives other than vengeance and delusions, together with tension experienced before the theft and pleasure after the theft.[19] In addition, kleptomania often involves depression and anxiety disorders. On the other hand, kleptomania involves law breaking, and it is not an automatic excuse for crime. The *DSM* Cautionary Statement reminds us that mental disorders do not automatically exempt from responsibility for breaking the law.[20]

Are kleptomaniacs gripped by irresistible impulses, so that it is unfair to hold them accountable? As Goldman writes, for most kleptomaniacs "stealing certainly *seems* or *feels* irresistible (or at least necessary), but it very likely is not—at least not all the time."[21] There is an important distinction between feeling that an impulse is irresistible and literally being unable to resist it. Kleptomaniacs will not steal if you place a police officer beside them. Their disorder makes it more difficult for them to avoid stealing, but it does not render them completely helpless to resist and to modify their impulses to steal. Indeed, therapy for kleptomania involves helping individuals accept responsibility for their conduct, rather than telling them they are helpless victims.

Accountability is one thing; appropriate punishment is another. Beth faces special obstacles which a judge or jury might take into account in meting out appropriate punishment. The law holds all adults to a minimum standard, regardless of the unlimited variations in how difficult it might be for a particular individual to resist an impulse to break the law. At the same time, humane laws make therapy available to offenders, either after they are imprisoned or as part of their sentences. In this way, therapeutic approaches complement rather than compete with punishment. The same is true regarding drug abuse and drug dependency.

Drugs and Drug Courts

Americans zigzag between moral and therapeutic perspectives on drugs, with the overall aim of reducing harm in cost-effective ways.[22] Moral perspectives view drug use as a choice for which individuals are responsible. Therapeutic perspectives view it as a sickness to be healed. Each perspective has many variations. Thus, moral perspectives range from permissiveness that would legalize all drugs, an attitude voiced by both libertarians and many participants in the drug culture, to harsh punitiveness that imposes severe jail sentences on drug users and traffickers. Therapeutic perspectives include both treatment and preventive approaches, such as education and public service ads.

Public support is growing for integrating moral and therapeutic approaches in combating drugs, even though it is often unclear how best to achieve that integration.[23] The citizen-generated Proposition 36 in California illustrates social experimentation to find an appropriate integration. Prior to July 1, 2001, a third felony conviction in California for possessing cocaine sent criminals to prison for life. After that date, individuals convicted of the same crime were given the option of entering therapy. Penalties for drug dealers, manufacturers, violent offenders, and traffickers remain unchanged. Proposition 36 is incoherent if we apply a morality-therapy dichotomy, but it makes sense once we abandon that dichotomy. By bringing drug users before the courts, Proposition 36 holds them accountable for a crime while acknowledging they have a health problem, requiring therapy, for which they are responsible.

Whether Proposition 36 succeeds remains to be seen. During the first six months after its implementation, 30 percent of individuals either did not show up for therapy or dropped out of programs.[24] Worse, subsequent budget crises threaten to allow individuals to escape both therapy and prison.[25] Such statistics might lead Californians to toughen penalties or, alternatively, to try decriminalizing drugs. I believe they would do well to expand the use of drug courts.

The drug court movement, dubbed "therapeutic jurisprudence," is heralded as the most important innovation in jurisprudence in a decade.[26] It began in 1989 in Miami, Florida, when President Ronald Reagan's punitive "war on drugs" failed to reduce drug use and proved too costly by overloading prisons.[27] An experimental drug court succeeded, and nearly a thousand drug courts were established within a decade. Although drug courts have many variations, typically a judge closely monitors whether individuals cooperate with their therapists, therapy groups, and social workers. Judges are selected based on their combination of caring, firmness, and flexibility. In most instances, they work closely with addicts for over a year, usually demanding more time and effort from drug abusers than is required by jail sentences. The combination of close legal monitoring and use of therapy yields a high cure rate. Forced therapy for drug addiction works.

Influenced by the morality-therapy dichotomy, critics charge that the rationale for the courts is self-contradictory: "To the extent that drug-taking is an illness, it cannot also be (in any common sense of the word) a crime."[28] This charge is defused, however, once we abandon a morality-therapy dichotomy. On the one hand, using illegal drugs is a choice and a criminal offense for which individuals should be brought before the courts. On the other hand, therapy is needed to overcome drug use. Certainly it is needed once drug addiction has taken hold and the individual can no longer avoid drugs by exerting normal levels of willpower. The *DSM* defines this loss of direct self-control in drug dependency as three or more of the following: tolerance, withdrawal, greater use than intended, failed efforts to cut down or stop, heavy involvement in getting and using drugs, damage to other important activities, and continued use despite knowing the likely problems.[29] Restoring self-control is a personal struggle of courage, honesty, perseverance, self-control, hope, and faith. In supporting this struggle, therapists typically downplay blame and guilt, for these emotions often reinforce drug abuse, but they also encourage their clients to accept responsibility.

To be sure, some moral approaches are linked to religious beliefs that oppose secular therapies. A noteworthy example is Teen Challenge, a Pentecostal ministry that operates the world's largest residential drug rehabilitation program. The program rejects the mainstream view that drug and alcohol addiction is a disease. Instead, it regards addiction as a problem of values. Substance abuse is a sin (not a sickness), and it is overcome by "students" (not "patients") who turn to Jesus.[30] "Drugs are not the root problem of the addict, but a symptom of a deeper internal problem" of sinfulness.[31] The solution is a moral and spiritual transformation in which value commitments replace drug abuse.

Teen Challenge appeals to many drug addicts precisely because of its moral and spiritual emphasis. In contrast, secular approaches derive their effectiveness largely from their nonjudgmental approach. How can this be? That is, how is it possible that accenting guilt is therapeutic for some individuals, while downplaying guilt is effective for others? The answer is that what matters most is a context of support, whether secular or spiritual, that is suitably matched to the basic values of individuals.[32] This support strengthens self-esteem and self-respect, and it releases guilt feelings through forgiveness. Naturally, different perspectives offer alternative interpretations of what occurs as individuals are helped with their drug addictions. Secularists see the placebo effect at work in what others call spiritual healing.[33] Secularists will note that Teen Challenge is engaging in therapy by including work therapy, group therapy, individual therapy, music therapy, and recreational therapy in its residency programs. In turn, religious observers see divine grace extended to nonbelievers who are helped in secular programs.

An integrated, moral-therapeutic perspective will attend to public health policy, as well as to individual therapy. As Eva Bertram and her coauthors in *Drug War Politics* emphasize, drug abuse and addiction are public health issues because of the enormous damage they inflict, and because they are influenced by the social environment as much as individual choice. This public health approach, however, is compatible with affirming personal responsibility for choices: "There is an element of choice at every point in drug use—in the decision to experiment, to engage in casual use, to engage in heavy use, and even to seek treatment in order to moderate or abandon drug use."[34] A moral-therapeutic public policy does not imply being "soft" on crime. As James Q. Wilson observes, "putting an addict in jail is certainly 'punitive,' but putting him in a treatment program, however benevolent its intentions, may be seen by him as no less 'punitive.'"[35] Thus, compulsion and punishment enter in offering addicts a limited set of unattractive options designed to change their behavior.

Serious Crime as Sickness

We cannot generalize from kleptomania and drug abuse to all serious crime.[36] Adrian Raine argues, however, that there is a basis for viewing most serious crime as clinical disorders, or at least as manifesting suboptimal health. His argument has empirical and conceptual components. The empirical component establishes the extent to which criminals differ from noncriminals in terms of variables from psychology, biology, and social background. Studies of linkages between genetics, neurochemistry, neuropsychology, brain imaging, cognitive deficits, family and social influences bolster the case for saying that serious crime suggests "impaired functioning," in a sense that enters into many definitions of psychopathology, thereby adding to the reasonableness in applying definitions of psychopathology to serious crime.[37]

The conceptual component of Raine's argument, which interests me here, seeks to establish that serious crime fits a plausible definition of pathology. Raine considers many definitions, aware that none is backed by a consensus. For example, he emphasizes that serious crime deviates from social norms and ideal mental well-being, manifests impaired social adjustment, and constitutes habits harmful to others and oneself. Especially important, he argues that most serious crime falls under the *DSM* definition of mental disorders as syndromes involving significant distress, disability, or increased risk of harm. Thus, most serious crime (for private gain) is a sign of impaired social functioning—defined, in accord with the *DSM*, in terms of overt conduct rather than underlying causes. Moreover, serious crime increases the risk of losing important freedoms through imprisonment, and in that sense fits the *DSM* definition. Moreover, the *DSM* already lists a large number of disorders defined by reference to criminal conduct. For example, in addition to kleptomania, the *DSM* lists antisocial personality disorder, conduct disorder, pedophilia, pyromania, intermittent explosive disorder, exhibitionism and some other paraphilias, and substance dependence and substance abuse (where the substance is an illegal drug). To a remarkable extent, the *DSM* interprets serious crime as a symptom of pathology.

Raine's comments about responsibility, unfortunately, are distorted by a morality-therapy dichotomy. Influenced by Menninger, he calls for a gradual replacement of punishment by therapy. Because currently we lack therapies to heal most of the "disorders of crime," he tells us, we must for now adopt a more flexible approach. He suggests retaining prisons while gradually reshaping them toward something like mandatory treatment centers in which individuals are given as much freedom as is safe and "at the same time minimizing all punitive aspects of the regime."[38]

Yet, nothing Raine says justifies abandoning punishment. To begin with, predisposing factors that add to the risks of criminal conduct do not force people to become criminals.[39] I suspect that Raine, like Menninger, mistakenly assumes hard determinism: if conduct is caused, then we are not morally responsible.[40] Certainly he assumes that sickness automatically lessens responsibility: "If we accept that crime is a disorder, then at least to some degree we also have to accept the fact that the offender is not completely responsible for his criminal behavior."[41]

Neither the law nor the American Psychiatric Association views mental disorder as an automatic excuse for crime, and neither should we. Pedophiles, pyromaniacs, and psychopaths all deserve punishment for their crimes, even though they are paradigms of sick individuals. In short, once we renounce the morality-therapy dichotomy, Raine provides a basis for viewing serious crime as both sickness and punishable wrongdoing.

Criminal Insanity and the Abuse Excuse

Severe disorders are relevant in meting out specific punishments, but most of them do not entirely exempt individuals from responsibility. The one exception is criminal insanity, which is a very special case indeed. The criteria defining criminal insanity differ by states, but two main approaches have been adopted: irresistible impulses and the M'Naghten Rule.

The "irresistible impulse" standard—exemption based on being incapable of resisting an impulse to commit a crime—is both vague and tends to inflate exemptions due to mental disorders. That standard, however, has largely disappeared since 1981, when it was used to find John W. Hinckley not guilty by reason of insanity for his attempted assassination of President Reagan. It was clear that Hinckley had several mental disorders, including a narcissistic personality and suicidal tendencies, throughout most of his adult life. The question was whether his mental illness caused him to behave as he did, such that at the time of acting he was unable to appreciate the wrongness of his conduct or was unable to conform his conduct to the law. Jurors listened to expert witnesses on both sides. Just two hours before the attack he had written a letter to the actress Jodie Foster, with whom he was obsessed, divulging his plan to kill the president, apparently providing evidence of a controlled and deliberate act. Nevertheless, the defense attorneys won their case for criminal insanity, and Hinckley continues to reside in a mental facility, even though psychiatrists testify he is no longer a danger to society.

Following the acquittal, the question shifted to whether Hinckley was sufficiently dangerous to warrant forced detention. Government prosecutors, who during the trial portrayed him as sane and responsible, were then forced to reverse, portraying him as dangerously ill and a threat to himself and others. Most Americans were convinced Hinckley simply beat the system, and some experts agree that Hinckley was a sociopath who skillfully faked the aspects of mental illness.[42] Sick, yes, but also responsible.

Public outcry over the Hinckley decision prompted a return to the more stringent, nineteenth-century, M'Naghten Rule: "To establish a defense on the ground of insanity, it must be clearly proved that, at the time of the committing of the act, the party accused was labouring under such a defect of reason, from disease of the mind, as not to know the nature and quality of the act he was doing; or if he did know it, that he did not know he was doing what was wrong."[43] Thus, "disease of the mind" is not enough. It must be shown that the disease makes persons unable to know what they are doing.[44] Using this standard, Hinckley would probably have been found guilty.

Whichever standard is used, the plea of criminal insanity is now rare, and it usually fails. There is no likelihood that widening our conception of mental illness will result in abuse of the insanity defense. If anything, just the opposite is true, as we realize that the overwhelming majority of mental disorders have nothing to do the M'Naghten Rule. This conclusion is fully supported by the American Psychiatric Association (APA). After the Hinckley case, the APA urged the courts to count as legal insanity only the most "severely abnormal mental conditions that grossly and demonstrably impair a person's perception or understanding of reality," and the APA explicitly ruled out personality disorders and intoxication due to substance abuse.[45]

Legal responsibility is not all or nothing. Many courts employ a conception of "diminished capacity" that takes mental disorders into account in making criminal charges and assigning punishment. Moreover, attorneys can and should try any line of defense that might help protect their clients. Critics of the therapeutic trend charge that therapeutic attitudes are undermining the legal system. For example, Alan M. Dershowitz warns that "the 'abuse excuse'—the legal tactic by which criminal defendants claim a history of abuse as an excuse for violent retaliation—is quickly becoming a license to kill and maim."[46] Dershowitz cites several high-profile cases—for example, the Menendez brothers, who killed their parents in cold blood and then tried to excuse themselves as victims of child abuse, a ploy that led to a hung jury in the first attempt at prosecution. He also assembles dozens of pathological syndromes that have entered into criminal defense cases, including attempts to excuse violence by appealing to the battered woman syndrome, posttraumatic stress disorder, and computer addiction.

If Dershowitz is correct, the therapeutic trend is undermining the justice system. Is he correct? James Q. Wilson shares the concern about juries' over-preoccupation with motives and past influences.[47] Nevertheless, he finds Dershowitz's claims greatly exaggerated. Juries make mistakes, but they do not excuse gross immorality at the mention of every new psychological "syndrome." They manage to find sick defendants guilty—for example, to convict drunk drivers, even though they have a substance abuse disorder. Even in the Menendez case, the jury was not deadlocked over whether the brothers were innocent but, instead, over whether they committed first-degree murder or manslaughter, and a second prosecution successfully convicted them of first-degree murder. Appeals to pathology and "abuse excuses" can be misguided, as can all excuses, but that does not make them invalid in all situations.[48]

To sum up, pathologizing serious crime does not by itself exempt from accountability. The courts demand more than pathology to remove or even to mitigate guilt. Typically, an attorney must show that the pathology was beyond the control of the individual. An integrated, moral-therapeutic perspective regards serious crime as the product of choices, and exempts from responsibility only in rare instances such as criminal insanity. Therapy-oriented rehabilitation is one component in a justified system of punishment, rather than an alternative to punishment. The next chapter develops this approach with regard to violence.

10

VIOLENCE AND EVIL

In calling terrorists evil, President George W. Bush invoked our most powerful moral epithet condemning murder, torture, rape, and other extreme cruelty.[1] Some observers found his rhetoric "too absolute" and demonizing. Others called the terrorists sick, seeing derangement in their wild or deadened eyes, even though psychiatrists report that few terrorists are mentally ill.[2] I will explore how violence—in the sense of cruel and unjustified physical injury—can be both pathological and evil. I begin by rejecting James Gilligan's attempt to replace morality with therapy. Next I turn to sociopaths as paradigms of simultaneous moral and mental disorder, and then I discuss collective violence. I conclude by commenting on attempts to abandon blame toward violent individuals.

Replace Morality with Therapy?

Psychiatrist James Gilligan contends that "it is time now to retire the moral way of thinking about violence for one capable of utilizing all the methods and concepts of the human sciences" (94).[3] In my terms, he adopts a morality-therapy dichotomy and uses it as the springboard for a replacement project. Gilligan merits attention because he studied convicted murderers for three decades as director of Harvard Medical School's Center for the Study of Violence and as director of psychiatric services for the Massachusetts prison system. One man he studied was a middle-aged husband-father who taught Sunday school, conducted a church choir, and raped and murdered a fourteen-year-old girl who sang in the choir (34–36). As a child, the man experienced impotent rage toward his mother for humiliating him before his peers, but the rage was so repressed that he felt only numbness when he murdered. A second man exploded in a murderous rage when his wife threatened to leave him for another man (128–131). Although he had known about the adultery for several years, he could not bear the prospect of being left alone or the shame in being so dependent and unlovable. A third man killed a police officer and was repeatedly violent during incarceration (120–123). He felt terror at the prospect of living alone and shame about his lack of self-confidence and desire to have others take care of him in prison.

In explaining the men's violence, Gilligan highlights their shame and self-hatred in response to felt humiliations, both as children and adults. Shame is a "germ" that operates within the mind, but it spreads socially as a "contagious disease," shaped by a host of economic and societal factors (105). It generates violence when several additional conditions are met: deep shame about one's shame, as being unmanly; absence of nonviolent avenues for regaining pride; and the lack of normal resources for inhibiting the violent impulses stimulated by the shame, especially respect for others and self-interested fears of punishment (113). Under these conditions, violence functions to reduce shame and to raise self-esteem by exercising power over others.

Gilligan's account does not explain all violence, even when shame is a factor. For example, no doubt shame played some role in motivating Timothy McVeigh, who exploded a truck bomb that killed 168 people and wounded hundreds of others at the federal building in Oklahoma City on April 19, 1995.[4] McVeigh was ashamed of his parents, his failure to achieve admission to the military's special forces, and his inability to get a good job when he returned from the Gulf War as a decorated officer. But McVeigh was also highly intelligent and resourceful, confident and dogmatic, paranoid and a racist. His pathology centered on fanatical hatred of the U.S. government, and it involved obsessions that unhinged his judgment, unbalanced his passions, and dissociated him from his victims. And when violence is more impulsive than McVeigh's, the emphasis should be on the failure to exercise self-control over violent impulses, regardless of whether the impulses are generated by shame.

Having said this, I agree that much violence manifests a cycle of shame, rage, and loss of control. The question is why Gilligan thinks this explanation provides a basis for abandoning morality. He has three arguments: morality is ineffective, otiose, and archaic. His first argument is that morality has been "singularly unsuccessful in reducing the level of violence" (94), and it actually increases violence by intensifying shame and guilt (239). Here Gilligan is speculating wildly. He provides no evidence that a cultural abandonment of shame and guilt would lead to less violence. Given the key role of these emotions as constraints on objectionable conduct, it is more likely their absence would increase violence overall.[5] In addition, his argument assumes that the only rationale for punishment is to deter crime, thereby ignoring punishment as deserved retribution for harming others.[6]

His second argument is that morality is otiose because it contributes nothing to understanding and preventing violence. Morality explains nothing; it merely evaluates and condemns (92). And condemning violence is as irrelevant as condemning cancer (25). To prevent violence we must explain it scientifically and attack its underlying causes. In reply, we can agree on the need for scientific understanding of the root causes of violence. But Gilligan reduces moral judgments to only one of their functions, the criticism of persons. Moral judgments are also used to praise people, express ideals, evaluate actions, and guide conduct. Indeed, insofar as they guide conduct, moral judgments partly explain actions in terms of reasons that motivate us. Furthermore, although shame can become pathological, it is difficult to understand self-respect and self-esteem without allowing some role for healthy forms of shame and guilt.[7] Finally, moral values identify the unjustified forms of extreme harm that require explanation and prevention in the first place.

Gilligan's third argument is that morality relies on "archaic, prescientific language" and values rooted in blame, shame, and guilt (239). It is "a force antagonistic to life and to love, a force causing illness and death—neurosis and psychosis, homicide and suicide."[8] Therapy is grounded in science, honesty, realism, and love. In reply, Gilligan portrays morality in a narrow, pejorative manner and then criticizes it as an immature outlook; then he smuggles in selected moral values (honesty, love) under the guise of nonmoral therapy. In any ordinary sense, love, caring, and honesty are moral values, as well as therapeutic values.[9]

Although Gilligan's arguments for his replacement project are unconvincing, I take seriously his suggestion that (much) violence is "a symptom of individual or group psychopathology," or at least suboptimal health, regardless of how "natural" or commonplace it is (98). An integrated, moral-therapeutic view takes a keen interest in the factors that predispose individuals to violence, interpreting these factors as influences and risks rather than as complete causal determinants. Moreover, an integrated outlook is realistic while retaining an optimistic, forward-looking emphasis on preventing and curing violence by improving mental health and applying ideals of both caring and fair punishment.

Sociopaths: Sick and Accountable

According to critics of the therapeutic trend, to pathologize evil is to trivialize it and invite excuses for it. Philip Hallie mocks, "if somebody's done some destructive work—sick, sick, sick—the person is thought of as a patient in a hospital. How can you blame somebody who is sick? How can you become angry at somebody who is sick?"[10] Contrary to Hallie, mental disorder sometimes underscores rather than trivializes the horror of violence. Using sociopaths (or psychopaths) as an example, let us see how violence can be both sickness and wrongdoing for which one is accountable.

John Gacy was a contractor who lured at least thirty young men and boys to his house with the promise of jobs and then raped, tortured, and suffocated them. Henry Lee Lucas murdered his mother, dismembered his wife, and confessed to committing hundreds of murders along a 500-mile highway from Texas to Florida. Jeffrey Dahmer added cannibalism to his list of horrors. Ted Bundy killed at least thirty-six young women, deriving erotic pleasure from playing out his morbid fantasies by exercising power in "hunting" and "owning" his victims. Sometimes he would have sex with the corpses of his victims, and once he suffocated a little girl by holding her face in the mud.[11]

These men are sick. They are sick in a colloquial pejorative sense—distorted, perverse. They are not motivated by moral reasons and emotions in anything like a normal way, whether in caring about people, exercising self-control, being responsible in love and work, or experiencing guilt and shame for wrongdoing. They are also sick in the technical *DSM* sense. They have anti-social personality disorder, a pervasive failure to respect the rights of others, as shown in at least three of the following: (1) repeated law breaking, (2) repeated deceitfulness for personal profit, (3) impulsivity and lack of foresight, (4) repeated physical aggressiveness (e.g., fights, assaults), (5) reckless disregard of safety, (6) repeated irresponsibility (in such matters as work and money), and (7) lack of remorse for harming others.[12]

Notice that the *DSM* definition relies on moral concepts—rights, irresponsibility, harm, remorse, and so on. In addition, as I have emphasized, the *DSM* Cautionary Statement blocks any automatic inference from disorder to excuse. Compatible with the *DSM*, the public and the courts hold sociopaths accountable.

Some philosophers, bewitched by a morality-therapy dichotomy, have denied that sociopaths are morally accountable. Recall, for example, that Peter Strawson said sociopaths are not accountable members of the moral community because they do not accept responsibility for their actions. We should treat them, he says, from an "objective" point of view, as objects to be controlled, manipulated, and medically treated.[13] Let us agree that many sociopaths, like infants and the insane, are not members of the *reciprocity-community*: the community of individuals who have the capacity to reciprocate other persons' moral respect and good will in normal ways. But sociopaths, as well as infants and the insane, are members of the *recognition-community*: the community of individuals who have moral worth and as such deserve moral recognition. Their membership in recognition-community, together with basic abilities to act, provides a basis for moral accountability. The alternative is to deny moral status to large segments of humanity: the *DSM* estimates that as many as 3 percent of males and 1 percent of females might be sociopaths.[14]

Herbert Fingarette has reworked Strawson's approach, while sharing his dichotomy between moral and therapeutic attitudes to sociopaths. Fingarette argues that it is pointless to blame sociopaths. Blame has the practical purpose of pressuring individuals to feel guilt for their wrongdoing and to make reforms and reparations. Because moral reform is not possible for sociopaths, blame is futile.[15] Yet, to the contrary, blame serves purposes beyond provoking reform, such as expressing resentment and demanding appropriate punishment.[16] Moreover, sociopaths do respond in various degrees to threatened punishment, albeit for self-interested reasons.

Jeffrie Murphy also reworks Strawson's approach. He understands moral community in terms of social contract theory, the view that morality is created through agreements among moral agents. Moral practices presuppose a general willingness to acknowledge and to try to live by those agreements. Because sociopaths lack this willingness, they are not part of the moral community and lack moral significance: "The psychopath, by his failure to care about his own moral responsibilities, his failure to accept them even if he recognizes them, becomes morally dead—an animal rather than a person. He has no rights."[17] Hence we have no moral obligations toward them, beyond those owed to animals—such as not torturing them. In my terms, Murphy slides from non-membership in reciprocity-community to nonmembership in recognition-community, and his view suggests we can treat sociopaths as animals. He is aware this slide is dangerous, and he tries to block abuses, in my view unsuccessfully. He tells us, for example, that we cannot be certain which individuals are sociopaths. In fact, often we can, and if we never could, then Murphy's discussion would be irrelevant. He tells us that treating sociopaths like animals might make us callous and eventually lead to treating political dissidents in the same way. But that is a dubious slippery slope argument, and the appeal to callousness seems to support the case for counting sociopaths as members of the recognition-community. He says we all share blame for creating a society that produces sociopaths, but that consideration applies to all criminals and has no obvious implications concerning punishment. Finally, he says that psychopaths might deserve some respect because they "may be like infants or the senile—not now persons, but potential or former persons." Yet, infants and the senile *are* persons with inherent moral worth and deserve moral respect, even though they are not currently moral agents, and the same is true of sociopaths.

We can now outline the positive case for viewing sociopaths as morally accountable members of the recognition-community. Granted, it would be unfair and pointless to require sociopaths to respond to moral reasons if they completely lack a capacity for doing so, but that is not what we do. Instead, we hold them responsible for meeting minimum standards of decency, whatever their reasons for doing so. Even when they lack capacities for love and loyalty, they have capacities to avoid killing and torturing. Fortunately, only a small percentage of sociopaths become murderers. Moreover, although sociopaths lack moral *concern*, most of them have some understanding of moral standards, and they also have capacities to restrain their conduct accordingly.[18] In varying degrees, their understanding is that of outsiders to moral practices. They are observers and mimickers of what moral agents care about. But they know they are violating the rules of society, and for that reason the courts regard them as legally sane.

From another direction, it would be psychologically unrealistic to blame most people for routine wrongdoing while not blaming sociopaths when they commit extreme evil. Our basic reactions need to cohere, morally and psychologically.[19] They cannot become so compartmentalized that the most extreme forms of evil are exempt from resentment and outrage. These emotions have evolved as integral to our genetic and cultural heritage, and they have important roles in motivating responsible conduct. They are liable to excess and require constraint within a legal system, but attempts to abandon them might cause far greater damage.

Sociopaths themselves need to be shown a rough consistency in society's attitudes. Although they do not respond in normal ways to moral reasons, they often do respond to self-interested reasons. They tend to be short sighted and impulsive, but they value their freedom. Our negative reactions give sociopaths a strong and clear message about what they can expect by way of sanctions. These consistent reactions also play a therapeutic role. There is no cure for sociopathy, but many sociopaths modify their destructive tendencies by the time they enter their forties.[20] Even if they only respond to self-seeking reasons, social attitudes can signal desirable directions for change.

Sociopaths vary considerably in moral deficiencies, which is another reason for not banishing them from the recognition-community. Consider a textbook example of a nonviolent sociopath.[21] Roberta, who is twenty years old, began at age ten to steal items from her family and from local stores. Well before entering her teenage years she developed a pattern of truancy that led to her expulsion from several schools. She would frequently buy clothes and cosmetics by writing bad checks and using her father's charge cards without permission. She broke her parents' rules about staying out late at night and frequently lied to them without remorse. Eventually she ran away from home and survived by taking temporary jobs. She had many casual sexual encounters with men for whom she felt no deep affection. She never developed long-term career plans or significant commitments in her relationships and work. She is a seriously damaged person, but a person nonetheless, and her parents continued to love her.

Robert Smith suggests that instead of regarding sociopaths as radical anomalies we should view them along a spectrum of amorality. Sociopaths manifest, in extreme forms, tendencies that permeate our society, including short-sighted pleasure-seeking impulse, shallow egotism that violates both prudence and morality, aggressiveness, failure to learn from mistakes, lack of deep commitments, and absence of shame and guilt.[22] Moreover, not all sociopaths are lone wolves. When they engage in wrongdoing they might act in concert with people who are not sociopaths.[23] Many of us share more with sociopaths than we like to think, suggesting an unsavory side to our fascination with them.[24]

Sociopathy is an extreme case, but for that very reason it provides a compelling example of why mental disorders do not render moral perspectives inapplicable. Personality disorders are not the only category of mental disorders that might manifest themselves in violence. Some violence is linked to mental retardation, attention deficit/hyperactivity disorder, schizophrenia and manic depression, organic personality disorder, temporal lobe epilepsy, posttraumatic stress disorder, substance abuse and dependency, depression, dementia, intermittent explosive disorder, and personality disorders such as conduct disorder, antisocial personality disorder, borderline personality disorder, and paranoid personality disorder.[25] But most violence involves none of these *DSM* disorders, and we must now ask whether therapeutic ideas have any broader relevance to immoral forms of violence.

Collective Violence and Preventing Violence

An integrated, moral-therapeutic perspective acknowledges that most violence is committed by otherwise normal and healthy individuals placed in abnormal situations. Abnormal situations include acute or prolonged stress—for example, within families or at the workplace—and they include situations of group violence, such as war. As James Waller emphasizes, "the cause of most extraordinary evil does not lie in a pathological or faulty personality. Rather, it lies in the truth that 'well-adjusted' people can be caught up in a tangle of social forces that may lead them to act in concert with their leaders to massacre opponents."[26]

The question, however, is whether normal people remain entirely healthy as they commit atrocities, or whether they take on abnormal, unhealthy mind-sets. Pathology and suboptimal health can be short-lived, contextual, and limited. In applying this approach to collective or group violence, I emphasize that attending to individual pathology does not deflect attention from deeper social causes, such as poverty, patriarchy, community breakdown, and conflicts among religions and ethnic groups.[27]

In *Humanity: A Moral History of the Twentieth Century*, Jonathan Glover paves the way for an integrated perspective on violence that is sensitive to social causes. Glover interweaves social explanations with explanations in terms of individual character and personality—in particular, the breakdown of normal moral restraints in an individual. He argues that what prevents most of us from engaging in violent acts is a combination of self-interest, including the fear of punishment and ostracism, and moral restraints such as respect for persons, sympathy for their suffering, and a sense of oneself as a "decent person." To some extent, most of us enjoy cruelty: "Deep in human psychology, there are urges to humiliate, torment, wound and kill people."[28] (Compare Nietzsche: "Seeing-suffer feels good, making-suffer even more so—that is a hard proposition, but a central one."[29]) This enjoyment does not by itself explain cruelty, however, any more than it provides a basis for saying cruelty is healthy. Echoing Gilligan, Glover suggests that many violent men are emotionally stunted. And, even more important, extreme social conditions can weaken moral identity and the humane responses of respect and sympathy. Those conditions include modern warfare, with its ability to create psychic distance from the enemy (My Lai, Hiroshima), tribal and ethnic hatreds (Rwanda, Bosnia), and ideological beliefs that degrade and reshape moral identities (Nazi anti-Semitism and Stalinism).

At three junctures, Glover closely links ethical principles and moral psychology—the psychology of the moral life and its distortions. First, irrational beliefs, perverse value judgments, and other cognitive distortions help us understand group violence. Psychologists help us understand how paranoid, bigoted, and other distorted beliefs are generated and promulgated. Psychologists also illuminate role-related illusions, for example, when a pilot tells himself he is just delivering bombs, not killing persons. Cognitive psychology complements and expands, rather than compete with moral explanations. Second, our understanding of violence is enriched by studies of how normal controls on irrational impulses break down, both in impulse control disorders and in more episodic failures. These studies are promising in understanding family violence, where people kill or maim people who mean the most to them. More generally, they help us understand weakness of will, greed, addictions, and immaturity. Third, studies of how moral identities become distorted have much to contribute. Hannah Arendt coined the phrase "banality of evil" to express how even the most horrific evil can emerge from otherwise normal individuals.[30] Since she wrote, numerous studies have shown how identities become fractured or compartmentalized in ways that facilitate violence.[31]

Robert Jay Lifton uses case studies to explore the pathological states of professionals acting in their roles within Nazi Germany and also those of terrorists, in particular the Aum Shinrikyo, which is the Japanese religious cult that in 1995 released nerve gas on five subway trains, killing eleven people and injuring about five thousand. In both instances, "normal" physicians, scientists, accountants, and other professionals played key roles in carrying out terrible evil. They engaged in *doubling*, which is "the division of the self into two functioning wholes, so that a part-self acts as an entire self. An Auschwitz doctor could, through doubling, not only kill and contribute to killing but organize silently, on behalf of that evil project, an entire self-structure (or self-process) encompassing virtually all aspects of his behavior."[32] Doubling is different from Freud's idea of dissociation, whereby part of the ego splits off, for the entire self acts in the social role while disavowing the meaning of and responsibility for what one does. The professionals also used *psychic numbing*, "a general category of diminished capacity or inclination to feel," especially to feel sympathy, compassion, and guilt for killing.[33] In addition to doubling and psychic numbing, Lifton explores how paranoid and megalomanic beliefs enter into group violence, as in the Nazi's anti-Semitism and Aum Shinrikyo's perversion of the Buddhist concept of *poa*, killing for the sake of your victims.[34]

Lifton's account is controversial, and I use it only to illustrate how conceptions of pathology can be applied to collective violence.[35] Lifton's view is compatible with Glover's insights into the perverted moral psychology (and character) typical of group violence, as well as compatible with social explanations of violence by appealing to economics, religion, and so on. Even so, it is difficult to see how doubling could explain the evil of the terrorists in their attack on the World Trade Center in New York City on September 11, 2001 (9/11). Their evil expressed personalities that were unified around a sick morality and a perverted religious faith. A sound integrated perspective will shun attempts to explain all evil in terms of one psychological mechanism.

An integrated perspective will support both individual therapy and public health approaches to preventing and curing violence. It does not envision a magic cure of violence. Experts approach violence contextually, striving to develop specific techniques that work on specific forms of it. For example, one expert sorts wife batterers into three main groups: sociopaths, overcontrolled, and cyclical/emotionally volatile.[36] For the sociopaths, there was little he could do. For the overcontrolled—that is, those spouses whose violence erupts after a long period of suppressed, seething rage—current therapies are helpful. The same is true for the cyclical/emotionally volatile: that is, those who manifest cycles of blaming and rage against their spouses unfold in recurring acts of violence. In both of the latter cases, the therapy consisted primarily of four months of group counseling. The ground rules for the counseling sessions centered on taking responsibility for violent acts and the willingness to engage in honest discussion about the acts with other members of the group. In other words, the therapy was moral-laden. Even the counselor would depart from a value-neutral stance to challenge any negative stereotypes of women voiced by members of the group, as well as to enforce the procedural rules.

Public health approaches seek to prevent violence without being able to predict which individuals will engage in it. Some obvious solutions, such as removing the easy availability of guns, are hamstrung by political controversies. Other solutions, however, center on strengthening community ties. Special programs are developed within schools and corporations, as well as support for troubled families. Administrators are trained in how to identify, control, and prevent individuals at risk because of excessive stress. Such programs and training are largely conducted by therapy-oriented professionals who also have training in basic security procedures. All these approaches implement morally responsible approaches in light of contemporary therapeutic understanding.

Revise Morality: Responsibility without Retribution?

I conclude by responding to the suggestion that we should stop blaming violent and sick individuals. A familiar suggestion is to redirect negative emotions and attitudes toward deeds rather than persons, to hate the sin but love the sinner. That suggestion is made by M. Scott Peck, a psychiatrist who converted to Christianity and who is one of the most popular writers on ethics in recent decades. Peck defines evil broadly as "the use of power to destroy the spiritual growth of others for the purpose of defending and preserving the integrity of our own sick selves."[37] Blending psychiatry with the Christian condemnation of pride, he portrays evil as a narcissistic personality disorder characterized by self-deceiving denials of responsibility. We are "responsible for the state of health of our souls" and for the evil we inflict.[38]

Peck sets forth an integrated, moral-therapeutic perspective, but not one I can endorse. Directly or indirectly, our attitudes of resentment, indignation, and hatred inescapably target persons, not disembodied actions. As with crime, there is an inherent tension between justice and love in thinking about violence. Nonetheless, the tension can be creative, and it should be resolved contextually. In contexts where we have opportunities to help a person who seeks improvement, we should try to constrain or suspend anger. But it is neither realistic nor desirable to abandon all blame of persons.

For more subtle reasons, Gary Watson suggests we should go much further in downplaying resentment.[39] He argues there is a kind of contradiction within morality between retribution and love. To illustrate, he has us attend to Robert Harris who, along with his brother was having difficulty hotwiring a car in the parking lot of a fast-food restaurant in San Diego, California. Harris decided to steal the car of two sixteen-year-olds who were eating at the other end of the parking lot. After kidnapping the youths at gunpoint, Harris drove to a remote canyon and released them with the promise they would not be hurt. As the teenagers walked away, Harris shot one of them in the back. Then he hunted down the other teenager and shot him four times. When he returned to find the first teenager still alive, he shot him point-blank in the head. Harris was having fun, and he was still jovial fifteen minutes later when he ate the hamburger of one of his victims. At the time, Harris was twenty-five and had a criminal record that included torturing animals and beating a neighbor to death during a dispute. His sister described him as having "no feeling for life, no sense of remorse."[40]

How does someone become so inhumane, so inhuman? Much of the answer is clear. Both his parents were alcoholics. His father beat him frequently when he was a child. His mother confesses she could never love him, and even when he was an infant she avoided physical contact, sometimes kicking him away when he attempted to touch her. He was raped several times at age fourteen while in a federal youth detention center. Psychiatric help was never provided, even though he was obviously disturbed. Unquestionably Harris had a tragic childhood and as an adult is sick, suffering from a "malformation of the self" that incapacitates him for normal moral relationships.[41]

As a result, according to Watson, we lack a coherent moral response to him, and to others like him. On the one hand, we appropriately respond with deep antipathy to Harris because of his heartlessness. On the other hand, we appropriately respond with sympathy because of the childhood that left him incapacitated for normal relationships. Our reactions of antipathy and sympathy clash in ways that "do not enable us to respond overall in a coherent way." We must view him both "as evil (and hence calling for enmity and moral opposition) and as one who is a victim (calling for sympathy and understanding)"; hence, "Harris both satisfies and violates the criteria of victimhood" in ways that reveal ordinary morality is incoherent.[42]

This conclusion does not follow. Ambivalence is not incoherence, and there is no contradiction in feeling both antipathy and sympathy toward him.[43] Nor should ambivalence paralyze our practical responses in punishing him for violating basic norms of decency. Jurors and judges should weigh his tragic childhood in meting out punishment, but his heinous crimes justify retribution. It is misleading to say that Harris both satisfies and does not satisfy the criteria for being a victim, for there are two topics. Harris fully satisfies the criteria for being a victim of a tragic childhood; he also fully satisfies the criteria for being a brutal victimizer of the people he murdered. His tragic childhood does not excuse his brutality, for terrible childhoods do not determine adult evil, as Watson admits. Indeed, Harris's siblings suffered equally abusive childhoods but did not turn to violence. Ultimately, the issue turns not on ambivalence but, instead, on whether it is just and fair to hold Harris, maimed as he is, to a standard of minimum decency that makes civilized society possible. Surely it is.

Watson shows that we can conceive of justice without retributive attitudes. Gandhi, Martin Luther King Jr., and Einstein all spoke for justice rooted in love without retribution: "They *stand up* for themselves and others against their oppressors; they *confront* their oppressors with the fact of their misconduct, *urging* and even *demanding* consideration for themselves and others; but they manage, or come much closer than others to managing, to do such things without vindictiveness or malice."[44] In this way, negative emotions can in principle be stripped away when judging moral responsibility for violence. Doing so is one tack in developing an integrated moral-therapeutic perspective. It is not the tack I would pursue, however.

Ideals of love should be kept prominent within an integrative project. Nevertheless, I find it unrealistic to abandon retribution altogether. A justified ethics will be psychologically realistic in its expectations.[45] An ethics of pure love, stripped of all retributive sentiments, might be suitable for saints, but most of us have retributive sentiments deeply embedded in us, arguably the product of evolution. Love for people we care about, as well as justice and self-interest, generates our resentment toward perpetrators of violence. Again, resentment is an essential motivator for most people in combating injustice and cruelty.[46] Trying to implement ideals of pure love might even increase hostility by frustrating basic human desires, thereby harming rather than promoting community.

To conclude, an integrated, moral-therapeutic perspective on (unjustified) violence must grapple with the tension between blame and compassion. As Watson makes clear, the tension is within morality itself, however, not between morality and therapy. Extreme and unjustified cruelty warrants the strongest moral condemnation, but it also invites using the full resources of therapeutic understanding and healing. The same is true of bigotry, to which I turn next.

11

ARE BIGOTS SICK?

Therapeutic images are frequently applied to bigotry: racism is a wound, misogyny is a sickness of the soul, antisemitism is a disease of society, and homophobia is a phobia.[1] Sometimes these images are intended as metaphors to highlight how bigotry—especially *shallow bigotry*, or prejudice based primarily on ignorance—injures and spreads like a plague and is easily overthrown by education and experience. Therapeutic language carries more literal meanings, however, when applied to *visceral bigotry*, which is my topic; this is prejudice involving deeply irrational beliefs and attitudes that are well entrenched in the personality and serve important needs such as elevating self-esteem and expressing frustration.[2] I make a case for viewing visceral bigotry as both sickness and wrongdoing.

Prejudice as Pathology

Therapeutic approaches to bigotry are currently out of fashion, but they are not without supporters, as the following event illustrates. In 2000, *Sports Illustrated* published an interview with John Rocker, a relief pitcher for the Atlanta Braves, in which Rocker slurred women, gays, Asian Americans, African Americans, and other minorities living in New York City.[3] Taking the interview as evidence that Rocker was emotionally unstable, the commissioner of major league baseball ordered psychological tests on him. The order caused as much controversy as Rocker's remarks. Most observers saw the issue as moral, not therapeutic, and insisted that Rocker immediately be fined and suspended (as he eventually was). Harvard psychiatrist Alvin F. Poussaint, however, praised the commissioner. For some time, Poussaint and other African American psychiatrists have lobbied to include "racist personality disorder" in the *DSM*. Their efforts were blocked, according to Poussaint, because mainstream psychiatry is insufficiently sensitive to racial issues: "If black psychiatrists had been in control of establishing what the diagnoses should be in the D.S.M . . . [then in] some way, racism would be in that book."[4]

Bigotry and psychopathology might be related in two ways, empirically or conceptually. First, they might be related empirically, such that bigotry is contingently correlated with currently recognized mental disorders. In this vein, we might ask whether Rocker was "off his rocker," in terms of a mental disorder currently listed in the *DSM*. The *correlation claim* is that bigotry is correlated with currently recognized mental disorders in statistically significantly numbers. Second, bigotry and psychopathology might be related conceptually, such that bigotry is a distinctive mental disorder. Thus, we might ask whether Rocker's bigotry itself constitutes a distinctive disorder that should be entered in the *DSM*. The *conceptual claim* is that the well-entrenched, need-serving, irrational attitudes characteristic of visceral bigotry constitute psychopathology.

An additional example will clarify the distinction. In August of 1999, Buford Furrow walked into a Jewish community center in Los Angeles and fired seventy bullets at young children and their caregivers. While fleeing, he murdered a postal worker because he was nonwhite and a government employee. At age thirty-seven, Furrow was described as "a frequently inept and mentally unstable bumbler," "a reticent isolated man whose rage would periodically consume him," and someone with very low self-esteem who would fluctuate between depression and rage.[5] During the preceding decade he formed ties with the Aryan Nations Movement, and for a while he was married to the widow of a slain leader of a neo-Nazi splinter group. Once he tried to commit suicide. Another time he served a prison sentence for assault. Twice in the previous year he entered psychiatric facilities.

Furrow is obviously sick, but how is his bigotry related to his sickness? Applying the correlation claim, we might see his bigotry as a symptom of currently recognized mental disorders that are defined without mentioning bigotry. Thinking along these lines, the psychoanalyst Peter Wolson says Furrow suffers from an impulse control disorder, the failure to control impulses in a normal manner. Furrow also has intermittent explosive disorder, manifested by several episodes of aggression disproportionate to any provocation. Wolson uses Furrow to illustrate the cultural shift from neurotic or anxiety disorders, which dominated clinical practice during the first half of the twentieth century, to the current predominance of impulse control disorders. In addition, Wolson suggests Furrow manifests general affective disorders, such as low self-esteem and paranoia, which he understands in psychoanalytic terms: "By identifying with the 'racially superior' Aryan Nations, he compensated for his inferior self-image, which he then projected onto Jews. In trying to kill Jews, Furrow was attempting to kill off the hated, disowned parts of himself."[6] Here Wolson makes a correlation claim about empirical ties between Furrow's bigotry and low self-esteem and impulse control disorders. More generally, bigots might manifest antisocial personality disorder, schizophrenia, substance abuse disorder, sexual identity disorder, and so on for the hundreds of other mental disorders currently recognized by psychiatrists.

In contrast, following Poussaint, we might understand Furrow's (visceral) bigotry as constituting psychopathology, as a distinctive syndrome. Parsed in this way, the question "Are bigots sick?" asks, Is it illuminating to pathologize prejudice per se, regardless of its connections with other mental disorders and regardless of its ultimate causes? The conceptual claim implies it is. I am primarily interested in the conceptual claim, aware that it blurs with the correlation claim when there are strong correlations exist between bigotry and current entries in the *DSM*.

Definitions of Psychopathology

A decisive argument for pathologizing visceral bigotry would establish that a canonical definition of psychopathology applies to it. As we have seen, there is no such definition. Nevertheless, bigotry might still be a sickness according to some influential definitions of psychopathology. I consider four such definitions: *DSM*, explicitly moral-laden, relativistic, and psychoanalytic definitions.

Bigotry as Dysfunction

The *DSM* defines mental disorders in terms of distress, disability (impairment), or increased risk of harm.[7] Poussaint believes that bigotry fits this definition, and hence he advocates adding racist personality disorder to the *DSM*. He also believes, however, that the *DSM*'s current entry for delusional disorders applies to much bigotry, thereby suggesting that bigotry might fit as a subheading of current *DSM* entries.[8]

Why did the *DSM* authors refuse to include bigotry? One reason is that bigotry does not always cause distress to bigots; there are many happy racists. Nor, typically, is there an increased risk to bigots. But what about impairment—in particular, in dealing with members of groups targeted by the bigotry? The *DSM* authors argued that racism is so widespread that it is a "normal" or "expectable" cultural response, rather than a dysfunction.[9] They granted, however, that racism is suboptimal health: racism is "a good example of a condition representing a non-optimal psychological functioning which renders a person vulnerable in certain environments to manifesting signs of disorder."[10] Today, its suboptimality is increasingly obvious, and saying racism is an expected cultural response seems weak grounds for calling it normal.

I agree with Poussaint that (visceral) bigotry fits the *DSM* definition of mental disorder. Bigotry is a dysfunction in responding to large segments of humanity. It constitutes impairment in responding in healthy and responsible ways toward targeted groups because of irrational hatred, fear, contempt, or other negative attitudes. This is true even when bigotry helps a person function effectively in other respects, as in thriving among other racists. For example, homophobia and antisemitism constitute emotional and cognitive impairments regarding particular groups of individuals.

Bigotry as Extreme Irresponsibility

Morally explicit definitions of psychopathology apply straightforwardly to bigotry. Consider Rem Edwards's definition of mental illness as "extreme and prolonged practical irrationality and irresponsibility."[11] Edwards set forth his definition in opposition to the therapeutic trend, and he would oppose pathologizing prejudice. Nevertheless, his definition applies to much bigotry: "extreme and prolonged" conveys entrenchment, "irrationality" conveys false beliefs resistant to evidence, and "irresponsibility" implies lack of responsible agency toward targeted groups.

In an essay on the Holocaust, Martin P. Golding calls bigotry a "moral pathology," and he might also have called it an immoral pathology. For Golding, extreme bigotry is morally dysfunctional: "It is the inability to choose or act for the good of the whole, of the society or the individual. . . . This inability *is* unhealth and injustice; and it is a moral defect."[12] Exactly. Golding points out that entire moral outlooks and systems, for example those of Nazi Germany, can become pathological, as well as individuals.

Bigotry as Socially Maladaptive

Relativistic definitions understand mental health as adaptation to society and its values and pathology as significant maladaptation. Mental health is the ability to cope in one's society without constant frustration, anxiety, or other emotional and behavioral difficulties.[13] Accordingly, whether bigotry is pathological depends on the society where it is found. When bigotry is widespread, it can be socially adaptive and hence healthy. Using this reasoning, Gordon Allport concluded that "much prejudice is a matter of blind conformity with prevailing folkways," rather than sickness.[14]

Relativistic definitions of mental health are problematic, however. What is the appropriate society: a nation's majority, a nation's laws, a group's dominant power, a subgroup within a nation, or the entire international community? A bigot might be sick relative to one group (e.g., the United States) but healthy relative to another group (e.g., the Ku Klux Klan). More important, by reducing health (and other) values to custom or socially sanctioned power, relativism makes nonsense of sound reasoning about values. It also fails to allow that an individual might be sick even though society values the sickness.

Consider Adolf Eichmann. Hannah Arendt applied a relativistic sense of health when she called Eichmann "terrifyingly normal," someone who illustrates "the banality of evil."[15] Eichmann was an utterly ordinary man, neither sick nor sadistic. He was a conscientious bureaucrat and loyal citizen who functioned effectively—in particular, in spearheading the deportation of Jews to concentration camps and crematoriums. Stanley Milgram's experiments also document a strong human tendency to cooperate with authorities in causing harm: "Ordinary people, simply doing their jobs, and without any particular hostility on their part, can become agents in a terrible destructive process."[16]

Arendt's and Milgram's influence led Holocaust historian George M. Kren to dismiss all attempts to pathologize antisemitism: "The attempt to apply medical labels—insane, 'criminal superego,' pathological—is an attempt to avoid confronting the unpalatable reality that these were ordinary people...[and that] most individuals would, if placed in such situations, act in a similar way."[17]

I disagree. Even if we grant that Eichmann and most other Nazis did not manifest currently recognized psychopathology in higher numbers than the general populace, the question remains whether their attitudes and conduct are signs of sickness, or at least suboptimal health. In my view, Eichmann's ability to distance himself from his horrific evil indicates suboptimal mental health, even though, as Robert J. Lifton says, the distancing relied on quite ordinary mental processes such as rationalization and psychic numbing.[18] It is one thing to say that normal people, using ordinary psychological processes, are drawn into extensive participation in genocide. It is another thing to say they remain entirely healthy once they became immersed in genocide.

As another example, consider Henry Ford, the great automobile entrepreneur. During the 1920s, when he was the wealthiest person in the world, Ford sponsored the most intense outburst of antisemitism in American history. He paid for a series of antisemitic articles that ran each week for almost two years in his own newspaper, the *Dearborn Independent*, articles that later formed the basis for the antisemitic book, *The International Jew*. The dominant theme was that Jews were pursuing a secret political conquest to govern the world. Ford did not engage in physical violence against Jews, but his enormous prestige helped make antisemitism respectable, thereby contributing to the climate that permitted the United States to downplay the Nazi persecutions of Jews. Albert Lee argues that Ford's antisemitism was caused primarily by populist sentiments against the large influx of intellectually oriented Jews, together with his personal hatred of (Jewish) financiers. Assume that is true. Nevertheless, his entrenched and virulent antisemitism distorted his personality and his character. Regardless of its ultimate causes, Ford's antisemitism was sick, even though it was in tune with the dominant attitudes of society. I should add that Lee himself uses therapeutic language when he portrays Ford as "infected with anti-Semitism" and as having a "Jew mania."[19]

Bigotry as Psychological Disharmony

Freud's definition of psychopathology was not entirely relativistic, and he allowed that some societies and even all of humanity might be neurotic in some respects.[20] Confronting a Victorian society where anxiety-creating attitudes toward sex and altruistic ideals were the statistical norm, Freud criticized these attitudes as unhealthy. He also believed in a continuum between mental health and illness. Most psychoanalytic definitions focus on harmony among basic drives and other aspects of the personality, while partly defining that harmony by reference to social adaptation, especially the ability to work and love in meaningful ways. Here is one typical definition: "The concept of normalcy refs to a condition of relative harmony between the various parts of the personality, and between the personality and the reality situation."[21]

Applying such definitions, many psychoanalysts regard bigots as sick, although in doing so they blur the conceptual and correlation claims. For example, when Theodore Rubin avers that "every anti-Semite is emotionally disturbed,"[22] he seems to make an implausible correlation claim to the effect that antisemitism is invariably the product of more general emotional problems. His view is more plausible, however, if it is interpreted as a conceptual claim about visceral bigotry. Indeed, he portrays the entrenched hatred and fear characteristic of antisemitism as "a nonorganic disease of the mind," a "psychiatric illness," a "symbol sickness" that involves making Jews symbols of virtually everything undesirable.[23] Paranoia, psychological conflicts, and defense mechanisms are often involved, but the defining features of the illness are the bigoted attitudes themselves.[24]

In her illuminating psychoanalytic study, *Anatomy of Prejudices*, Elizabeth Young-Bruehl contends that prejudice has no special connection with psychopathology, but in making this claim she relies on a relativistic definition. Thus, she agrees with Hannah Arendt, her former teacher, that Eichmann was "terrifyingly normal" in that he functioned adaptively within the bureaucracy of the Third Reich.[25] Nevertheless, Young-Bruehl notes that prejudice often serves the same functions as sickness: "Many people have prejudices *instead of* the conventional forms of various pathologies, somewhat as people have perversions instead of neuroses if they act on their forbidden desires rather than repressing them." Moreover, she is willing to speak of racist groups and societies as having "social pathologies" that function as "social mechanisms of defense."[26]

I find it odd to say that societies are sick but not the individuals instantiating the relevant syndrome. If we abandon relativistic definitions, and use more traditional psychoanalytic definitions of psychopathology, Young-Bruehl's main themes are in tune with the conceptual claim. In particular, in exploring the underlying hatred, fear, and anxiety produced by inner conflicts, Young-Bruehl insightfully distinguishes several different kinds of prejudices.

"Ethnocentric prejudices" arise from the universal tendency to form and preserve cultural groups based on economic, political, and social ties, and to set themselves in opposition to other groups. In contrast, "ideologies of desire" are prejudices rooted in worldviews and structured by shared desires. They target victims across cultural groups based on "marks of difference" in human form and identity.[27] Interestingly, Young-Bruehl gives pathology-sounding labels to the various ideologies of desire: obsessional, hysterical, narcissistic, and homophobic. Obsessional prejudice, for example antisemitism, centers on "fixed ideas," such as conspiracy theories about demonic enemies, which enable the prejudiced person to behave sadistically. Hysterical prejudice, such as racism, involves projecting one's repressed sexual and aggressive desires to another group. Narcissistic prejudice, such as sexism, centers on self-elevation and intolerance toward people significantly different from themselves, anatomically or in terms of gender. Homophobia combines obsessions, sexual desires, and narcissistic gender prejudices.[28] In my view, these ideologies of desire are also pathologies of desire.

Objections to Pathologizing Prejudice

Poussaint suggests that psychiatrists' opposition to pathologizing prejudice is based on racial insensitivity, but surely much else is also involved. We need to respond to four objections. To pathologize prejudice is (1) incompatible with holding bigots responsible, (2) politically regressive, (3) unnecessary, and (4) simplistic.

The first, and most important, objection is that viewing bigots as sick is incompatible with holding them morally responsible. According to Naomi Zack: "If racists are judged to be emotionally disturbed simply because they are racists, this lifts their moral responsibility for harm done."[29] Zack targets what I call the conceptual claim: racists are emotionally disturbed "simply because" they are racists. Her objection is that sickness automatically excuses, whereas racists must be held accountable for the harm they cause and for their bigotry itself. Clearly, Zack assumes a morality-therapy dichotomy, such that sickness is an automatic exemption from responsibility. Once we reject that dichotomy, however, we can understand bigotries as *DSM*-type patterns of behavior, emotion, and belief for which individuals can be responsible. With bigotry, as with other disorders, we have responsibilities for our health and for preventable harm caused by our sickness. These responsibilities need to be understood contextually. Persons raised in a racist group might have little responsibility for initially forming racist views, but they are responsible for changing when opportunities arise.

The second objection is that pathologizing bigotry is politically regressive and would leave us without effective ways to oppose bigotry. Zack notes that "there are few, if any systematic programs of psychological therapy for classic racists.... [and] most racists do not consider their racism to be an emotional illness, so they are unlikely to seek such help."[30] Similarly, Ann E. Cudd argues that psychoanalytic approaches to bigotry are "politically paralyzing": "Psychoanalytic theories generally locate pathologies, including the social pathology of oppression, in personal failings. This also makes the prospects of a solution [to prejudice] bleak, for it would have to be psychotherapeutic and thus individual, rather than political and collective."[31]

Zack and Cudd force us to choose between moral and therapeutic ways of combating bigotry. Yet, as an analogy, there is nothing politically paralyzing about viewing alcoholics as sick—just the opposite. True, alcoholics usually do not view themselves as sick until their addictions cause great damage. When they finally do seek help, they are often "converted" into thinking of their problem as a sickness by attending Alcoholics Anonymous, but a central part of therapy is helping them accept responsibility for their drinking. Or, if they already regard their problem as a disease, it is because society has conveyed that outlook to them. Quite possibly, something similar might occur if society came to view prejudice as pathological. In addition, new therapeutic approaches might be developed if society came to view bigotry as pathological. The therapy need not be lengthy psychoanalysis but, instead, the currently favored shorter versions of cognitive-behavioral therapy.

Cudd's worry about coercion is also excessive. Although most of the health care community views alcoholics as sick, our society does not force them to enter therapy, at least until they cause serious harm to others. A similar approach to bigotry would make therapeutic help available and socially encouraged, but coercion would not be involved until the bigot causes direct injury. Indeed, mandatory "diversity" and "sensitivity training programs" are already used by employers and others as part of imposed penalties for causing harm, in addition to preventive measures for all employees. Furthermore, overthrowing bigotry can play a part in therapy for many other problems brought to therapists. As Gordon Allport notes, "while it is safe to say that a patient never comes to a therapist for the express purpose of changing his *ethnic* attitudes, still these attitudes may assume a salient role as the course of treatment progresses, and may conceivably be dissolved or restructured along with the patient's other fixed ways of looking at life."[32]

Most important, individual therapy is only one component of a therapeutic outlook on bigotry. Public health approaches are equally important. As a society, we are making progress in treating alcoholism, smoking, problem gambling, and a host other problems as public health issues. In addition to individual therapy, public health approaches shape public opinion through formal education, the media, and self-help books. They also include taking preventive measures in the form of public policies designed to discourage the problematic activities—for example, restrictions on advertising cigarettes and alcohol. All these approaches have moral and therapeutic aspects, as would making bigotry a public health issue.

A moral-therapeutic perspective can also illuminate why bigotry is so deeply entrenched in individuals and societies, thereby increasing effectiveness and realism in combating it. As I noted, the widespread adoption of the therapeutic term "homophobia" helps combat that insidious form of bigotry. A moral-therapeutic perspective alerts us to the need to provide healthier outlets for the fears and desires that underlie bigotry. Such a perspective also reminds us that blame easily becomes excessive and self-defeating. There are appropriate occasions for blaming bigots, but when blame merely arouses defensive maneuvers against perceived hostility, anxiety, and guilt, we should seek ways to express moral convictions without inflaming hostility. For this reason, Jody David Armour attempts in his law classes "to move the discussion away from fault and blame" and "to approach it [racism] as a public-health problem in which we are *all* responsible for the cure."[33]

Turning from political strategy to everyday life, therapeutic strategies can help us confront bigotry in our families and friends, our employers and colleagues, and indeed ourselves. For example, the co-authors of *Encountering Bigotry* apply therapeutic approaches in opposing bigotry, without turning away in silent embarrassment or contempt, while maintaining relationships that are "respectful and egalitarian."[34] Their suggestions include focusing on the interaction itself (e.g., an invitation to laugh at a racist joke) rather than being drawn into discussing generalizations about the maligned group; meeting other persons as they are, rather than trying to change their character on the spot; expressing our view honestly but without unnecessary inflammation; being sensitive to the context and the relationship with the individual; hoping for "good enough" handling of the situation, without expecting an altogether happy outcome.

The third objection to pathologizing prejudice is that doing so is unnecessary. Bigotry can be fully understood in terms of "normal" psychological factors such as ignorance, fear, and everyday cognition and economic-sociological factors. Thus, Cudd explains bigotry in terms of everyday patterns of cognition, together with differences in wealth and power. Prejudice simply manifests ordinary reasoning that involves distortion, exaggeration, and simplification of information, as well as the formation of in-groups versus out-groups designed to bolster self-esteem. In explaining the entrenchment of bigotry in the personality, Cudd notes how stereotypes are self-fulfilling in ways that generate vicious cycles. Stereotypes are stable structures that, once formed, are used to integrate new information. Sometimes they are even embraced by members of victimized groups, thereby fostering feelings of shame, inferiority, hopelessness, and prejudice toward members of their own group. This leads them to acquiesce to their status as victims, thereby confirming oppressors' view of them as inferior. Bigotry is best opposed by attacking harmful stereotypes, exposing hypocrisy and false consciousness, and fostering new in- and out-groups based on interests rather than race.[35]

In reply, I agree that the psychological literature on normal cognitive functioning greatly enriches our understanding of bigotry. Nevertheless, psychological explanations do not by themselves settle whether bigotry is pathological. That issue turns on the definitions of health and sickness. Henry Ford's antisemitism is sick even though it might be explained as the product of familiar patterns of reasoning, together with economic biases. Furthermore, cognitive psychology, at least in Cudd's version, does not completely explain bigotry. Paul Wachtel better explains bigotry by leaving room for two broad types of psychological explanations of racism: need-based and cognitive-based.[36] *Need-based prejudice* serves important desires (beyond those involved in cognition); it enters into one's self-conception (explicitly or implicitly); and it is well-entrenched so that marshalling evidence about its irrationality does not easily overthrow it. Examples of important desires include desires for money and economic security, social power and status, sex and aggression, and self-esteem. *Cognitive-based prejudice*, by contrast, is prejudice based on patterns of perception and reasoning that operate in all areas of life. It is prejudice rooted in faulty reasoning and false information received from parents and peers or from limited exposure to diversity. Wachtel is hopeful that cognitive-based racism can be overthrown by broadened experience and education, but need-based prejudice poses greater challenges.

The last objection to pathologizing prejudice is that it fosters simplistic thinking. It lumps together all bigotry, as if it were one homogeneous phenomenon. It also leads us to apply stereotypes of mental illness to bigots, including dismissing them as mentally deranged and inferior beings.

In reply, this objection is better understood as cautionary rather than conclusive. On the one hand, we need to attend to differences among forms of bigotry in terms of their meaning, causes, and suitable therapeutic responses. Obviously there are differences among targeted groups; for example, homophobia targets gays and racist personality disorder would target race-based bigotry. There might also be differences in the psychodynamics of different kinds of bigotry, as Young-Bruehl suggests. Rather than being simplistic, a therapeutic perspective might alert us to these significant differences. On the other hand, in pathologizing prejudice we need to avoid stereotyping persons with mental disorders. No stereotype is more harmful than thinking that mental disorders render a person sick in every way. No matter how severely prejudice infects a personality, it remains one dimension of a person. Ethicists also lapse into stereotypes. In particular, Jean-Paul Sartre's *Anti-Semite and Jew*, perhaps the most famous philosophical discussion of prejudice, demonizes bigots as inhumane in every area of their lives. Their "passion" of fearing freedom is not limited to any one sphere.[37] Demonizing bigots in this way is psychologically unrealistic because character is invariably speckled, a mixture of vice and virtues in varied combinations.[38]

To conclude, we can understand (visceral) bigotry as pathological without altering our conviction that it is immoral. Doing so allows us to appreciate how overcoming bigotry can be both a moral and a therapeutic process. At the same time, pathologizing prejudice (as with crime) carries risks in the current social climate where sickness is often assumed to be an automatic excuse. We need to ensure that justice remains a key component in an integrated, moral-therapeutic perspective.

Part IV
HEALTHY MORALITY AND MEANINGFUL LIVES

Psychology is not just the study of disease, weakness, and damage; it also is the study of strength and virtue. Treatment is not just fixing what is wrong; it also is building what is right.

Martin E. P. Seligman, "Positive Psychology,
Positive Prevention, and Positive Therapy"

Philosophy heals human diseases, diseases produced by false beliefs. Its arguments are to the soul as the doctor's remedies are to the body. They can heal, and they are to be evaluated in terms of their power to heal.

Martha Nussbaum, *The Therapy of Desire*

12

DEPRESSION AND IDENTITY

Although I occasionally return to wrongdoing, the focus in Part IV is the connection between meaningful lives and positive health—that is, biopsychosocial well-being, in addition to the absence of mental disorders. Meaningful lives embody defensible values (objective meaning) and are enlivened by a sense of worthwhileness (subjective meaning). The therapeutic trend has led psychotherapists to explore all aspects of meaningful lives, including everyday moral issues concerning love, work, community service, happiness, and authenticity. In discussing these and other topics, my aim is to illustrate how therapeutic insights complement and advance understanding, rather than replacing morality with something else. In addition, chapter 14 applies my integrated, moral-therapeutic perspective to philosophical counseling, a movement that sometimes wrongly sets itself at odds with psychotherapy's emphasis on mental health. I begin by discussing depression, the most ubiquitous concern about meaning brought to psychotherapists.

According to psychiatrist Michael Miller, "depression has overtaken anxiety as our presiding discontent."[1] As a contributing factor to suicide, drug addiction, alcoholism, troubled relationships, damaged careers, and much plain misery, depression is a fundamental source of self-diminishment. Hence we should celebrate the powerful new treatments for it, both pharmaceutical and psychotherapeutic. Nevertheless, critics of the therapeutic trend worry that we have gone too far in medicalizing everyday depression: that is, low moods involving a sense of lessened self-worth and meaning. Depression can be an ally as well as a threat in meaningful lives, and a knee-jerk resort to "mood brightening" drugs undermines its contributions in stimulating insights, accepting defeats, and fostering change.

Mill's Moral Malady

One approach to understanding depression relies on the morality-therapy dichotomy: each instance of depression is either pathological (a mood disorder), in which case a therapeutic perspective applies, or healthy (a normal mood), in which case a moral perspective might be relevant. I reject this dichotomy because many instances of depression simultaneously raise moral and health issues, as illustrated by a famous episode in John Stuart Mill's life.

At age twenty, following a remarkable education that had him reading Greek and Latin before age ten and mastering logic and economics by age fourteen, Mill fell into a depression that continues to intrigue philosophers and psychologists alike. At the time he was working very hard, taking on increased responsibilities at his job in the Examiner's Office of the East India Company and editing a five-volume work by Jeremy Bentham. Sheer exhaustion does not explain his depression, however, if only because he always managed a Herculean work load. In his autobiography, Mill presents his depression as a crisis in his intellectual and moral development. Moral ideas permeate his account of the cause, content, cure, and consequences of the depression.

First, Mill was raised to believe in the utilitarian ethic espoused by his father James Mill and their frequent household guest Jeremy Bentham. One day he asked himself whether he would be happy if he achieved all his present goals, including changes in social institutions. When he answered no, his "heart sank within." His self-questioning precipitated a severe depression lasting most of a year and causing months of "irremediable wretchedness" before gradually subsiding. The occasion for the self-questioning is noteworthy: "I was in a dull state of nerves, such as everybody is occasionally liable to; unsusceptible to enjoyment or pleasurable excitement; one of those moods when what is pleasure at other times, becomes insipid or indifferent; the state, I should think, in which converts to Methodism usually are, when smitten by their first 'conviction of sin.' "[2] It seems that when he posed his fateful question, Mill was already in a mild depression characterized by unhappiness and perhaps guilt, given the allusion to sin.

Second, the six months of unrelenting suffering included a dramatic loss of meaning and moral commitment in which he felt there was "nothing left to live for." His despair was not a *feature-specific depression*, focused on one or two aspects of his life.[3] At least, he was not aware of being depressed about any particular misfortune or suffering from despair about a specific activity or relationship. Instead, he experienced a *non-feature-specific depression*, a general hopelessness in which all his activities and relationships seemed futile and worthless, even though he managed to carry on in a dispirited manner.

Third, Mill needed moral support, perhaps from a friend or loved one in whom he could confide. Sadly, no one was available, least of all his father, whom he was certain would find his depression mystifying. What did help, eventually, were works of literature dealing with moral values and relationships. Hope came when he found himself crying as he read a memoir about a family's grief in response to the death of the father. The tears confirmed that he was still capable of feeling, and later the poetry of Wordsworth deepened his emotions and sustained the recovery.

Fourth, Mill's depression led to significant changes in his moral outlook. He came to believe that the ethical theories espoused by his father and Bentham were seriously incomplete. Personal happiness must be pursued indirectly by finding enjoyment in other things, not directly as he had been taught. Furthermore, moral commitment must be rooted in something more enduring than artificial conditioning, especially within a life of philosophical analysis that constantly challenges and erodes assumptions created by that conditioning. A sound education would establish natural ties between pleasures and goods such as love, aesthetic appreciation, and the community well-being. This insight led him to emphasize higher pleasures, what we might understand as intrinsically better enjoyments derived from worthwhile activities and relationships, contrary to Bentham's belief that quantity of pleasures is all that matters.[4]

In these four ways, Mill depicted his depression as a moral and intellectual crisis. A closer look, however, uncovers medical references as well. Mill says he yearned for a "physician who could heal" his "mental malady," and he called Wordsworth's poems "medicine for my state of mind." He also says "the words of Macbeth to the physician often occurred to my thoughts": "Canst thou not minister to a mind diseased. . . ." Actually, he alluded to these words without quoting them, as if doing so might render the nature of his suffering all too clear. As a stiff-upper-lip Victorian, Mill found his illness embarrassingly "egotistical" and "in no way honorable" and hence did not dwell on his symptoms; but he knew he was sick.[5]

Indeed, Mill meets the *DSM* criteria for a major depressive disorder, which occurs when five or more of the following symptoms are present nearly daily over at least two weeks: (1) a depressed mood (e.g., feeling sad or empty), (2) markedly reduced interest and pleasure in most activities, (3) loss or increase in appetite or weight, (4) insomnia or excessive sleep, (5) psychomotor agitation or retardation, (6) fatigue, (7) feelings of worthlessness or inappropriate guilt, (8) inability to concentrate, (9) recurrent thoughts of death or suicide.[6] Mill clearly met five of these criteria:

(1') He underwent six months of what Coleridge described as "a grief without a pang, void, dark and drear."

(2') The "cloud" of dejection was carried "into all companies, into all occupations."

(4') Sleep failed to refresh and brought only "a renewed consciousness" of having nothing to live for.

(6') He could only carry on "mechanically."

(7') He disparaged his life and even his own depression as "in no way honorable."

He may have met two additional criteria.

(8') He could later "remember next to nothing" about the speeches he delivered during the depression.

(9') Suicidal thoughts are suggested when he reports frequent self-questioning about whether to continue living, concluding that "I did not think I could possibly bear it beyond a year."[7]

Depression takes mild, moderate, and severe forms, and apparently Mill's depression was severe. Even if there are doubts that he suffered a major depressive disorder, the *DSM* identifies further categories that might apply. Thus, the *DSM* distinguishes depression as a single episode and as a chronic or recurrent problem. (Mill indicates the depression recurred, with some relapses that "lasted many months," although never again so severely.) Again, the *DSM* lists some half-dozen forms of bipolar disorder (formerly called "manic-depression") in which depression alternates with states of abnormally elevated, expansive, and excited states.[8] And dysthymic disorder has symptoms that are less severe but more chronic— specifically, two or more of the following symptoms during most hours or most days over a two-year period: poor or excessive appetite, either insomnia or sleeping too much, fatigue, low self-esteem, poor concentration, feelings of hopelessness.

Mill knew his depression was both a medical and a moral concern, even though he highlighted the latter when he wrote his autobiography. In general, much depression has both health and moral dimensions. Depression is a moral matter when it is a potentially meaningful encounter with troubled relationships, activities, values and self-respect. It is a therapeutic matter when it is a clinical syndrome of mood disorder, cognitive dysfunction, low self-esteem, and chemical imbalance. Yet, therapists and ethicists alike have had difficulty in acknowledging as much. Let us begin with the therapists.

Therapists' Morality-Therapy Dichotomy

Psychoanalytic treatments for depression are now overshadowed by cognitive-behavior and chemical-neurological treatments, discussed later. Nevertheless, psychoanalytic explanations remain relevant to understanding the causes and meaning of depression. Freud interpreted depression (melancholia) as aggression turned against oneself, motivated by unconscious conflicts and ambivalence. This self-devaluation is rooted in "reproaches against a loved object which have been shifted on to the patient's own ego."[9] Later, Freud reconceptualized this process as the unconscious part of the superego channeling aggression toward the ego as punishment for the id's socially unacceptable aggressive impulses.[10] Hostility is repressed because we find it intolerable to hate people whom we also love.

Applying this psychoanalytic framework, A. W. Levi insists Mill's crisis had nothing to do with dissatisfaction over Bentham's utilitarian theory: "The real cause was . . . repressed death wishes against his father, the vague and unarticulated guilt feeling which he had in consequence, and the latent, though still present dread that never now should he be free of his father's domination."[11] Mill revered his father as the parent who oversaw every detail of his upbringing and education. Yet his father was a severe disciplinarian who made excessive demands accompanied by implicit threats of punishment for any failure. As a result, the young Mill experienced intense ambivalence toward his father, mingling conscious love and respect with unconscious fear and resentment. The conflict paralyzed his emotions and led to depression. It is no coincidence, then, that the literary passage precipitating Mill's recovery was a scene in a memoir describing the impact of a father's death on his son. The passage resonated with Mill's filial ambivalence, evoking (conscious) sadness and (unconscious) pleasure in the thought of his father's death. This psychoanalytic account can be extended further. As discussed in chapter 3, Freud located the cause of depression and anxiety in the unrealistic moral standards of the Victorian era in which Mill lived. Just as he criticized Judeo-Christian ideals of loving everyone as oneself, he would object to Mill's ideal of impartially promoting the good of all as psychologically unrealistic.

Mill's moral account and Levi's therapeutic explanation differ considerably, but must they be opposed? There is a third possibility: acknowledge that depression has both moral and health dimensions. Mill's depression had multiple causes, including those he cites and the ones Levi identified. Indeed, Mill's emotional rebellion against his father's dominance and his intellectual rebellion against his father's philosophy would naturally accompany each other.

Turn now to pharmacological treatments of depression. How would Mill fare if he sought help from today's drug-oriented psychiatry? Contemporary therapies are enormously varied, and their outcomes depend on the interpersonal dynamics between particular patients and therapists.[12] Still, we can imagine John Mill encountering something like what John Moorehead encountered. Moorehead was in his forties and working as the provost at a Jesuit college when he began to experience severe mood irregularities: sadness, anxiety, irritability, listlessness, and general loss of capacity for enjoyment. Normally enjoying abundant energy, he found himself unable to perform the simplest tasks without enormous effort. He also suffered loss of appetite, disruption of sleep patterns, inability to concentrate, and severe self-blame. Alarmed by persistent thoughts of suicide, and encouraged by his sister to seek help, he went to the psychiatrist Peter C. Whybrow.

In early therapy sessions, Moorehead explained his depression in terms of his religious tradition. His problem arose from laziness, spiritual pride, and moral weakness, the affliction the Catholic Church once called "acedia" and regarded as an occasion for spiritual self-scrutiny.[13] Whybrow dismisses this self-diagnosis as a medieval excrescence that misidentifies pathology as wrongdoing: "John Moorehead, struggling to explain his changing mental state within the terms of his own experience, had missed the mark; he was suffering not from sloth but the medical illness of severe depression." [14] To understand his illness we need to consider synapses, not sin: Moorehead's condition was a "disturbance in the dynamic regulation of the neurotransmitter messenger systems that sustains communication among the neuronal centers of the limbic alliance."[15] The cure is pharmacology rather than spiritual insight.

Once again, we are offered one-sided interpretations that neglect the possibility that much depression is about both values and biology. Moorehead neglects earthy moral matters about his personal relationships, community tensions, and stress. For his part, Whybrow avoids crass biological reductionism, acknowledging multiple biopsychosocial factors.[16] Nevertheless, he introduces a sharp contrast between Moorehead's moral-religious explanation, which he rejects wholesale, and a biological explanation in terms of serotonin-disrupting stress. In fact, Whybrow's clinical account of the sources of stress is compatible with a moral understanding of Moorehead's depression as linked to disrupted relationships of trust, collegiality, and mutual support. During the prior year he was involved in a major upheaval at his college. The conflict centered on whether Jesuit colleges like his should recruit distinguished non-Jesuit professors in order to raise the quality of the colleges, as a solution to declining enrollments. Moorehead led the opposition that lobbied for the new recruitment policy. In doing so, he lost the friendship of the college's chief administrative officer who, as a father figure, had mentored him during his career (echoing Mill's relationship to his father). He accepted the trustees' offer to become the provost but quickly became isolated from his colleagues, including those who backed him during the conflict. Alienated, self-doubting, and cut off from usual support systems, he was in a crisis that had moral, spiritual, and biological dimensions. Evidently, medication helped him improve to the point where he could make this discovery for himself. In that way, curing Moorehead's depression required adjustments in moral relationships and serotonin levels alike.

Does introducing moral language invite blame, which would be therapeutically self-defeating? Most pathologically depressed persons are already unreasonably hard on themselves; indeed, their excessive self-denigration is one of their primary symptoms. The denigration might begin with dismay over a particular event, but it quickly expands to the entire self: I am worthless; my life means nothing; there is no hope. Negative moral judgments merely intensify irrational self-depreciation. Whatever moral responsibility Moorehead shared for his strained personal relationships, his self-blame was inflated. In general, therapy is a special context of support aimed at healing, and appropriate professional distance requires suspending negative moral judgments.

Nevertheless, therapists seeking to empower clients might at times use moral terms—for example the need to accept responsibility, to care about oneself, to muster courage, and to forgive oneself. In doing so, they understand responsibility as accepting forward-looking obligations to deal appropriately with difficulties, not backward-looking blame for shortcomings. Thus, Whybrow underscores the need for patients to accept personal responsibility for their recovery, although he does not say this is a specifically moral responsibility. And he admits that restoring understanding and trust with colleagues was the culmination of Moorehead's therapy, even though he casts these matters in terms of health rather than morality.[17]

Ethicists' Morality-Therapy Dichotomy

For their part, ethicists worry that reducing depression to neurochemical imbalances eclipses the relevance of moral values in understanding it. Depression is singularly important in stimulating insights because it centers on self-worth, self-respect, identity, hope, and meaning. Thus, after acknowledging that depression can take pathological forms, Robert C. Solomon suggests that depression is a "window to the soul"; it can be "our most courageous attempt to open ourselves up to the most gnawing doubts about ourselves and our lives"—courageous because it requires responding to the threat of radical self-diminishment.[18] Unlike sadness or grief, serious depression is an emotional signal that we have doubts about the basic structures in our lives, including our values. Solomon captures an enormously important truth, although he overstates it and risks romanticizing melancholia, as did the nineteenth-century Romantics.[19]

Ethicists have opposed attempts to regard Mill's depression as pathological, fearing that doing so eclipses its moral significance in transforming his ethical theory and his personal character. Thus, George Graham suggests Mill's depression was not pathological at all. By "drawing valuable insights from depression and using such insights to build a better life," Mill illustrates how depression can be justified, rational, and prudent, as well as morally creative.[20] Graham worries that the medical model of depression eclipses the valuable functions of justified depressions, as in shaping Mill's insights. Influenced by a morality-therapy dichotomy, Graham contrasts "depression as deep vision or insight and depression as sickness or illness," as if we must choose between mutually exclusive options.[21] To the contrary, Mill's crisis illustrates how both can be involved in the same case.

Graham implies there was no pathology involved because pathology implies harm to oneself, whereas Mill reacted to the depression in a positive way that led to a valuable or "adaptive" outcome. But that is like arguing that a heart attack is not a matter of pathology if it motivates a person to adopt a healthier life style. Much sickness has positive results, and the creative potential of even severe disease to provoke insights is a familiar theme in fiction, biography, and clinical studies.[22] In any case, we should distinguish between (a) thoroughgoing harm to oneself and (b) elements of harm mixed with wider benefits. Mill benefited overall from a pathological depression, but he also suffered a harm.

In addition, Graham distinguishes between depressions that are biochemical eruptions and those that are "intentional," in the phenomenological sense of having an object—that is, of being about something. Intentional depressions can be justified or unjustified, according to whether the beliefs, emotions, and desires they embody are appropriate. In contrast, chemically produced non-intentional depressions, like a viral infection, cannot sensibly be said to be appropriate or inappropriate. Graham says his distinction parallels psychiatrists' distinction between depressions that respond to the environment (reactive, exogenous) and those caused by physiology alone (biochemical, endogenous).[23] I believe, however, that he conflates *objects* of moods with their *causes*. Nearly all depressions have objects; they are "intentional" in that they are about something, if only about ourselves and our lives as a whole—even when they are caused neurochemically. Likewise, psychiatrists conflate causes with objects, but the primary point of the exogenous-endogenous distinction is to distinguish two types of causes: biological versus environmental.[24]

I would recast Graham's distinction. Some depressions are feature-specific in that they are focused on specific aspects of our lives (relationships, activities, events, etc.); other depressions are non-feature-specific in that they have no such focus. Both kinds can be intentional in targeting our lives as a whole, but feature-specific depressions have additional intentionality directed to particular aspects of our lives. Using this distinction, we can agree that the beliefs, emotions, and desires embedded in either type of depression might be justified or unjustified. They are justified when beliefs (e.g., that some bad event has occurred) are true or well-supported, when emotions (e.g., misery, hopelessness) are appropriate to the situation, when desires (e.g., to withdraw from social interactions) express good judgment, and when the patterns of reasoning involved are warranted. Both feature-specific and non-feature-specific depressions might be valuable or harmful, healthy or sick, a window to the soul or the soul's prison, or some combination of all these things.[25]

Solomon and Graham worry that therapeutic approaches to depression undermine explorations of values, as if prescribing Prozac to Mill would have impeded the history of ethics. But a humane morality encourages therapy for sickness, where therapy is itself rooted in moral values of caring and respect. Moreover, therapeutic responses to depression are far more varied than simply drugs, and usually drugs are combined with psychotherapy. In principle, insight-oriented therapies, including psychoanalysis, existential therapy, and cognitive therapy are compatible with Graham and Solomon's insight-oriented concerns. I agree, however, that there is need for caution. Much therapy narrowly targets symptoms, especially when it is funded by insurance programs willing to pay only for quick fixes, often shunting aside insight-oriented value inquiries.

Additional problems arise when psychologists writing for a popular audience use the word "depression" to suggest pathology. For example, Aaron Beck, a pioneer of cognitive therapies, is well aware there are many normal and healthy moods of feeling blue, unhappy, empty, or lonely.[26] But in his books he uses the word "depression" to mean unhealthy states characterized by illogical thinking patterns such as overgeneralization ("I never succeed at anything"), magnification ("I will never find another job"), and personalization ("It's all my fault"). Intended or not, the message conveyed to the public is that all depression is pathological.

Identity: Chemicals and Character

Peter Kramer coined the expression "cosmetic psychopharmacology" to refer to medicines used as mood elevators rather than cures for pathological conditions. Despite his exaggerated celebration of Prozac in *Listening to Prozac*, Kramer raises important issues about the continuum between unhealthy and normal forms of depression, and he grapples with how depression interferes with identity and autonomy.[27] Had he discussed Mill, he would no doubt highlight the impairment of agency during the worst six months of the depression. Had he discussed Moorhead, he would attend to how the depression distorted self-understanding. But let us consider Tess, the first patient Kramer treated with Prozac.

Tess was referred to Kramer by a psychologist who had helped her confront many painful aspects of her life, including sexual abuse in childhood, a father who died when she was twelve, a mother who suffered from unremitting depression, becoming the surrogate parent for nine siblings, suffering through an unhappy marriage, and surviving several abusive relationships. The therapy did not, however, alleviate her deepening unhappiness, fatigue, low self-esteem, and suicide wishes. Kramer first prescribed imipramine, a long-proven anti-depressant, but it brought only mild relief. Next he tried Prozac, recently approved by the Food and Drug Administration. Within two weeks the drug transformed Tess, healing her depression and dramatically altering her personality, making her "better than well." She became more relaxed, energetic, and self-confident in ways that improved her work and her relationships with men. Eventually Kramer weaned her from Prozac, but after eight months she requested to take it again because of lowered mood and lessened energy. Kramer obliged, this time prescribing Prozac not for depression but instead because Tess insisted she was not "herself" without the drug.

The case raises several fundamental issues about meaningful life: impaired autonomy, self-identity, the health-illness continuum, and self-knowledge.

Impaired Autonomy

Pathological depression damages autonomy, in varying degrees. It does so by reducing energy, enthusiasm, concentration, hope, optimism, self-esteem, and self-respect. It is naive, sometimes even dangerous, to call for a severely depressed person to just "snap out of it!" In addition, depression can disrupt normal assessment of risks, either by misjudging risks or by lowering capacities to care about particular risks in the manner of healthy persons.[28] "Pharmacological Calvinists," like Graham and Solomon, object to the widespread use of antidepressants, warning that pill-popping reduces openness and tolerance to difficult emotions and unpleasant realities. Kramer acknowledges this danger, but emotional self-crippling was not what he observed in his patients.[29] Antidepressants empowered them to live with greater courage, optimism, and openness to experience.

Self-Identity

Autonomy has a role in personal decisions about the identity we affirm. Kramer observes that drugs can substantially alter a personality, thereby raising the question, "Whose autonomy are we out to preserve?"[30] Given our traditions of valuing individuality, presumably individuals have the right to make their decisions about whether to use legally prescribed drugs. After all, much is at stake for them, not only in shaping their commitments but also in responding to social pressures that favor particular identities or "selves."

The "selves" at issue are not givens. They are normative constructions of identities as esteemed or devalued, regarding both specific and overall features. The construction is never achieved once and for all. It is an ongoing struggle within the framework of one's past, social present, and projected future. Questions about authenticity arise when individuals passively accept society's mandates, yet none of us lives in complete independence from those mandates. Our society favors outgoing, friendly, nondepressed personalities, and Prozac highlights this cultural preference.[31] We are not inauthentic because we aspire to have socially affirmed identities or because we respond to social pressures. What matters is how we respond: autonomously or unthinkingly?

Autonomy is tied to authenticity. An essentialist view of authenticity says there is one true self for each of us, typically a higher self defined in terms of a favored value perspective (such as a particular religious viewpoint). A more plausible process view acknowledges that we can shape ourselves in many different directions. We are authentic insofar as we choose honestly and autonomously. To be sure, some persons have sufficiently focused talents and opportunities that their authenticity aims unilaterally at many junctures in their lives. Thus, it may seem obvious that Moorehead's authentic identity consisted in restoring him to his place in the Jesuit community from which his depression had isolated him. Yet he had additional options, and his postdepression choice to return to the community was very much an autonomous decision that therapy helped him to make.

Health-Illness Continuum

Health and illness form a continuum. Each of us participates in distinguishing what is healthy or sick with regard to ourselves, especially in the large middle ground of suboptimal health that falls short of full-blown mental disorder. Insofar as the concept of mental health is normative, individuals have a right to participate in determining when depression is pathological.

The social bias against mildly dysthymic individuals can pressure them into using medication.[32] David A. Karp highlights this pressure in *Speaking of Sadness*. He contends that much of what psychiatrists "call mental illness is nothing more than a political designation sold as science." In particular, rather than a psychiatric disorder, depression is a manifestation of the breakdown of community. As such, it can be "a normal response to pathological social structures," and we should change those disintegrating community structures rather than "cure" normal emotional responses to them. Karp argues convincingly that "depression arises out of an enormously complicated, constantly shifting, elusive concatenation of social circumstance, individual temperament, and biochemistry."[33] Some confirmation for his views can be found in a cross-cultural study that locates low incidence of depression in Taiwan and high incidence in Beirut and Paris.[34] Yet, in decrying the breakdown of community that contributes to depression, Karp leaves us with little hope for immediate cure, apart from a concluding sympathetic nod toward spirituality. Depression can be "normal," in the sense of an understandable and expected response to harmful social structures, and yet have pathological aspects that disrupt our ability to carry on with our lives. And we cannot wait until community problems are solved before dealing with suffering.

Self-Knowledge

Finally, Kramer challenges any general assumption that depression, healthy or unhealthy, offers privileged access to insights into personal identity and the human condition. Studies suggest that depressed persons tend to be more accurate in some assessments of their abilities and of the problems they confront.[35] But perhaps depressed individuals are blocked from deeper truths about the joys to be found in commitments and relationships undermined by the depression.[36] Why should we assume the depressed pessimistic self is more genuine than the chemically brightened self?

Kramer does not settle these issues. He concludes by conveying uncertainty, ambiguity, and ambivalence that clash with his overall optimism about Prozac. Depression can be a creative source of insight and self-transformation, or it can constitute a problem that undermines insight and impedes autonomy. My discussion adds to these complexities by accenting how depression can be simultaneously pathological and insight-provoking, how therapeutic and moral values are interwoven, and how the continuity between health and sickness enmeshes all of us in a therapeutic morality.

To conclude, it is not surprising that depression has become our "presiding discontent," given our preoccupations with identity and self-worth amid rapid social change, eroding community, and increasingly many ways in which our lives are subject to forces over which we have little control. For good reason, depression is receiving attention within many disciplines. A century ago, William James suggested that religious experiences, including "religious melancholy," have both neurological and value dimensions.[37] In a similar spirit I have urged that therapeutic perspectives complement and merge with moral perspectives, rather than replacing or diluting morality.

13

SELF-DECEPTION AND HOPE

Ever since Socrates pronounced the unexamined life not worth living, ethicists have linked meaningful life and honesty with oneself.[1] Similarly, therapists regard honesty with oneself as integral to healing, and they regard contact with reality as a criterion for positive mental health. Some recent psychologists, however, suggest that self-deception and unrealistic optimism might be good for us. I agree with them that self-deception sometimes contributes to hope and love, and thereby to meaningful life and healthy functioning. It does so in a limited way, however, and not to the extent that justifies abandoning contact with reality as a criterion for mental health. Even when self-deception advances psychological health, there is no fundamental clash between therapy and morality, for all the values involved—hope, love, and honesty—are both moral and therapeutic values that are sometimes in tension. By reaffirming truthfulness within a moral-therapeutic perspective, morality and mental health once again emerge as interwoven.

Vital Lies

"The life-lie, don't you see—that's the animating principle of life," proclaims Dr. Relling in Ibsen's *The Wild Duck*.[2] Life lies, or vital lies, are self-deceiving beliefs based on unfounded optimism, unwarranted hopes, and rationalizations about our failures. We rely on them in order to cope and to maintain happiness and health: "Deprive the average man of his vital lie, and you've robbed him of happiness as well."[3] Dr. Relling fosters inflated self-images in his patients. In particular, he encourages Hjalmar Ekdal to believe he is on the verge of a revolutionary discovery in photographic technology, when actually he is tinkering with a bunch of useless gadgets. Ekdal is a cooperative patient who is already prone to self-deception. He believes he is the sole provider for his family, yet his wife balances their household budget by relying on large subsidies from the former business partner of Ekdal's father. Ekdal also assumes he is the father of Hedvig, his greatest joy, when in fact she is the offspring of the former business partner.

The son of the former business partner, Gregers Werle, calls for complete honesty and encourages Ekdal to abandon his illusions about work and family. Yet Werle's moralizing is self-righteous and neurotic, motivated by unconscious hatred of his father and shame at his extramarital affair and illegitimate child. When Ekdal learns that Hedvig is not his biological daughter, he immediately becomes estranged from her. Feeling disowned by the father she adores, the emotionally fragile Hedwig sinks into depression and kills herself. At least in this instance, honesty is apparently self-destructive, undermines love, and has dubious motives.

Most of us do not need a Dr. Relling to prescribe our vital lies. As self-deceivers, we have ample resources within. Like Ekdal, we need reinforcement from family and friends, but usually they are willing to indulge illusions that keep us buoyant with optimism—assuming we reciprocate. Beyond these social dimensions of self-deception, what mental activities and states are involved in deceiving ourselves? The question has generated a substantial literature in philosophy and psychology.[4] The central issue is whether the paradigm, garden-variety, cases of self-deception involve *purposeful evasion* of truth. Or do they instead consist entirely of *motivated irrationality*—biased beliefs that are false and contrary to the evidence? I believe both kinds of self-deception exist and are commonplace.

To begin with motivated irrationality, we are all familiar with how biases, such as self-esteem and happiness, filter what we see and think. Thinking along these lines, Stanley Paluch concludes that "self-deception" is a metaphor for false and unsupported beliefs formed by biased assessments of evidence.[5] More recently, Alfred Mele says that self-deception consists in forming false beliefs that go against the evidence, and doing so under the influence of a biasing desire or emotion.[6] There is no intention to evade reality or to embrace a falsehood. Suppose, for example, my physician informs me that I have a fatal and untreatable cancer, giving me six months to live. My doctor is well-qualified, and a second opinion confirms her diagnosis; on balance, I have every reason to believe my chances are slim. Yet, hoping against hope, I believe I will beat the odds. My belief is influenced by a desire to live and a fear of dying, but there are various possibilities. One possibility is honest hope, whereby I struggle to believe I will survive even though I am painfully aware of the evidence to the contrary. The other possibility is motivated irrationality, in which I downplay the contrary evidence ("What do doctors know, anyhow?") and highlight positive evidence. Self-deception occurs when I lose my grasp of what the evidence indicates.

I believe there is another possibility, however: purposeful evasion. Paluch and Mele reject this possibility because they believe it involves modeling self-deception on lying to other people, which generates two paradoxes. First, when I lie to another person, I know (or believe) something unpleasant and get the other person to believe the opposite. By analogy, when I lie to myself it seems I know (or believe) one thing and simultaneously get myself to believe the opposite. But that seems impossible, for my knowledge would prevent me from acquiring the false belief. Freud offers one solution to this paradox: the unpleasant belief is kept unconscious, and the opposing belief is held consciously. A different solution is that the unpleasant knowledge is held at a less-explicit level of consciousness and ignored.[7] I believe self-deception can involve either unconscious beliefs or disregarded beliefs. Most purposeful evasion, however, does not involve self-contradictory beliefs at all, but instead one belief formed by evading unwanted evidence or its implications.

Turning to the second paradox, when I lie to another person I intend to mislead them. By analogy, when I lie to myself it seems I must be aware of an unpleasant truth and use that awareness to form an intention to flee the truth. But that is a psychological impossibility, except perhaps in cases of dissociative identity disorder (multiple personality). Here the solution is to specify that my intention is to evade a reality and its evidence, rather than (a muddled) intention to believe what I know is false. In addition, the intention is formed and acted on spontaneously rather than self-reflectively. As a self-deceiver, typically I have some suspicion of an unpleasant reality and use the suspicion to ignore the reality, discounting evidence contrary to what I want to believe.[8] Selective attention, willful ignorance, and distorted use of evidence suffice to explain purposeful self-deception, without postulating a conscious intention to believe what I know is false. As Herbert Fingarette writes: "The crux of the matter . . . is that we can take account of something without necessarily focusing our attention on it. That is, we can recognize it, and respond to it, without directing our attention to what we are doing, and our response can be intelligently adaptive rather than merely a reflex or habit automatism."[9] For example, we write on a computer without thinking about the specific motions of our fingers across a keyboard, and we drive a car while taking account of many details in the environment without attending to them, much less attending to our patterns of attention. Similarly, in self-deception we take account of unpleasant truths and evidence without attending to them. We do so as part of "a purposeful and skillfully pursued policy" in which typically we "secretly do know" or suspect the unpleasant truths and evidence.[10]

To sum up, self-deception includes both purposeful evasion and motivated irrationality. Both kinds might be involved in the same case, and often are. And both kinds are relevant to understanding the interplay of honesty and hope, as well as morality and mental health.

Healthy Self-Deception: Honesty versus Health?

Some recent psychological studies echo Ibsen's insight that self-deception contributes to vitality and happiness.[11] For example, an anthology of essays adopts the theme that "self-deception is a normal and generally positive force in human behavior."[12] Again, Jonathon Brown cites an extensive body of psychological studies, including his own, showing that healthy, well-adjusted individuals "possess unrealistically positive views of themselves."[13] And in *Positive Illusions: Creative Self-Deception and the Healthy Mind*, Shelley E. Taylor argues that "unrealistic optimism" promotes mental and physical health: "Normal human thought and perception is marked not by accuracy but by positive self-enhancing illusions about the self, the world, and the future."[14] I focus on Taylor's book because, by presenting the experimental literature to a wide audience, it enters into the therapeutic trend. Because she avoids moral language, she does not explicitly affirm mental health over honesty, but clearly she implies as much.

Taylor groups healthy "positive illusions" under four headings: egocentricity, illusions of control, illusions of progress, and self-fulfilling beliefs.

> *Egocentricity.* We are heroes in our own dramas, interpreting the world through a subjective lens. In doing so, we cast our actions, talents, achievements, and prospects in a favorable light in order to maintain self-esteem, hope, and happiness. We selectively ignore unpleasant evidence that goes against what we want to believe about ourselves. Failures and setbacks are conveniently forgotten, and painful events are affirmed as positive learning experiences.
>
> *Illusions of Control.* Typically we exaggerate the control we have in our lives, thereby manifesting unrealistic optimism about the role of chance and external influences. Most gamblers, for example, think they can beat the odds and that they have skills in areas where pure luck dictates the outcome. They roll the dice gently when they want low numbers and more vigorously when want high numbers. Again, most drivers—about 90 percent in one study—believe they are above average in skill, including drivers who have caused major accidents. And we blame victims of all kinds by holding false stereotypes about them, thereby creating the illusion that we are protected against dangers because we are more careful than them.
>
> *Illusions of Progress.* Most of us are optimistic about progress in our lives (as distinct from progress in the world). For example, in a study of college students enrolled in a special program that promised increased study skills and better grades, students reported dramatic improvements. Even when they failed a test they would reinterpret the failure as progress in learning how to do better next time. In fact, no differences in results were found between students enrolled and not enrolled in the program.
>
> *Self-Fulfilling Beliefs.* Belief in the prospects of achieving a specific goal tends to bring about favorable results by strengthening motivation and bolstering hope. A familiar example is the placebo effect, which is any positive therapeutic impact due to patients' beliefs about medical procedures. This includes sugar pills given to patients who believe they are taking an active drug, and it includes beliefs in the effectiveness of health professionals and their institutions. The extent of placebo effects is controversial, but many researchers believe it affects about a third of us. Positive beliefs and attitudes also encourage others to support our efforts.

Citing a wealth of studies in the preceding areas, Taylor concludes that self-deceptive positive illusions are healthy: "Increasingly, we must view the psychologically healthy person not as someone who sees things as they are but as someone who sees things as he or she would like them to be." The mentally healthy person has a positive self-image and abilities to be happy, to care about others, to work productively, and to continue to grow.[15]

Taylor vastly overstates her case. She does so because she equivocates between two senses of "positive illusions": unproven beliefs and irrational beliefs.[16] *Unproven beliefs* are beliefs not shown to be true by the evidence, and which might be true or false. Using this sense, Taylor defends optimism: unproven positive beliefs in the form of hope, faith, and optimism promote mental health. This is an important insight, but hardly revolutionary. Common sense tells us that positive attitudes promote our ability to maintain self-esteem and to cope with work, personal relationships, and ambitious projects. *Irrational beliefs*, in contrast, are false beliefs contrary to the available evidence. In using this sense, Taylor successfully defends only some, not most, self-deception as healthy because it promotes hope, coping, and self-esteem. For example, she claims that irrational, self-deceiving beliefs are "normal" because most of us believe we are above average at everyday tasks such as driving.[17] In fact, these studies merely show that unproven beliefs are ubiquitous. Drivers who hold unwarranted beliefs are not necessarily evading evidence about their rankings as drivers, for they are not provided with such evidence. The drivers *value* (affirm) their driving skills, endeavors, and future prospects, without having hard data about how to accurately *evaluate* (rank) them.

Sometimes Taylor says that positive illusions are false beliefs, but other times she suggests they can simply be unproven beliefs that cast reality in a positive light.[18] Now, there is no basis for counting all unproven beliefs illusions—"unproven" does not mean "proven false." Why, then, did Taylor count unproven beliefs, whether true or false, as illusions? I suspect she borrowed the deviant usage from Freud's *Future of an Illusion*. Freud writes: "What is characteristic of illusions is that they are derived from human wishes. . . . Illu-Illusions need not necessarily be false—that is to say, unrealizable or in contradiction to reality."[19] Freud's odd notion that illusions can be true contributed to the polemical tone of his book in denigrating religion. In turn, by conflating unproven and false beliefs, Taylor greatly exaggerates the health benefits of self-deception.

Truthfulness and Mental Health

The tendency to perceive accurately and to maintain justified beliefs is a traditional criterion for mental health, as we saw in chapter 2. The criterion is embedded in Freud's "reality principle," the norm of living in tune with reality. It is equally central to cognitive psychologists' emphasis on realistic cognition. And Marie Jahoda assumed that "as a rule, the perception of reality is called mentally healthy when what the individual sees corresponds to what is actually there."[20] In explaining the caveat "as a rule," however, Jahoda emphasized the plurality of reasonable interpretations of the world. Equally important, she said mental health requires only "relative freedom" from distortion by our desires, together with a disposition to test reality to check whether it conforms to our wishes. Likewise, Taylor's arguments should lead us to qualify, not abandon, truthfulness as a criterion for mental health.

Although Taylor's main interest is in positive mental health, she devotes a chapter to psychopathology, focusing on pathological depression and mania. Mild depression and low self-esteem involve fewer positive illusions and more accurate beliefs than healthy states, an idea called "depressive realism." Taylor suggests that therapy should encourage positive illusions.[21] Once again, however, her suggestion is marred by ambiguity. Is she saying that the absence of self-deceptive beliefs contributes to depression, so that therapists should encourage self-deception in their clients? Or is she saying that the absence of unproven positive beliefs contributes to depression, so that therapists should encourage hope? The first claim is a Dr. Relling–like prescription for untruthfulness; the second claim is a morally responsible endorsement of honest hope.

Depression involves loss of caring about ourselves and our world. Depression is primarily a diminished valuing of ourselves, other people, relationships, activities, and life itself, regardless of whether it involves unwarranted evaluation. Accordingly, when therapists cure depression they are not encouraging untruthfulness. They are helping patients value themselves and their world by restoring honest hope, faith, and caring.

Taylor discusses mania more briefly, again focusing on mild cases. Mania is rarer than depression, and usually it is connected with bipolar disorder (manic depression). Mania interests Taylor as the exaggeration of normal positive illusions. Frequently, it contributes to the work of the creative artist, the daring leader, and the religious innovator. In discussing these ideas, she again fails to distinguish unwarranted evaluations from positive valuing. Either might be involved, of course, but blurring them exaggerates the contribution of self-deception to creativity. And by stipulating that mania is an excessive illusion that differs from "milder" positive illusions, she neglects how self-deception sometimes contributes to psychopathology.

Moving to more serious disorders, a few writers believe self-deception enters into psychosis, but for the most part self-deception is a different phenomenon than involuntary hallucinations, psychotic delusions, and other complete breaks with reality. Even so, there are continuities, not absolute differences, between psychosis and ordinary self-deception. Families immersed in untruthfulness breed pathology.[22] Self-deception also plays a role in personality disorders, such as narcissistic and histrionic disorders defined by grandiose views of one's talents, worth, and entitlement.

Addictions provide a more straightforward example of how self-deception contributes to pathology. Indeed, Alcoholics Anonymous portrays alcoholism as the disease of denial. And addiction specialist Abraham J. Twerski exposes the rationalizations used to maintain optimism about how much one drinks ("I am a social drinker"), about the degree of one's self-control over the addiction ("I can stop at any time"), and about the desirability of using drugs ("They help me cope and cause minor problems at most").[23] Addicts might also deceive themselves about their diminished self-respect and gradually lose a sense of who they are.[24]

Self-deception also enters into the neuroses, understood as the result of psychological defense against anxiety, although defense can also serve healthy ends.[25] Thus, defense might undergird an artist's fanatical devotion to her work, but only in the workaholic might pathology be involved. Psychological defense is often interpreted as self-deception, even though Freud rarely used the term "self-deception."[26] Yet, psychological defense can be understood in two ways, paralleling the two varieties of self-deception. Sometimes Freud described repression, denial, projection, and other defense mechanisms as motivated biases that operate unconsciously and without any activity by the person. Other times he described psychological defense as purposeful and intentional activities. Most likely, he thought defense might involve either or both. Moreover, defense ranges from activities that are partly conscious and preconscious (available to consciousness) to processes below the level of mental contents available to consciousness without special help from a therapist.[27] Either way, removing repression can lead to both more realistic cognition and better coping.[28]

Finally, pathological self-deception is not an automatic excuse for wrong-doing. When we have, or should have, good reason to believe that unconscious motives are distorting moral understanding, we are obligated to take special precautions to ensure that we are meeting our responsibilities.[29] Unconscious motivations are not automatically excuses, and they often lead to culpable negligence. The same is true of self-deception involving conscious activities. Here again, the therapeutic trend does not replace morality but instead integrates it with therapeutic understanding.

Moral Values in Tension

If self-deception were always dishonest, then Taylor's psychological studies would support a morality-therapy dichotomy: honesty condemns self-deception; health celebrates self-deception. Some philosophers do in fact condemn all self-deception as dishonest. Kant wrote: "By a lie a man makes himself contemptible—by an outer lie, in the eyes of others; by an inner lie [i.e., self-deception], in his own eyes, which is still worse—and violates the dignity of humanity in his own person."[30] Jean-Paul Sartre condemned all self-deceivers as cowards and scum.[31] And Daniel A. Putman says that "self-deception always works to destroy a fundamental virtue, integrity. Self-deception isolates part of the self and prevents that part from being integrated into consciousness."[32]

These absolute condemnations are too extreme, however, for not all self-deception is immoral. Despite its enormous importance, honesty is one virtue and one obligation among others, and it is not paramount in all situations.

Thus, an instance of self-deception might be untruthful and yet justified by other moral values that promote meaningful lives—for example, hope and faith, self-esteem and self-respect, and love and friendship. Hence, the therapeutic contributions of some self-deception do not threaten morality in its entirety. To return to an earlier example, suppose I am a self-deceiving cancer patient who distorts the evidence about my condition. Untruthful, yes, but the self-deception might be embedded in a pattern of other virtues. Faced with great danger, including the danger of collapsing from fear, I might be courageous in keeping hope alive.[33] Doing so manifests self-respect in trying not to fall apart, in struggling to carry on with dignity, integrity, and self-respect. It also helps my family cope with a difficult situation. Honesty and hope are sometimes in tension, but they are connected within a complex web of virtues.[34]

Not surprising, the occasional tension between honesty and hope parallels tensions between realistic cognition and coping as criteria for mental health. On the one hand, truthfulness and healthy cognition largely overlap; indeed, truthfulness is the primary moral ideal guiding realistic cognition. By definition, truthful persons care about truth: they try to perceive accurately, reason cogently, respond rationally to evidence, and expand understanding in light of new information. On the other hand, truthful persons need hope and mental health. Hope overlaps with healthy coping, social adaptation, and self-esteem. Because moral values are embedded in mental health, we might expect wide congruence between healthy and morally permissible self-deception.

Finally, an instance of self-deception might be healthy in one respect, by contributing vitality or happiness, but unhealthy in other respects, by distorting reality. Perhaps that is true of Hjalmar Ekdal. This complexity parallels the moral complexity of self-deception. Hope, in many (though not all) forms, is just as much a moral value as honesty, and the tensions between them are as much moral as therapeutic.

To conclude, I have suggested that moral and therapeutic values are not inherently at loggerheads with regard to honesty, hope, and self-deception. The complexity revealed by therapeutic perspectives parallels and is interwoven with the complexity within morality itself. Self-deception, both motivated irrationality and purposeful evasion, does sometimes advance mental health, but it also advances moral values such as hope and love. Even so, self-deception is less beneficial than suggested by Taylor and others who conflate unproven beliefs and irrational beliefs, and frequently it is linked to unhealthy evasions of reality. And the tensions between honesty and hope reveal tensions internal to morality and mental health alike, not a basis for a morality-therapy dichotomy.

14

PHILOSOPHICAL COUNSELING

Philosophical counseling applies ethical perspectives, critical think-ing, and other philosophical resources to help individuals pursue meaningful lives and cope with personal problems. Still a fledgling movement, it began in 1981 when Gerd B. Achenbach opened a private practice in Germany, although it has precursors in Stoic and Epicurean philosophy. From the outset philosophical counselors embraced a morality-therapy dichotomy in order to distinguish their moral-oriented endeavors from the health-oriented work of psychotherapists.[1] I suggest that philosophical counseling becomes more coher-ent by embracing an integrated, moral-therapeutic perspective centered on the themes of healthy morality, responsibility for health, and moral-laden mental health.

Goals in Helping

Lou Marinoff's *Plato, Not Prozac!* provides a useful focus because it is the first general-audience book inviting Americans to embrace philosophical counseling as an alternative to psychotherapy. In the title, "Plato" symbolizes ethics and "Prozac" symbolizes psychotherapy. Ironically, then, the title introduces a di-chotomy between ethics and therapy that Plato would renounce, as we saw in chapter 1. Marinoff inveighs against both the therapeutic trend and against mainstream psychotherapy (11).[2] He mocks the *DSM* for pathologizing unde-sirable behaviors, emotional disturbances, and character faults (18). And he sympathetically cites Thomas Szasz's view that mental illness is a myth (16, 27–28). The vast majority of people who seek counseling, according to Marinoff, need moral reflection and dialogue, not healing (4, 6). Their problems concern moral values and decisions about staying in a love relationship, coping with a divorce, overcoming unhappiness with a job, exploring a religious crisis, ac-cepting sexuality, and struggling to find meaning in life (3). Yet surely these problems pertain to mental health as well as moral values, and Marinoff would do well to acknowledge as much.

Consider a case study involving depression, which Marinoff borrows from his another philosophical counselor, Ben Mijuskovic. A thirty-seven-year-old man, who had been a monk since he was seventeen, sought Mijuskovic's help because he was experiencing " 'symptoms of major depression,' fatigue, sleeping problems, feelings of hopelessness, helplessness, and suicidal ideation."[3] Mijuskovic judges that the monk's depression was not a pathological depression or otherwise a health issue. Instead, the monk suffered from a value conflict rooted in two decades of religious service that precluded sexual intimacy and family involvement. The man faced a choice between reaffirming his vows as a priest and abandoning his vows in order to begin a new life outside the monastery. As such, according to Marinoff, he faced a crisis of meaning and values, not a health problem. During six months of counseling, Mijuskovic and the monk discussed writings about religious conversions, such as those of St. Augustine and Søren Kierkegaard. A turning point came when Mijuskovic asked the monk whether his depression caused the loss of meaning, or instead the loss of meaning caused the depression (218). The monk immediately affirmed the latter, thereby initiating a resolution of the crisis. Eventually the man left the monastery but retained his religious faith.

Now, I agree that issues of meaning are central in the case, but mental health is also involved. The major depression and loss of meaning are not two entirely different things, one causing the other. Instead, they are intertwined: the loss of meaning is manifested as depression, and the depression is experienced as an absence of meaning. As we saw in chapter 12, much depression concerns both mental health and moral values, and only a morality-therapy dichotomy could make Marinoff think otherwise.

This dichotomy leads Marinoff to set forth an implausible view of when depression is pathological.[4] He distinguishes four types of depression, according to whether the underlying problem is (1) a genetic brain abnormality, (2) an induced brain abnormality due, for example, to drug or alcohol abuse, (3) an unresolved childhood trauma or other problem in the past, or (4) "something acute happening in one's current life," such as a divorce, a problem at work, or broader moral issues (33). The first two types, he claims, are illnesses requiring the help of physicians; the third type can benefit from psychology and sometimes from philosophical counseling; for the fourth and most common type, "philosophy would be the most direct route to healing" (33). Marinoff's last claim on behalf of philosophy is unsubstantiated, and it conflicts with both psychiatry and common sense. Psychiatrists define pathological depression in terms of patterns of behavior, belief, and emotion, not in terms of their causes. The criteria include feeling depressed most of the time, losing interests in usual activities, incapacity for pleasure, insomnia or hypersomnia, and persistent fatigue.[5] It is common for everyday events to trigger pathological depressions, as probably occurred in the case of the monk.

To return to broader issues, I suggest that although his book is structured by a morality-therapy dichotomy, Marinoff is not consistent. He frequently invokes therapeutic language. Without explanation, he calls philosophical counseling a form of "talk therapy," and he speaks of philosophical counselors "healing" depression by exploring moral values (33, 21). He admits that some individuals need both medication and moral exploration (10), and he urges that philosophical counselors deserve reimbursement from health insurance companies for their services (24). Finally, he refers to philosophical counseling as "therapy for the sane" (11). This interesting expression raises a dilemma. If "sane" means completely healthy, then the term "therapy" is inappropriate. If "sane" means "not insane," then most psychotherapy is also therapy for the sane, and hence the phrase fails to identify anything distinctive about philosophical counseling.

For the most part, when Marinoff wants to distinguish philosophical counseling from psychotherapy, he denies that philosophical counselors engage in therapy. But when he celebrates the contributions of philosophical counseling, he implies that healing is involved. His view would be more coherent and illuminating if he renounced the morality-therapy dichotomy and moved toward an integrated, moral-therapeutic perspective. In doing so, he would do well to replace his narrow, negative definition of health (as the absence of maladies) with a positive conception of mental health (as well-being).[6] Positive conceptions, such as those used by Plato, the Stoics, and the World Health Organization, would enable Marinoff to say that the issues faced by all counselors have health dimensions, even when they do not involve pathology. According to positive definitions, mental disorders and optimum health are not exhaustive categories. There are intermediary states of suboptimal health involving habitual anxiety, rage, envy, difficulties in relating to people, lack of self-control, and smoking and drinking immoderately. There are also intermediary states between pathological and normal depression. A positive conception of health allows us to say that even if the monk was not clinically depressed, he was certainly not in peak mental health when he sought help.

I am not suggesting that philosophical counselors need to share any one conception of positive health, any more than psychotherapists do. They should, however, acknowledge the interconnections between moral values and mental health.[7] Of course, not all problems brought to philosophical counselors have therapeutic dimensions. Some clients simply want to study philosophy outside university settings, and for them philosophical counselors function much like private tutors. Other clients seek moral advice—for example, about whether to have an abortion or how to implement justice at the workplace—and philosophical counselors might then function as sounding boards and even offer advice (3, 194–198). More often than not, however, health matters are involved in some way.

As we have seen, morality and mental health are interwoven conceptually. Mental health is partly defined in terms of moral values that affirm some psychological conditions as desirable and others as undesirable. Typical criteria for positive mental health are paired with moral values: for example, self-esteem and self-respect, realistic cognition and truthfulness, coping and responsibility, and integration and integrity. Mental health and moral character are also connected causally, such that well-being and growth are influenced by moral values. And philosophical counselors can help their clients understand how confused and irrational values often foster suboptimal mental health.

Methods and Results

As with goals, the methods and results of philosophical counseling and psychotherapy have both moral and therapeutic dimensions. Whether philosophical or psychological, counseling is a human interaction centered on dialogue. Here we might ask, How is it possible for literally hundreds of different kinds of psychotherapy and counseling, including philosophical counseling, to promote positive health and coping? The answer is that generic factors in counseling often have a greater impact than particular techniques have. Carl Rogers identified three common features of effective counselors: genuineness, caring, and empathetic understanding. Genuineness ("congruence") means that therapists present themselves to clients openly and "without facade." Caring ("unconditional positive regard") means conveying to clients a deep concern for them as individuals. Empathy means accurately understanding what clients are experiencing and then skillfully communicating that understanding to them.[8] Regardless of a therapist's theoretical framework or specific techniques, these three features are catalysts for personal growth. They provide a context of support and trust in which clients can solve problems, achieve greater self-acceptance, and become more open to experience.

Although not all aspects of Rogers's hypothesis have been substantiated, his "common factors approach" to understanding counseling has won support. In particular, Jerome Frank conducted studies suggesting that specific doctrines and techniques often matter little. Therapies succeed because of four factors: (1) an emotionally charged relationship with a caring therapist, (2) a healing setting in which clients believe the therapist has expertise and feels safe in opening up emotionally, (3) a rationale that provides a plausible explanation of the patient's symptoms, and (4) a procedure that both the therapist and the client believe will lead to healing.[9] Most likely, much of the effectiveness of philosophical counseling also resides in these generic factors.[10]

Next, consider two overdrawn contrasts that philosophical counselors use to differentiate their methods from psychotherapy. The first contrast is between causes and reasons. Marinoff, echoing Mijuskovic, says that philosophical counselors focus on immediate reasons for actions, whereas psychotherapists are preoccupied with the distant causes of problems—in particular, the unconscious causes rooted in infancy (17–18, 26). In contrast, philosophical problems concern values about which the person is able to exercise reflection and make choices.[11] Now, it is false that all psychologists focus on distant causes of problems and ignore values. That is a preoccupation for psychoanalysts but not for all psychotherapists. Similarly, the emphasis on complete causal determination applies only to some therapies, such as psychoanalysis and behaviorism. Because those forms of therapy were dominant just prior to the emergence of philosophical counseling, it is understandable that early philosophical counselors were preoccupied with them. Today, however, psychoanalysis has declined in influence, behaviorism has been reworked and connected with cognitive psychology, and health care insurance now funds only short therapy programs that preclude extensive exploration of childhood influences. Moreover, popular cognitive therapy is closely related to philosophical counseling—both emphasize values and patterns of thinking about problems. Again, Albert Ellis's Rational Emotive Therapy is close kin to the rational dialogue employed by philosophical counselors.[12] And most psychotherapists are interested in their clients' current values, as embedded in attitudes and patterns of conduct and reasoning.[13]

In any case, there is no necessary link between identifying causes and finding cures. Problems spring from many factors, and even when a current event triggers a problem the event might connect with one's upbringing, genetic makeup, and brain chemistry. These influences might enter into the explanation of why some of us explode in rage to an insult at the workplace while others quickly laugh it off. Again, regardless of the particular cause of a depression, many forms of counseling might help. Philosophy is not always the best way to tackle a personal crisis involving values.

The second overdrawn contrast is between emotions and values. Marinoff claims that most psychotherapy never progresses beyond "validating the emotions," whereas philosophical counselors explore the underlying values that structure emotions and cause distress (38). This is a false stereotype, fitting some but not all types of psychotherapy. Precisely because emotions are not separable from values, the prototypical therapeutic question to clients, "How do you feel about that?," elicits nuanced expressions of values. Those values can then be explored, as part of solving problems, and unhealthy emotional tendencies modified. Indeed, Alan C. Tjeltveit suggests that in practice a psychotherapist often functions as a quasi-ethicist, in the sense of "a person who reflects on, has convictions about, and/or attempts to influence others about ethical questions and issues."[14] It is easy for psychotherapists to be unaware of this function, for their professional code of ethics requires them to be nonjudgmental and to avoid directly imposing their personal values on clients. Nevertheless, within the bounds of respect for client autonomy, therapists do influence clients' values. Moreover, there are limits to value-neutrality, and sometimes an explicit goal is to change the behavior of a child molester, as part of court-ordered therapy.

Furthermore, some psychotherapists adopt philosophical approaches aimed at reasoning about values explicitly. That is true, for example, of existential psychotherapists, whose approaches emerged from the writings of Martin Heidegger and Jean-Paul Sartre. Existential psychotherapy understands clients' problems as centered in unhealthy responses to anxieties linked to fundamental features of the human condition—death, freedom, isolation, the need for personal responsibility, and the threat of meaninglessness.[15] As such, much existential psychotherapy and philosophical counseling overlap.

Philosophical Counseling,
Philosophy, and Truth

Can we go further and say that the therapeutic aspects of philosophical counseling essentially make it a form of psychotherapy? The answer depends, of course, on what counts as psychotherapy. If it is restricted to psychology-based and psychiatry-based counseling, then philosophical counseling is not psychotherapy. But if psychotherapy is understood more broadly as therapies aimed at promoting positive health and meaningful life, then philosophical counseling can be regarded as a new form of psychotherapy. I prefer to say that philosophical counseling is a form of counseling that has therapeutic dimensions.

In any case, acknowledging the therapeutic aspect of philosophical counseling does not threaten its distinctiveness. Philosophical approaches explicitly and extensively focus on values, explore worldviews, clarify concepts, identify hidden assumptions, and emphasize cogent reasoning. Philosophical resources include readings, insights, and perspectives from the history of philosophy that express the substantive views of philosophical thinkers. And philosophical interests include a search for important truths, justified values, solution of conceptual perplexities, and exploration of worldviews. These resources and interests provide fresh approaches in counseling.

A more interesting question is whether philosophical counseling is a form of philosophy and philosophical ethics. Many academic philosophers know nothing about philosophical counselors, and those who do have tended to be critical of it.[16] Unfortunately, philosophical counselors have sometimes exacerbated tensions with academics by denigrating mainstream academic philosophy. Thus, Marinoff dismisses academic philosophy as "mental gymnastics having nothing to do with life" (8). More constructively, Ran Lahav acknowledges the importance of applied or practical ethics, which has flourished in academia since the 1960s.[17] Applied ethics tackles topics as earthy as sex and love, work and professional standards, philanthropy and politics. It has produced a rich literature that provides valuable resources for philosophical counselors to draw upon, just as counselors provide applied ethicists with new resources.

There are, of course, significant differences between what goes on in university courses on applied ethics and what occurs in the offices of philosophical counselors. Whether theoretical and applied, academic philosophy is a branch of the liberal arts. Most professors attempt to connect readings and assignments with students' practical interests, but usually not in response to the specific life problems each student brings to the classroom. Because of these different goals, academics and counselors adopt different techniques. Academics assign extended readings on opposing sides of issues, and they grade essays and tests with an eye to inculcating high standards in the pursuit of understanding. Does this mean that philosophical counseling is a mere simulacrum of philosophy? I see no reason to think that. Philosophical inquiries take many different forms, and it would be elitist to accept only its academic versions as the "real thing."

Another objection is that philosophical counseling distorts genuine philosophy by subsuming truth to expediency. Counselors work with people who seek help with specific problems and who might view the wider pursuit of truth secondary to immediate coping. In particular, although Marinoff speaks of drawing on "timeless insights" from the history of philosophy, in practice he draws on any philosophical idea he thinks will help his clients live a better life (9). He compares philosophical counselors to matchmakers, linking their interests and needs to particular philosophical perspectives that help them flourish (50). For example, in helping a woman who is excessively self-sacrificing, Marinoff recommends reading Ayn Rand, who reduces morality to maximizing self-interest. Even if he only intended Rand as a corrective for a given excess, rather than as providing the basis for a sound ethics, we might fear that when philosophy becomes narrowly focused on solving immediate problems it compromises its search for truth.

The danger of subsuming truth to therapeutic efficacy was discussed long ago by Aristotle in critiquing Plato's integration of morality and therapy. Aristotle pointed out that health care has little interest in exploring many different views on ethics, given its primary goal of healing. In contrast, philosophical ethics requires exploring alternatives, if only to counter the influence of blinkers and biases in a search for broader truths. As Martha Nussbaum reminds us, Aristotle was concerned that therapeutic orientation invariably dilutes the philosophical search for truth.[18] In contrast to the virtues (excellences) of health care, which are aimed at healing, the virtues of ethical inquiry are valued for themselves, as part of the goal of pursuing truth. The risk in thinking of ethics as therapy is that clarity of thought, cogency of reasoning, and commitment to truth become secondary to health and are thereby corrupted. Nussbaum herself cautions that a "passion for health" "might subordinate truth and good reasoning to therapeutic efficacy."[19] Despite their rigor, Stoic and Epicurean philosophers were sometimes tempted to elevate healing and practical problem-solving over philosophical understanding.

In reply, I note that most forms of therapy have a focus in practical problem solving in ways that limit what can be done in a short amount of time and with limited resources. That does not mean that philosophical counseling cannot combine genuine philosophical inquiry into truth with a concern for positive health. Some philosophical counselors, notably Ran Lahav, make a sustained effort to keep problem solving secondary to the broader search for meaning, "a never-ending search, an endeavour of creative openness to new horizons rather than an attempt to produce solutions and ultimate theories."[20] The danger of distorting truth in the name of immediate helping can be confronted and managed.

Finally, Aristotle's rejoinder to Plato reminds us that the aims and procedures of philosophical ethics have always been controversial. Assuming there is a willingness to engage alternative perspectives, the disagreements promote the development of philosophy. Philosophical counseling began by setting itself against both the therapeutic trend and academic ethics. Perhaps in the future it will enrich academic ethics by exploring new ways to integrate morality and mental health.

15

HEALTHY LOVE

In Plato's *Symposium*, Aristophanes imagines human ancestors as rolling creatures with double appendages, gendered in one of three ways: male-female, male-male, and female-female. When these powerful creatures offended Zeus, he cut them in two and forced them to wander in search of their other half, driven (respectively) by heterosexual, gay, and lesbian desires. Erotic love is a symptom of a wound, a source of suffering, and often diseased. Yet it can also heal: "Love is born into every human being; it calls back the halves of our original nature together; it tries to make one out of two and heal the wound of human nature."[1] For Plato, love is both a therapeutic and a moral phenomenon, and so it is for us. We eagerly embrace therapeutic approaches that promise to improve viable relationships, minimize damage in ending unwanted relationships, and even help in understanding what love is. I begin by illustrating how love can simultaneously involve sickness and immorality, using examples of jealousy, unrequited love, and sadomasochism. Next I outline a virtue-oriented conception of healthy love, illustrating how moral and therapeutic conceptions of love overlap. I conclude by replying to Robert Bellah's criticisms of the therapeutic trend regarding love.

Sick Love

Judith Shklar recommends putting cruelty first in thinking about morality.[2] If this seems odd advice in connection with the ethics of love, we need only bring to mind family violence, vicious divorces, and the sometimes murderous passions of sexual jealousy and unrequited love. Let us begin, then, with the modest hope that lovers stop killing each other.

Consider Othello, who asks to be remembered as "one that loved not wisely, but too well."[3] In fact, he loves without minimum decency; when he murders Desdemona, he is both sick and culpable. Indeed, psychiatrists sometimes refer to morbid sexual jealousy as the Othello Syndrome, a subcategory of "Delusional Disorder, Jealous Type," in which the delusion, based on implausible and unwarranted inferences, is that one's spouse is unfaithful.[4] Othello is deluded, for even Iago's skillful machinations do not justify his extreme jealousy. Even without delusion, his morbid jealousy is an obsessive-compulsive disorder: "disturbed behavior associated with distressing irrational thoughts and disordered emotions, all of which show an underlying dominant theme of consuming preoccupation with the partner's sexual unfaithfulness."[5] Othello's obsession is a monomania in which one set of motives (desires, beliefs) dominates all others, generating a radical imbalance of character.[6] Perhaps additional pathologies are involved. Arthur Kirsch suggests that his insecurities as a middle-aged man, newly married to a woman half his age, are compounded by lack of self-esteem and self-respect.[7]

Eryximachus, the self-assured physician in the *Symposium*, tells us that "the love manifested in health is fundamentally distinct from the love manifested in disease."[8] Yet, there is no sharp line between healthy and unhealthy love, with regard to jealousy or any other aspect of love, and an instance of love might be healthy in some ways and unhealthy in others. Moreover, jealousy can be a healthy and morally desirable aspect of love insofar as it signals that love is at risk. Within limits, jealousy is love's friend.[9] Or is it? Since the 1960s, sexual jealousy has been suspect for many, and it "is now regarded . . . as unhealthy, as a symptom of immaturity, possessiveness, neurosis or insecurity."[10] The therapeutic trend played a part in pathologizing sexual jealousy, as therapists challenged traditional romantic myths. Equally important, changing moral outlooks led to sweeping critiques of monogamous relationships in the name of sexual liberation, autonomy, and authenticity. Indeed, the distinction between healthy and pathological jealousy turns on moral values embedded in therapeutic perspectives. Insofar as we value long-term committed relationships, at least as one valid ideal of love, we will acknowledge a role for healthy jealousy in preserving them. Even so, healthy jealousy shades into the extreme possessiveness that suffocates love, as quite literally occurs when Othello kills Desdemona.

Unrequited love is a second area where love can become unhealthy, and where a continuum between healthy and sick love exists. In the *Symposium*, Alcibiades declares his life was enriched by loving Socrates, despite the pain and sadness from not having his love returned. Not everyone handles things so well. As Oscar Wilde retells a biblical story, Salome falls deeply in love with John the Baptist. She requests, then pleads for, then demands a kiss from John, but the prophet curses her. (Without blaming the victim, we might wonder whether John could have handled things more diplomatically.) Shortly afterward, Salome performs the dance of seven veils for Herod in return for John's head delivered on a silver shield. When her trophy arrives, Salome seizes it and roughly kisses John's lips, proclaiming her unity with him in death.[11]

Salome's sickness and cruelty illustrate, says Helen K. Gediman, how "the desire to dominate, to insure possession, to merge, can result in the most extreme pathological outcomes."[12] Clearly, moral values have a role in distinguishing between healthy and unhealthy responses to unrequited love. Salome also illustrates the continuum between healthy and sick responses in love. Salome perverts the normal and endearing fantasy to merge with her beloved at death. These love-death (*Liebestod*) fantasies are familiar in art—for example, in depictions of Romeo and Juliet, and Tristan and Isolde. They are commonplace in everyday life as well. Literal fusion would undermine love by destroying the lovers' individuality, but fantasies of union are powerful expressions of love.

Othello and Salome illustrate the attitudes and actions of one partner in relationships. As an example of dual pathologies, consider sadomasochism: taking pleasure in aggression toward one's partner (sadism) and enjoyment in one's own suffering (masochism). In healthy relationships, aggression and submission are relatively mild and balanced, but once again there is a health-sickness continuum. In D. H. Lawrence's *Women in Love*, Gerald and Gudrun's marriage begins with mild sadomasochism that grows extreme. As a powerful industrial magnate, Gerald is accustomed to controlling human beings, but the death of his father unhinges him. For her part, Gudrun is frustrated in her career as an artist. The relationship begins by releasing "pent-up darkness and corrosive death" and quickly unravels with Gerald's first infidelity. Gudrun rationalizes the affair as natural for a powerful male, but she also tries to regain control over him. Soon they are at war: "Always it was this eternal see-saw, one destroyed that the other might exist, one ratified because the other was nulled." In the end, Gerald strangles Gudrun, interpreting her desperate resistance as a sign of pleasure in being dominated. Releasing his grip just before she would have died, he wanders in a daze until he falls to his death.[13]

Death again. The prominence of this motif leads Denis de Rougemont to conclude that romantic love is inherently pathological, a "twin narcissism." It is based on an illusion, a "love of love itself," rather than a genuine caring for the beloved, that conceals the ominous unconscious passion of desiring death: "Passion and marriage are essentially irreconcilable."[14] Let us hope that an integrated, moral-therapeutic perspective can promise more.

Jealousy, unrequited love, and sadomasochism are only a few areas where love can become sick, but they suffice to overthrow any general morality-therapy dichotomy. Here, as elsewhere, health and sickness allude to moral values, and in none of the examples does sickness exempt from responsibility. Let us now illustrate how morality enters into healthy and mature love.

Healthy Love and the Virtues

Therapy helps couples preserve and deepen their love. As a commonplace example, consider psychoanalyst Deborah Anna Luepnitz's depiction of Karl and Daphne, who entered therapy with her on two different occasions.[15] On the first occasion, Daphne's sister was living with them following her divorce. She gave Daphne someone to talk with, especially when their mother died, but her presence caused friction with Karl. After several months of therapy, the sister moved out and Daphne became increasingly unhappy with Karl. Their marriage had always been volatile, but it survived major difficulties, including Karl's excessive gambling (which Gamblers Anonymous helped him overcome) and Daphne's longing for a better-educated husband than Karl (who never attended college). The present tensions centered on allocating homemaking tasks and deciding how to spend leisure, with Karl enjoying television and sports and Daphne preferring cultural events. The therapy concluded successfully about the time their first child was born.

On the second occasion, three years later, Karl and Daphne called Dr. Luepnitz from a hospital where Daphne was being treated for a severe panic attack related to new problems over Daphne's desire for a second child and Karl's opposition. Their battles escalated, Daphne repeatedly threatened to leave Karl, and the turmoil was upsetting their young daughter. Therapy disclosed that Daphne's preoccupation with a second child was linked to her need for personal security, and Karl's fears about additional children involved legitimate financial concerns. Dr. Luepnitz deflects their arguments about a second child by getting them to explore together their dreams, thereby applying a tool from classical psychoanalysis to couple therapy. This reestablished communication and paved the way for a calmer discussion of their primary disagreement. Daphne returned to work, and she and Karl decided to postpone a decision about the second child.

Luepnitz cites Jessie Barnard's dictum that a marriage is really two marriages, his and hers, or as a Chinese proverb puts it: "Same bed, different dreams." Luepnitz also contrasts Aristophanes' myth about romantic union with Schopenhauer's tale about porcupines. Two porcupines, caught in freezing weather, move closer for warmth but then quickly move apart as their quills inflict pain on each another. Gradually they achieve a relatively stable equilibrium between warmth and the pain of intimacy, sustained by periodic readjustments. Love is a thorny affair.

Love is also a committed affair, as Daphne and Karl illustrate, and commitment involves the virtues.[16] Genuine love centers on caring for the beloved as irreplaceably dear, and this caring is structured by virtues such as faithfulness, respect, honesty, and fairness. Additional virtues enable love to flourish: courage, perseverance, self-respect, sexual fidelity, and responsibility. Love encompasses myriad ways in which couples interpret and implement these constitutive and enabling virtues. Although therapists do not fully agree about the criteria defining healthy relationships, the following criteria recur: intimacy, balance, communication, self-esteem, independence (autonomy), trust, stability, and marital quality.[17] These criteria interweave, respectively, with caring, fairness, honesty, self-respect, mutual respect, trustworthiness, responsibility, and mutual fulfillment. Moral understanding is often enriched by therapists' insights into these virtues.

Intimacy and Caring

Intimacy means emotional closeness and deep caring, as well as sexual compatibility. In addition to avoiding cruelty, caring implies a willingness to give oneself, emotionally and morally. Rarely is caring entirely selfless, for love merges with and redefines self-interest. But love contains significant elements of altruism—concern for the good of the beloved for his and her sake. Good therapists help us understand desirable mixtures of giving and receiving. They help couples develop skills in expressing love, managing conflicts, and responding to threats to relationships.

Balance and Fairness

Balance implies sharing, mutual give and take, compromise. In addition, it implies fairness in the distribution of benefits and burdens, power and opportunities. Fairness pertains to the sublime (fulfilling careers, children) and to the mundane (money, sharing household chores), and under the influence of feminism it has become a key virtue in most relationships. Yet, fairness can be elusive and pull in different directions. Fairness calls for balance in terms of power, opportunity, resources, and emotional involvement. The balance is measured by both substance and process: by objective standards in distributing benefits and burdens, and by autonomously negotiated arrangements. These measures can conflict, reflecting wider social disagreements about marital love.[18] A familiar example is the couple who chooses a traditional relationship in which the husband works for money and the woman works as a homemaker, mother, and community volunteer. Some feminists insist this arrangement is inherently unjust and emerges from psychologically internalized oppression within patriarchal societies, so that women do not act autonomously when they choose traditional roles. Other feminists reject such generalizations as patronizing and disrespectful of women's autonomy.[19]

In any case, therapists help couples with their negotiations. Peter Kramer notes that fairness is a recurring topic in the daily practice of therapy.[20] The majority of his clients come with questions about whether to leave or stay in relationships that have become unbalanced and unfulfilling. Kramer notes that psychotherapy theories have said little about fairness (with the exception, I would add, of feminist family therapies[21]). The moral complexities of fairness in love need to be addressed within an integrated, moral-therapeutic perspective.

Communication and Honesty

In therapeutic contexts, the word "communication" is used honorifically to mean good or effective communication. That implies honesty in expressing feelings and in listening to one's partner. Honesty cannot be understood in isolation from other virtues. Unlike ruthless, malevolent candor, honesty is constructive truthfulness and trustworthiness aimed at supporting caring relationships. Communication skills were once touted as the single most important factor in improving troubled relationships. More recently, psychologists question whether good communication is sufficient to improve relationships, without underlying moral commitments and caring.[22] In turn, philosophical conceptions of honesty would benefit from taking communication skills seriously in thinking about love. As a moral excellence, truthfulness requires learning and exercising skills of communication within a framework of caring.

Self-Esteem and Self-Respect

Positive self-esteem of partners contributes to healthy relationships. As we have seen, health-defining self-esteem is not the morally neutral idea of having a positive attitude toward oneself. Instead, it is having an affirming attitude toward oneself within limits set by self-respect. Failing to value oneself highly enough shows a lack of self-esteem, and irrational self-elevation is the disorder of narcissism.

Independence and Mutual Respect

Therapists underscore the need for partners to maintain significant areas of independence and self-expression. Clarifying exactly what that means is the stuff of everyday negotiations between couples. Therapists can help by providing tools to help resolve conflicts. But the moral virtue at stake is clear enough: respect for each other's autonomy.[23] At the same time, love transforms autonomy. Robert Nozick reminds us that "love's bond" is formed not only by the pooling the lovers' self-interest, but by pooling their autonomy, so that "decisions will be made together about how to be together."[24] Nozick had in mind shared decisions about where to live, which friendships to cultivate, whether to have children and how many, travel plans, and what to have for dinner. In addition to guiding shared projects, the shared decision-making includes how to be apart, when and how to give each other some "space." The skills of negotiation, compromise, and emotional adjustment can sometimes be improved by therapy or self-help resources.

Family therapists emphasize cultural variations in what autonomy and mutual respect mean, noting that in many cultures greater stress is placed on loyalty to the wider family.[25] But there are limits. Feminists challenge family therapists to avoid complete relativity of values, especially to confront violent husbands and fathers.[26] These debates over permissible variations concern both morality and therapy.

Trust and Trustworthiness

Love's interdependencies render partners vulnerable. As Annette Baier eloquently summarizes, love is "fraught with risks—risks of mutual maiming, of loss and heartbreak, of domination, of betrayal, of boredom, of strange fashions of forsaking, of special forms of disease and of disgrace." Baier also notes that these risks are inseparable from "the promise of strengths united, of new enthusiasms, of special joys, of easy ungloved intimacy, of generous givings and forgivings, of surprising forms of grace."[27] Baier explores the role of reasonable trust and trustworthiness (honesty) in dealing with the dangers and difficulties of love. But she also calls for courage, the willingness to take risks in pursuing the relationship, and the ability to trust in ways that Othello could not.

Stability and Responsibility

Marital love typically involves the desire for stability and permanence. In conducting their experiments, psychologists define commitment operationally as the willingness to tolerate stress and adversity—either within the relationship or from pressures outside. A moral-therapeutic perspective will emphasize responsibility: accepting the obligations created by commitments made to one's partner. Stability is not stagnation, and responsibility implies flexibility and responsiveness in solving mutual problems and making readjustments. When problems become unmanageable, the responsible thing might be to seek help, either from couple therapists, self-help literature, or a good friend.

Responsibility implies faithfulness—the sincere effort to do what is needed to make the relationship work. Faithfulness is distinct from sexual fidelity. Thus, traditional marriage vows distinguish the promise to love (constancy) from the promise to forsake all others (sexual fidelity). For most couples, sexual fidelity is a way to establish the symbolism that makes the expression "making love" more than a euphemism for sexual intercourse. Sexual fidelity also reduces the danger that outside relationships will destroy the marriage.

Marital Quality and Mutual Fulfillment

Marital quality is the level of satisfaction of partners with the relationship. Typically, satisfaction is measured using self-reports, but various quantitative measuring tests are used to pinpoint sources of distress in relationships. Humanistic psychologists also invoke somewhat vaguer but powerful ideas such as partners' growth and fulfillment. Self-fulfillment is a traditional moral value (if not exactly a virtue), as well as a therapeutic one, but happiness is a closely related moral value, as well as a prudential one. Healthy relationships contribute to personal growth and happiness. They do so in part by redefining the self in terms of the relationship, and in part by reorienting activities around shared pleasures, hopes, and endeavors.

Love and marriage interweave self-fulfillment with an array of additional moral values. A couple becomes a "we," in which their interests are intimately linked—often shared in the sense that partners have desires for the same things, and otherwise a strong tendency to be willing to affirm the other's deepest desires even when one does not fully share them.[28] The features I have discussed identify preferences within Western therapeutic outlooks, and they need to be adjusted to other cultural traditions. Nevertheless, the interweaving of virtues and healthy relationships is clear enough.

Reply to Bellah

Robert Bellah and his coauthors of *Habits of the Heart* contend that therapeutic attitudes distort moral meanings of love. They see Americans oscillating between two understandings of love: "a traditional view of love and marriage as founded on obligation" and "the therapeutic attitude, based on self-knowledge and self-realization" (93, 98).[29] Where Bellah et al. see confused ambivalence, I see attempts at integrating moral and health perspectives. As I noted in chapter 5, Bellah et al. block a moral-therapeutic integration by stereotyping morality as obligations and therapy as self-oriented. On the one hand, by reducing morality to obligations these authors fail to appreciate the language of the virtues used by interviewees in characterizing their partners, relationships, and aspirations in love.[30] For example, one interviewee describes his wife as "really good," "special," someone he cherishes (104–105). Almost grudgingly, Bellah et al. admit that this language reaches beyond narrow self-seeking, but they insist that only the language of obligation can make sense of love as more than mere personal preferences (106). Another interviewee offers a virtue-oriented conception of marital love as "founded on mutual respect, admiration, affection, the ability to give and receive freely" (5). Because the man justifies the relationship in terms of self-fulfillment, however, Bellah et al. say he thinks in terms of "idiosyncratic preference" (6). A more sympathetic interpretation is that these individuals talk about love as a virtue-structured relationship that contributes to mutual self-fulfillment.

On the other hand, by reducing therapy to self-absorption, Bellah et al. lump together an enormous variety of therapeutic attitudes. Some therapy is narrowly self-oriented, including both some 1960–1970s outlooks and the "co-dependency" literature that became popular after *Habits of the Heart* appeared. Consider this passage from the co-dependency guru Anne Wilson Schaef: "The Ideal American Marriage is based upon mutual dependency: neither partner can function without the other. The lives of the married couple are totally intertwined.... After a while in this kind of arrangement, neither *can* leave because neither can function without the other. This is addiction!"[31] What Schaef calls addiction includes committed love, and hence Bellah et al.'s criticisms apply against her. But when Bellah et al. set "the" therapeutic attitude in opposition to commitments and responsibilities, they eclipse how sound therapeutic outlooks support love.

Again, although Bellah et al.'s interest is in the wider social effects of therapeutic outlooks, rather than critiquing professional therapists, they fail to note the wide variation in therapeutic models. Marriage counselors and couple therapists, like Luepnitz, adopt relationships, rather than one partner, as their focus. In order to help, therapists adopt a stance of neutrality, especially in avoiding taking sides between combating spouses, at least within wide limits—until, for example, a violent individual endangers his spouse.[32] But therapists are also attuned to the (reasonable) values of a couple in order to help their relationships flourish. Those values transcend self-preoccupation. Indeed, the tensions between individual needs and mutual sharing and responsibilities are the mainstay of most therapy. The (limited) value-neutrality of the therapist does not mean the therapeutic endeavor is itself morally neutral, for it remains rooted in respect for clients' autonomy (within bounds set by minimum decency) and caring about their well-being as, in large measure, they define it.

Ann Swidler, one of the co-authors of *Habits of the Heart*, reasserts the morality-therapy dichotomy in a later book on love. She also continues to stereotype "the" therapeutic outlook as narrowly self-oriented, although she describes it in terms that fit some moral conceptions: "The therapeutic ethic helps individuals discover their true selves, so they can make authentic choices that reflect what they 'really' want . . . freed of the inauthentic residues of family pressures, social roles, or others' expectations."[33] Swidler sounds a new chord, however. She emphasizes that Americans are discriminating in how they use therapeutic ideas. Instead of being muddled and oscillating willy-nilly between conflicting perspectives, couples listen to therapists or health experts and appropriate what they find useful for their own purposes, setting the rest aside.[34] These purposes often include moral and religious aims in sustaining committed love relationships. In my terms, Swidler confirms that couples weave together moral and therapeutic elements from a culture that has many conflicting strands, some superficial and others enriching.

To conclude, far from being inherently opposed to morality, therapeutic perspectives on love embody an array of virtues, including honesty and fairness, respect and self-respect, caring and responsibility. Problems arise when these virtues are concealed and create the false appearance of value-neutrality, or when they are appealed to uncritically in isolation from other relevant moral values. That occurred, for example, when psychoanalysts pronounced normal or "mature" love as heterosexual and patriarchal. It also occurred when psychiatrists characterized healthy femininity as a sacrifice of "masculine ambitions" for the role of wife-mother.[35] Things have improved. Today the health care community is ahead of conventional morality on many issues, including in urging full respect for gay and lesbian relationships. Yet there remains the need for greater clarity about the strong overlap between morality and mental health in understanding love.

16

MEANINGFUL WORK

The promise of the global economy is matched by its perils to meaningful work: increased layoffs, extended unemployment, job stress from longer working hours and demands for increased productivity, and preoccupation with money in every area of life. An integrated, moral-therapeutic perspective cannot remove these threats, but it can help us cope with them. To illustrate some therapeutic contributions in dealing with moral matters concerning stress and alienation, I begin with Herman Melville's short story, "Bartleby." Then I turn to positive conceptions of mental health in thinking about meaningful work—work that combines ethics with excellence.

Alienation

"Worker alienation" is the absence of meaning in what we do for a living.[1] In its psychological aspect, it is a pained or numbed lack of identification with work, a sense that our work does not express who we are and what we value. In its moral aspect, it is degradation in being reduced to an interchangeable and replaceable cog. These aspects coalesce in Marx's famous conception of worker alienation. Alienated work "is *external* to the worker" rather than a personal expression, and hence the worker "does not fulfill himself in his work but denies himself, has a feeling of misery rather than well-being, does not develop freely his mental and physical energies but is physically exhausted and mentally debased."[2] In addition to alienation from the activity of working, there is alienation from the products of labor, from co-workers, and from human beings in general. Marx believes all these forms of alienation are inevitable in capitalism. Yet, capitalism takes many forms, including kinder and gentler forms that establish reasonable safety nets, and its ruthless aspects can be tempered by healthy workplaces and humane government.

In "Bartleby," Melville portrays worker alienation as a combination of un-healthy work and unhealthy workers. The story's narrator, an unnamed law-yer, hires Bartleby to hand-copy legal manuscripts and then, working with a colleague, to check the copy for accuracy, word by word. Bartleby is adept and conscientious at this dull work, and the lawyer prizes his calm demeanor and constant presence at the workplace. One day, however, when the lawyer asks him to help proofread copy, "Bartleby, in a singularly mild, firm voice, replied, 'I would prefer not to'" (112).[3] Disconcerted, yet willing to accommodate the eccentricities of his staff, the lawyer indulges Bartleby's "passive resistance" (or passive aggression) (115). A crisis ensues, however, when Bartleby refuses to do any work at all and, after being fired, refuses to vacate the premises. Strangely affected by Bartleby's plight, the lawyer is reluctant to call the police. In a surreal gesture, he moves his company, leaving Bartleby to haunt the former offices. Subsequently he learns that Bartleby, in jail for trespassing and va-grancy, starves himself to death.

The lawyer provokes Bartleby's fatal refusal to work when he searches his desk for clues explaining his odd behavior. He discovers that Bartleby sleeps at night in the office and saves his earnings in his desk. Initially the lawyer responds with compassion, but he quickly dismisses this response as the mel-ancholy musings of "a sick and silly brain" (120). Reversing himself, he con-cludes it is Bartleby who is sick, "the victim of innate and incurable disorder" (122). The lawyer's compassion is replaced by repulsion: "When at last it is perceived that such pity cannot lead to effectual succor, common sense bids the soul be rid of it" (121–122).

Usually the story is interpreted as a critique of capitalism, denigrating the attorney as an exploitive manager and celebrating Bartleby as an existential hero (or anti-hero).[4] That interpretation is implausible. Bartleby is well-suited to his work. And far from being a callous representative of amoral capitalism, the lawyer manifests a father-like kindness toward him. Dan McCall concludes that we, like the lawyer, must confront a tragedy transcending the dark side of capitalism: "The deepest question in the story is what you do with Bartleby. The deepest answer the story provides is that you can do nothing."[5]

Therapeutic optimism challenges McCall's abandonment of hope as premature. Even when work is boring, the workplace can be made more stimulating. Con-temporary therapies might also help. A key question is whether Bartleby is sick or willfully rebellious. A morality-therapy dichotomy forces us to choose: either Bartleby acts voluntarily and hence is accountable, or he is sick and not ac-countable. This dichotomy underlies the lawyer's confused responses, as Maurice Friedman points out: the lawyer "oscillates between seeing Bartleby as a free and voluntary agent and as a helpless victim of an incurable disorder." As readers, we share this difficulty because "Melville has intentionally placed at the very heart of his story the question of whether Bartleby's 'sickness' is to be understood as involuntary compulsion, willful self-isolation, or both." Friedman concludes that Bartleby is both sick and accountable: "He retains responsibility for his will, but it is . . . the will of the man who is sick in his relations to others and to himself."[6]

What exactly is Bartleby's malady? It has been diagnosed as chronic depression, obsessive-compulsive disorder, attention deficit disorder, schizophrenia, catatonic disorder, and anorexia (given his austere eating habits and self-starvation[7]). I suspect he had schizoid personality disorder, a malady characterized by pervasive solitariness, detachment from others, lack of enjoyment, flattened affectivity, and dramatically restricted range of emotions.[8] Whatever the proper diagnosis, his avoidance of meaningful human interaction is both a moral and health concern. His signature utterance, "I would prefer not to," serves to limit human interaction, as seen in his refusals to share in proofreading, run errands requiring human contact, and answer questions about his past. Despite his malady, Bartleby remains responsible for doing his job.[9] That does not mean we should blame him. Like the lawyer, we are "strangely disarmed" by him. We are also amused by his "preferring not to," for we too have such preferences. Most important, his suffering precludes anger as a final response to him. His plight reveals how suboptimal health interacts with unhealthy workplaces to generate alienation, to which we are all vulnerable.

A moral-psychological concept of alienation is at home within an integrated, moral-therapeutic perspective that underscores the importance of self-respect and self-esteem. Meaningless work tends to demean, although sometimes it is redeemed by money and other perquisites. To be sure, one-sided therapeutic outlooks might be misused to deflect attention from the social structures that foster alienation, offering superficial remedies that manipulate workers into continuing to work under dehumanizing conditions. Indeed, pathologizing the unhappy worker is often a way to blame the victim of frustrating and futile work. Nevertheless, "Bartleby" is a cautionary tale which shows that alienation sometimes says as much about the worker as the work.

Coping

For many of us, stress is the primary threat to meaningful work. Managing stress is essential to maintaining positive health. "Coping" is a value-laden term referring to desirable ways of pursuing worthwhile activities and relationships. Coping requires managing our emotions in response to stressors, including colleagues, which generate anxiety, depression, anger, hatred, shame, and envy. This coping shifts our attention to the lawyer's attempts to cope with Bartleby's odd behavior. Could therapeutic understanding help the lawyer?

In *Toxic Coworkers*, Alan Cavaiola and Neil Lavender point out that individuals with schizoid personality disorder "can be quite self-sufficient. They are able to work with minimal amounts of supervision. This makes them excellent candidates for working alone or at home," and with "things rather than people."[10] Although personality disorders are extremely difficult to alter, even an "innate and incurable disorder" like Bartleby's can sometimes be worked around. Cavaiola and Lavender recommend accepting the greater needs for privacy that individuals with schizoid personality disorder have. The lawyer intuited as much about Bartleby, and it was only his ill-fated search of Bartleby's desk that undermined his earlier accommodations.

Managing our emotions is an important part of managing other people. The lawyer oscillates between compassion and pity, rage and resignation, confusion and grief, according to whether he views Bartleby as sick or irresponsible. On occasion, he wants to injure Bartleby—his "millstone" and "incubus"; at such times, he regains self-control only by bringing vividly to mind the Christian commandment to love our neighbor (115, 129). Throughout, he tries to understand and restrain his emotions in order to be professional and to be caring.[11] Today, a cottage industry of self-help books and workshops discuss "anger management," "diversity training," and myriad other emotional skills. Typically, these programs are presented under the guise of value-neutral psychology; in fact, they assume moral values.

A good example is the Emotional Intelligence Program popularized by Daniel Goleman. Goleman discusses pathologies such as depression and impulse control disorders, but he emphasizes ideals of positive health and maturity.[12] These ideals imply some twenty-five "emotional competencies" clustered around five "dimensions of emotional intelligence": (1) self-awareness—discernment of one's emotions, accurate self-assessment, and self-confidence which includes a strong sense of self-worth); (2) self-regulation—self-control, trustworthiness, conscientiousness, adaptability, and innovation; (3) motivation—achievement drive, commitment to group goals, initiative, and optimism; (4) empathy—understanding others, helping others develop, service orientation, cultivating opportunities made possible by diversity, and awareness of political dynamics within groups; and (5) social skills—influence, communication, conflict management, leadership, change catalyst, building bonds, cooperation, and team capabilities.[13] Many of these emotional competencies either are or imply virtues, for example, self-control, trustworthiness, and cooperation. In asides, Goleman admits as much: "There is an old-fashioned word for the body of skills that emotional intelligence represents, *character*."[14] Greater moral explicitness would make it clear that Goleman sets forth an integrated, moral-therapeutic perspective.[15]

Most psychology-based management approaches lack moral explicitness, increasing the risk of abuses. Arlie Hochschild shows how management seeks to manipulate "emotional work," the labor involved in managing emotions, by institutionalizing "feeling rules" and expectations. She studied flight attendants who are expected to maintain a constant caring, supportive, and cheerful demeanor. Because continual pretense will give itself away, self-manipulation of feeling is required. For example, training programs for flight attendants get them to fault themselves for feeling anger at rude passengers. Their anger shows they are "oversensitive, too touchy," and not seeing things from the passengers' point of view.[16] Taken to an extreme, this "commercialization of feeling" causes alienation. Goleman suggests that Hochschild tells only half the story. The presence or absence of alienation depends largely on whether workers identify with and value the work that requires emotional self-management.[17] Insofar as flight attendants or nurses value their work as a personal expression of who they are, the self-managed and other-managed heart can benefit workers. Even so, Hochschild pinpoints genuine dangers that disguising and diluting the virtues reduces them to manipulative tools of management. A more explicit virtue-oriented approach highlights the moral content of emotional intelligence, and it encourages individuals to ground their work in moral commitments.

Some psychologists acknowledge how moral virtues enter into therapeutic perspectives. Especially noteworthy, in heralding a "positive psychology," Martin Seligman identifies six core virtues present in all major moral traditions: wisdom, courage, love, justice, temperance, and self-transcendence (identification with communities).[18] In the abstract, these virtues are difficult to study scientifically, but much of their meaning can be conveyed in operational definitions in terms of specific "strengths." Thus, wisdom is manifested as curiosity, love of learning, open-mindedness, ingenuity, social intelligence, and perspective; courage as bravery, perseverance, and honesty; love as kindness, generosity, and personal caring; justice as loyalty, fairness, and leadership; temperance as self-control, prudence, and humility; and self-transcendence as appreciation of beauty and excellence, gratitude, hope, spirituality, forgiveness, humor, and enthusiasm.

In applying this perspective to work, Seligman cites polls showing that half of lawyers (to update "Bartleby") are dissatisfied with their work.[19] Although Seligman does not make happiness a defining feature of mental health, lawyers' unhappiness bears indirectly on their mental health, including their markedly higher-than-average rates of depression, alcoholism, and illegal drug use. Seligman discovered several causes of their unhappiness: the tendency to adopt pessimistic attitudes that explain bad occurrences as permanent, pervasive, and beyond their control; the large percentage of legal work that is high-stress and allows little latitude in decision-making; and the adversary legal system that ensures one side will have an unhappy result.

Seligman also recommends ways to alleviate the unhappiness of attorneys and other workers. One possibility is to seek less-stressful aspects of law (as did the lawyer in "Bartleby"). Other possibilities include pursuing aspects of law that allow greater personal control (such as library research), fostering more optimistic attitudes in their personal lives, and finding ways to exercise individual talents and strengths at the workplace. No individual possesses all the strengths that contribute to the six core virtues, but each of us has "signature strengths" we can emphasize in our work.

Meaning and Identity

Critics of the therapeutic trend charge that it focuses narrowly on adjusting workers to their fate, thereby eclipsing moral issues about job stability, decent income, integrating work with family and leisure, and meaningful life. As Joanne B. Ciulla writes, "excellence in work consists of creating a good product, the skill and expertise and high standards used in making the product, and a worker who is morally excellent, or virtuous." Ciulla dismisses therapeutic perspectives: "For those who are grappling with a philosophic, not an emotional, problem, the therapeutic and pop psychology avenues fail because they focus either on alleviating the symptoms of the question (such as depression or discontent) or on providing packaged answers."[20] Contrary to Ciulla, however, I believe that linking excellence and ethics requires attention to positive mental health and psychological realism. A sound moral-therapeutic perspective understands work within the wider context of a meaningful life. Such a perspective encourages incremental improvements in the health and morality of organizations, professions, and individuals.

Consider individuals. Ilene Philipson, a psychotherapist specializing in work problems in Silicon Valley, reports that her clients have emotional lives dominated by troubled work.[21] A typical client—whether a "dot.com" executive, legal secretary, or retail worker—might feel overwhelming hatred for being laid off after years of devoted service to a company, major depression because of being criticized by an adored boss, or recurring anxiety and panic attacks after moving into a new area of technology at a company. Adopting a moral-therapeutic perspective, Philipson understands work-related issues broadly, in terms of suboptimal health, moral values, and wider economic forces. After granting the importance of economic insecurity and compulsive consumerism, she decries excessive emotional involvements with work that threaten important relationships with family, friends, and community. When there is less to go home to, work takes up the slack. In addition, many jobs in the professions are engaging and exciting. The dual forces—exciting work and frustrating families—pose a double threat to families.[22] By linking individual therapy with public health concerns, and unifying both within a framework of moral values, Philipson challenges her clients to abandon their self-absorption and undertake new commitments.

The early therapeutic literature discussed work-family imbalances under the heading of addiction. The term "workaholism," modeled on "alcoholism," originally meant choosing excessive involvement work at the expense of other important values and relationships.[23] (The term does not apply to individuals whose sheer survival requires exhausting hours at work.[24]) Commitment to the job and career enters at the core of individuals' identity—sometimes creatively, and sometimes in unhealthy ways.[25] Because of the centrality of commitment, the analogy with addiction is strained. Indeed, the term "workaholic" now has favorable connotations among many workers, as well as employers. Nevertheless, overinvolvement with work has become a threat to meaningful lives. (Even Bartleby's problems stem in part from the absence of supportive relationships in his personal life.)

Excessive consumerism is a related topic of interest to therapists. A frustrating job or an unsatisfying career easily leads to excessive spending on material goods and entertainment. An endless cycle of getting, spending, and debt provides superficial satisfactions to compensate for the absence of deeper meaning.[26] Therapists write much about pathological buying, wealth addiction, and, more playfully, "affluenza": "a painful, contagious, socially transmitted condition of overload, debt, anxiety, and waste resulting from the dogged pursuit of more."[27] Understanding such patterns as unhealthy, compulsive consumerism can lead to greater self-control.[28] In addition, therapeutic understanding helps stressed-out professionals overcome other addictions, such as alcoholism and drug dependency.[29]

I have focused on individuals, but therapeutic insights contribute to wider social issues about work. For example, Howard Gardner and his co-authors of *Good Work* are concerned with how market pressures tend to erode professional standards in ways that undermine character by generating anxieties, exhaustion, frustrations, and "demoralization." They adopt a "person-centered perspective" that encourages individuals to understand their work in a broader social context.[30] Gardner's group explicitly embraces moral values at several junctures. One juncture is in specifying their topic: good work is excellent in terms of both technical standards and ethical desirability. Ethical desirability is understood in terms of both professional ethical values and socially responsible contributions. Another juncture is in embracing "stakeholder theory," the view that corporations have responsibilities to an array of constituencies which include clients, the community, and other workers, in addition to stockholders.

Professionals are more likely to find their work meaningful when the relevant forces shaping their work are "well-aligned." The forces include the commitments of the individual professional, the standards of the entire group of professionals, the owners or stockholders of the corporation in which one works, and the general public affected by the work. When these forces are misaligned—as, for example, in contemporary journalism—professionals are systematically pressured to compromise standards of excellence and ethics in order to maximize profits. The upshot is frustration, alienation, and anomie.[31]

To repeat, a sound moral-therapeutic perspective helps us understand and cope, but it cannot stop the economic transformations taking place. Instability and the need to change jobs or professions are making it increasingly difficult to pursue a continuous career within a profession, as the economy now forces abrupt changes in core job skills. As sociologist Richard Sennett observes, the motto, "no long term" is taking hold, in a way that threatens long-term commitments within professions. Professionals become disposable parts in a global economy, in ways that erode their sense of being needed by others and their ties to community: "'Who needs me?' is a question of character which suffers a radical challenge in modern capitalism. The system radiates indifference."[32]

Sennett offers no solution to this "corrosion of character," but he appreciates how moral-therapeutic understanding can help in coping with loss of jobs. He describes a group of laid-off IBM computer professionals with whom he met over several months. Initially they perceived themselves as betrayed and victimized by their company. Then they saw themselves as victims of the global economy. Finally they came to accept responsibility for becoming overly dependent on the company, for not making earlier career moves to expand their range of skills. Their "ethical act" of taking "responsibility for their life histories" culminates a process that is simultaneously moral and therapeutic.[33] It is a process involving communication, in the morally resonant sense that involves honesty and community, aimed at finding constructive ways to deal with failures and misfortunes, rather than victim-oriented self-indulgence.[34] This same role of dialogue and narrative—that is, telling a meaningful story about one's life—is what good therapy provides through dialogue with a counselor.[35]

To conclude, rather than stereotyping therapeutic outlooks as self-absorbed and dismissing them as superficial, we should identify the moral assumptions embedded in them. Then we can refine the best therapeutic outlooks in light of moral understanding. The overall aim will be to attach personal meaning to wider community values—exactly what critics of the therapeutic trend call for. A similar aim pertains to philanthropy, the final topic I explore.

17
COMMUNITY SERVICE

Philanthropy is voluntary giving for public purposes, whether the gift is money, time, or talent, and whether the purposes are humanitarian, environmental, civic, religious, scientific, artistic, or other goods for communities.[1] Critics of the therapeutic trend claim that it erodes America's vibrant philanthropic tradition by replacing altruism with self-seeking, virtue with subjective feeling, and community participation with pursuit of self-fulfillment.[2] To the contrary, I outline how an integrated, moral-therapeutic perspective on philanthropy emphasizes the confluence of self-interest, community service, and the virtues. Although all virtues contribute to philanthropy, I focus on compassion, gratitude, hope, and justice.

Compassion

When asked why they engage in philanthropy, Americans report feelings of satisfaction and self-fulfillment. To my mind, these reports suggest genuine caring, not self-absorption, which is not to deny that self-interest plays a major role. Indeed, exemplary philanthropists have always linked self and community, self-interest and morality, individualism and compassion, and self-fulfillment through service to others. Jane Addams is a good example, because she voices these themes as part of a health-oriented approach to social problems. As a young woman, Addams witnessed a decline in caring—that "healthful reaction" to suffering—and a diminishment in the "moral health" shown in harmony between professed values and actual conduct.[3] For eight years after graduating from college, she deferred acting on her own humanitarian commitments, trapped in a self-deceptive "snare of preparation."[4] Then, on a trip to Europe in 1888, she attended a bullfight in which five bulls and many horses were killed. Stunned by her apathy at the bloodshed, she began to confront the gap between her principles and practice. Within months she and a friend established Hull House in Chicago, an inner-city center that for decades would provide child care, education, emotional support, access to the arts, and other services to immigrant families.

Addams was a "wounded healer" whose suffering contributed to her effectiveness in helping.[5] Her mother died when she was a child, and the death of her father precipitated eight years of anxiety and depression. Healing came when she began to connect her life to people in need. Later she discovered the limitations of private giving, given the scale of suffering, and she became an advocate of public health approaches to social problems. She also became a public intellectual who, as a pioneer in social work and a participant in the Progressive Movement, influenced law and public policy to improve living conditions for immigrants. Her writings interweave themes of compassion, commitment to community, and self-fulfillment: "Nothing so deadens the sympathies and shrivels the power of enjoyment as the persistent keeping away from the great opportunities for helpfulness and a continual ignoring of the starvation struggle which makes up the life of at least half the race."[6]

Robert Wuthnow cites Addams to illustrate Americans' distinctive blending of compassion and individualism. He agrees with Addams that the primary value of philanthropy is to sustain networks of caring beyond the sphere of family and friends, not to replace government in solving vast social problems (3).[7] Compassion "enriches and ennobles us . . . because it holds forth a vision of what a good society can be, [and] provides us with concrete examples of caring that we can emulate" (308–309). Wuthnow also offers a nuanced assessment of the therapeutic trend, or what he calls the "therapeutic motif"—the preoccupation with feelings, the avoidance of explicit moral language, and an emphasis on taking care of one's own needs before helping others (100).

On the positive side, the therapeutic motif strengthens philanthropy by insisting that it should be healthy. Unhealthy philanthropy creates undesirable dependencies, rather than supporting recipients' autonomy and their efforts to solve their own problems (205). It fosters dominance and emotional exploitation on the part of donors. It expresses personal insecurities, such as neurotic "savior complexes" that elevate donors rather than empower recipients. And unless reasonable limits are set, helping can lead to burnout ("compassion fatigue") (193). In contrast, healthy self-love promotes effective helping. Wuthnow praises the therapeutic motif for reinforcing individualism, in all its meanings: freedom, self-assertion, desires for success, standing up for one's convictions, having a personal style, inner strength, a clear sense of identity, and personal growth (114). Again, the therapeutic motif facilitates helping by emphasizing nonjudgmental attitudes and appreciation of diversity (30). In many ways, donors combine obligations to others with a therapeutic sensibility. For example, some individuals contribute their time and resources to self-help/mutual aid groups (29). Others volunteer in child abuse and sexual assault clinics (109). Still others devote hours to religious-oriented service organizations that combine morality and spirituality with a health-oriented sensibility (100).

On the negative side, Wuthnow says the therapeutic motif blurs our understanding of the justification, demands, and desirable motives for philanthropy

(100). He raises objections which by now are familiar: the therapeutic trend encourages a subjective view of values and reinforces selfishness at the expense of community. His objections are insightful but overstated.

To begin with, Wuthnow says that philanthropy is at risk when feeling good becomes the primary rationale for philanthropy. Good feelings derive from innumerable sources beyond compassion, including money, power, and fame (292). Genuine compassion needs to be conceptualized as altruism, as caring about others for their sake (45). By avoiding explicit moral language, the therapeutic motif disguises the moral significance of philanthropy and reinforces the view that values are mere subjective preferences. In reply, I agree that justifications that stop with feelings eclipse the moral reasons for philanthropy, the virtues manifested in philanthropy, and even the justification of the feelings themselves. Philanthropy is valuable because it helps people, and the "good feelings" it generates have moral value because they manifest beneficence, compassion, and other virtues.[8] There is nothing objectionable, however, about Americans' ready resort to the language of feelings as a first expression of why they engage in philanthropy. Feeling good in helping others is a presumptive sign of genuine caring. And reluctance to parade one's virtues as justification can be a mark of humility and social decorum, as Wuthnow notes (76). Moreover, a sound moral-therapeutic outlook renounces the view that feelings are detached from activities or "free floating," so that one positive feeling is as good as any another.

Next, Wuthnow says the therapeutic trend encourages selfishness. The trend overemphasizes self-interest as a motive for giving (77). It accents multiple motives for any given act of helping—for example, a mixture of enjoyment, self-esteem, approval of others, a sense of power, and personal growth, as well as a concern for their well-being—thereby eclipsing caring and compassion (59). And it rejects moral ideals of self-sacrifice (103). In reply, I share the concern that society continually conveys the message that people are exclusively self-oriented. Not only does the message permeate business, but it is reinforced by academic disciplines as varied as economics, psychology, political science, and sociobiology, as well as parts of the therapeutic community.[9] The view that humans are entirely self-interested threatens loyalties that make communities possible.[10] It also belies the power of philanthropy to express caring for others, for their sake. Nevertheless, mixing moral and self-interested justifications need not mean losing moral understanding. Our motives are almost always mixed, and our needs for self-affirmation are deep and legitimate.

In sum, although Wuthnow begins with a sympathetic approach to the therapeutic trend, he misses an opportunity to develop an integrated, moral-therapeutic perspective on philanthropy. Philanthropy provides opportunities to express and enlarge who we are by putting our values into action and by creating caring relationships. A moral-therapeutic perspective emphasizes that the self is social in nature; that the reasons justifying philanthropy are not reducible to "feeling good" about ourselves; and that the justification centers on the values that, when acted upon, generate self-affirming feelings. Our emotions, interests, and identities, turn in part on the values we manifest in our relationships and activities. To have a character at all is to have a set of relatively enduring desires, concerns, projects and relationships—in which the virtues are embedded.[11] To the extent that we are invested in valuable philanthropic projects, we express and affirm our identity and interests, as we promote the good of others.[12]

Gratitude

Like compassion, gratitude combines moral concern and self-interest to provide a powerful motive for philanthropy. Gratitude is a positive response to the benevolence shown to us by our family, teachers, and innumerable strangers. As a virtue, gratitude is not merely appreciating gifts; it is appreciating the giver's caring for us, as manifested in the gift.[13] Appreciating this caring generates a desire to give back. To be oblivious to the caring is to be prone to selfishness, envy, and rancor.

Gratitude is prominent in the life and thought of Albert Schweitzer, a physician-philosopher who, like Addams, made therapeutic themes prominent in his diagnosis of society's pathologies.[14] Raised in a relatively privileged family, Schweitzer's appreciation of his good fortune developed early. As a college student, he was convinced that he "must not accept this good fortune as a matter of course, but must give something in return."[15] He resolved to pursue his own interests until he was thirty, at which time he would fully commit himself to a life of service. By then he had earned doctorates in theology and philosophy and distinguished himself as a scholar. Yet he kept his resolve and retrained as a physician in order to serve at Lambarene in the (Belgian) Congo during the next fifty years.

Schweitzer calls gratitude a "mysterious law of existence" that provides a wellspring of moral motivation.[16] Nearly all of us are helped by the beneficence of parents, teachers, health professionals, and soldiers. It is wrong to take this beneficence for granted, worse still to reduce it to self-seeking or to merely doing one's duty.[17] Often we cannot help those who help us. Perhaps they are dead, perhaps we do not know who they are, or perhaps the appropriate expression of gratitude is a simple and heartfelt thank you. But we can help third parties in the same spirit of caring and compassion. In this way, invisible roots unite individuals within communities.[18]

Similar themes are familiar in religious writings on "spiritual health," and health psychologists are also beginning to explore them.[19] Therapists caution about the abuse of gratitude, and more generally about unhealthy ways of helping—cautions that are as much moral as therapeutic.[20] They also emphasize that the extreme absence of appropriate gratitude is pathological, whether as a symptom of narcissism, depression, hatred, envy, or greed. More positively, therapists highlight the contributions of gratitude to mental health. For example, the humanistic psychologist Abraham Maslow portrayed "self-actualized" individuals as manifesting gratitude and capacities to appreciate what is good in life.[21] Psychologists are exploring how gratitude fosters self-affirmation and a sense of well-being. Gratitude signals appreciation that people care about us and thereby contributes to self-esteem. In turn, active expression of gratitude is itself self-affirming by heightening a sense of well-being. In one set of studies, college students were asked to keep a log of their emotions, physical symptoms, and health-related behavior.[22] Some students were also asked to write down things for which they were grateful, and others were asked to write down either minor or major annoyances. Students whose attention was drawn toward experiences of gratitude felt better about themselves and their lives.

Hope

Hope manifests mental health, as do faith and optimism. That was the view of William James in calling for a "healthy-minded" morality.[23] The good in our lives depends significantly on positive attitudes: "This world is good . . . since it is what we make it,—and we shall make it good."[24] To be sure, hope, faith, and optimism might be aimed at immoral ends. Nevertheless, hope as a virtue significantly overlaps with hope as health-manifesting. And as psychologists increasingly appreciate, the goals that hope motivates include benefits to others, not merely goods for oneself.[25]

Anne Colby and William Damon identify "positivity" as a central feature in nearly all the philanthropists they studied. Positivity is a combination of enjoyment in helping and optimism in the form of faith (trust without proof in some anticipated good) and hope (active desire for a good what we believe is possible though not certain). The faith and hope are neither naïve nor sentimental. Positivity was rooted in a realistic appraisal of problems while reframing the problems as challenges and opportunities. Jane Addams and Albert Schweitzer are good illustrations, but Colby and Damon studied less well-known individuals. For example, Cabell Brand is a business person who, in addition to running his family's business, developed innovative ways to fight poverty by providing "a hand up, not a handout." He created a nonprofit organization to help people get work, stay in school, and earn college scholarships. Brand's programs were developed in response to specific needs and subsequently expanded when they proved successful. Another example is Virginia Durr, who spent three decades working to overthrow the poll tax that prevented impoverished women and black people in Southern states from voting. Her endeavors involved sacrifice and risks to her family, but Durr showed courage and "fierceness" in the pursuit of justice.[26]

Martin Seligman studies optimism as a pattern of cognition. Optimists tend to see setbacks as temporary and also as due primarily to people and factors in the situation other than themselves. Pessimists, by contrast, tend to think that bad things will endure and are largely their own fault. Seligman notes that optimism tends to increase, and depression decrease, as we find meaning in larger groups. Selfishness, by contrast, tends to breed a pessimistic style of explanation that shuts us off from life-affirming groups. Although Seligman speaks as a therapist, he voices moral criticisms of some aspects of the therapeutic trend. Americans have become too narrowly self-focused, romanticizing individualism at the expense of the common good. He recommends greater involvement in community activities, including direct giving to individuals and volunteering. Echoing Jane Addams, he insists that compassionate engagement deepens the meaning in our lives. He also agrees that some therapeutic outlooks erode personal responsibility. In affirming an integrated, moral-therapeutic perspective, he balances care for others with care for oneself.[27]

Social Justice

As we saw in discussing crime and bigotry, justice poses special challenges to developing a moral-therapeutic perspective, and we might expect similar challenges regarding philanthropy in the pursuit of justice. Consider women's rights. Therapy-oriented attitudes, with their emphasis on compassion and downplaying blame, might seem to dilute demands for equal opportunity and justice. Feminists' hostility to Freud might suggest additional opposition to the therapeutic trend. In fact, historically the women's movement allied itself with the therapeutic trend. It borrowed heavily from the therapeutic ideas and ideals of humanistic psychology. Justice was invoked on the grounds of equal opportunities for self-fulfillment, more than abstract rights, and injustice was attacked by exposing the psychological damage it causes. To a surprising degree, the feminist adage "the personal is political" implies that the psychological is political.

Two decades before her *Feminine Mystique* ignited the 1960s feminist movement, Betty Friedan was a psychology major at Smith College. During those decades she continued to study the humanistic psychology of Abraham Maslow, Carl Rogers, Erich Fromm, and Rollo May.[28] These thinkers, with their integrated, moral-therapeutic approach to personal growth as a fundamental human drive, provided a conceptual framework for renouncing the cultural assumption that homemaking suffices to fulfill most women. Especially in her chapter "The Forfeited Self," Friedan applied humanistic psychology to defend women's pursuit of self-fulfillment: "It is surely as true of women's whole human potential what earlier psychological theorists have only deemed true of her sexual potential—that if she is barred from realizing her true nature, she will be sick."[29] For women, creating an authentic self requires pursuing opportunities to engage in meaningful and fairly paid work, just as it does for men. It also requires consciousness raising in which women learn to trust their voices and engage in "talk therapy" (honest communication) within self-help/ mutual aid groups.

Friedan applied humanistic psychology to critique Freudian psychology, reminding us that the therapeutic trend is not a monolithic movement. More recently, feminist therapies and feminist spirituality forged new links between morality and mental health. In *Revolution from Within: A Book of Self-Esteem*, Gloria Steinem embraces the self-esteem movement, linking it to meditation and spiritual practices. Citing Gandhi and other political-spiritual leaders, she suggests that self-esteem provides a new "prism" through which to view social causes: "Self-esteem plays as much a part in the destiny of nations as it does in the lives of individuals," and "self-hatred leads to the need either to dominate or to be dominated."[30] Self-esteem and self-respect constitute an important dimension of social justice, as well as personal fulfillment.

The therapeutic trend had a role in other rights movements during the twentieth century. Eva S. Moskowitz, who is generally critical of the therapeutic trend (as noted in the introduction), acknowledges the valuable contribution of therapeutic outlooks to social activism. She documents, for example, how the therapeutic trend influenced the civil rights movement. The National Association for the Advancement of Colored People (NAACP) relied on psychological studies in pressuring changes in the courts. Most notably, it successfully lobbied in support of *Brown v. Board of Education*, convincing the Supreme Court that forcible segregation damages black students by creating feelings of inferiority and self-doubt. As early as 1939, psychologists and sociologists began to document subtle damage to the self-esteem of black children when they identify with white rather than black dolls. And activists in the Black Power movement, such as Eldridge Cleaver, relied on Frantz Fanon's *Wretched of the Earth* to explore how colonization created a social-wide "inferiority complex." Such examples led Moskowitz to envision the need for "a politics and a therapeutics that are not mutually exclusive. . . . We must be wary of vapid public therapies offered while remaining open to the possibilities of a therapeutic politics that enhances social life."[31]

Meaningful lives have innumerable forms, but philanthropy has an important role in many of them by connecting personal meaning with the needs of community.[32] In igniting the therapeutic trend, Freud neglected community and stereotyped morality as unhealthy ideals. Then, in attacking the therapeutic trend, Rieff downplayed self-fulfillment and stereotyped therapy as self-absorbed. By setting morality and therapy in opposition, both thinkers obscured as much as they clarified. An integrated, moral-therapeutic perspective enables us to appreciate the confluence of morality and mental health in meaningful lives of service.

EPILOGUE

Culture Wars

America's therapeutic trend in ethics—the tendency to approach moral matters in terms of mental health—was politicized by America's culture wars during the second half of the twentieth century. Whether in thinking about addictions, crime, homosexuality, or self-esteem in education, liberals tended to embrace health-oriented approaches to moral issues, and conservatives tended to be alarmed by them. There were major cross-currents, however. Civil libertarians, concerned about therapeutic tyranny, sided with cultural conservatives in opposing the replacement of punishment with therapy. So did some liberals who believed the self-oriented bent of therapy diluted the stringent demands of social justice. Conversely, some conservatives borrowed heavily from therapeutic ideas in refashioning new forms of spirituality and religious practice. Often unheard were the voices of moderates who discerned promise and peril on both sides of the controversy.

The legacy of the culture wars is a polarized, confusing, and yet creative context for exploring Plato's proposal that morality and mental health are intimately connected in their meaning and reference. Although my interest is philosophical rather than political, I conclude by commenting on the political resonance of my three themes: healthy morality, responsibility for health, and mental health as moral-laden.

The first theme, healthy morality, is usually associated with progressive, re-form-minded liberals, those initially inspired by Freud but today oriented to the cumulative contributions of psychology, psychiatry, and the social sciences. Their concern was that traditional moral emphases on guilt, blame, punishment, and unrealistic other-worldly ideals were obstacles to human fulfillment. A few liberal-minded therapists, such as Karl Menninger and James Gilligan, called for replacing morality with therapy—replacement projects that I reject as muddled and dangerous. In the main, however, the public eagerly embraced the idea that moral standards should be psychologically realistic, rooted in authentic com-mitments, and supportive of self-fulfillment. Humanistic psychologists like Erich

Fromm and Abraham Maslow wrote popular books integrating moral values with therapeutic insights. The same occurs today, as "positive psychologists" more explicitly discuss moral matters in therapeutic terms, communicating their approaches to the public through a massive self-help industry that is sometimes superficial and other times illuminating.

The second theme, responsibility for health, is usually associated with conservatives. They emphasize obligations to shun harmful addictions and to accept responsibility for unhealthy habits. Cultural conservatives like Philip Rieff and the communitarian Robert Bellah object that the therapeutic trend makes virtually all forms of irresponsible conduct into sickness, which is then perceived as a basis for excusing wrongdoing or mitigating blameworthiness. In response, I argue that responsibilities for health, as grounded in Kant's basic duties of self-respect, can be taken seriously without opposing the main currents in the therapeutic trend. Rather than stereotyping "the" therapeutic stance as self-absorbed, conservatives should build on the attitude expressed in the *DSM*'s Cautionary Note: sickness is not an automatic excuse for wrongdoing. This attitude grows in importance as the catalogue of unhealthy behaviors continues to expand, driven in part by the *DSM* definition of mental disorders as patterns of behavior and emotion (emphasizing distress, disability, and dangers) whose etiology sometimes involves choices as well as genetic and environmental causes.

At the same time, I argue that responsibility for causing and curing health problems needs to be examined contextually. Sometimes sickness does exempt from responsibility—especially a serious mental illness that has been caused by organic incapacitations which individuals cannot reasonably be expected to avoid or to overcome without help; other times we are responsible, in various degrees, for the harm caused by our unhealthy habits and pathologically destructive conduct; still other times the exact interplay of bad habits, bad environment, and bad genes is morally indecipherable. A caring society will be wary of unjust and uncompassionate blaming of victims of illness, insensitivity to their social burdens, and stigmatizing the mentally ill. It will provide necessary assistance for individuals, as resources permit, and establish public health measures to support healthy and responsible conduct. But it will also take a firm stand against violence, bigotry, and oppression in which sickness may be present but does not excuse. A humane society will also emphasize that accepting personal responsibility is as central to healing as it is to moral involvement in communities.

The third theme, that moral values are embedded in mental health and psychotherapy, provides common ground for all sectors of the political spectrum, albeit with differing emphases. Civil libertarians rightly caution that disguising moral assumptions in therapeutic approaches can lead to therapeutic tyranny, to oppression disguised as science. Conservatives can derive inspiration from Plato, filtered through various religious traditions, that virtue is the health of the soul. And liberals ground progressive changes in conceptions of positive health that accent self-worth and self-fulfillment. All these groups rightly demand greater explicitness about the moral values embedded in concepts of mental disorders and positive health, as well as in particular therapeutic techniques and goals.

My themes provide ammunition for liberals and conservatives alike, but its main payoff is for pragmatic moderates who give balanced emphasis to all three themes. My sense is that most Americans are somewhere in this middle ground, and hence I am generally optimistic about the creative direction of the therapeutic trend. Even so, cogently integrating morality and therapy will require greater clarity in public debates. We must learn to avoid seductive but simplistic attitudes—for example, that sickness is an automatic excuse (overlooking the *DSM* Cautionary Statement), that morality is essentially about blame for violating obligations (neglecting the virtues), and that therapy is morally neutral (confusing nonjudgmental helping with amorality).

As citizens, we can participate in public debates about what healthy morality is, the extent of personal and societal responsibilities for health, and which moral values should enter into conceptions of mental disorders and positive health. Even more in our personal lives, we can articulate and act on our moral outlooks as they pertain to mental health. These freedoms are central to democratic pluralism. Not all views are equally justified, of course, and here, as elsewhere, sound moral reasoning is essential.

Whether in politics or private life, we should be prepared to ask three sets of questions about specific aspects of the therapeutic trend. First, regarding healthy morality: Are moral values and mental-health approaches integrated in clear ways, or is a muddled attempt under way to replace morality with mental health? Is it understood that mental health is moral-laden, rather than an amoral value incommensurate with the virtues? Are false stereotypes and constricted views of morality (as nothing but guilt and blame) and therapy (as nonmoral and deterministic) introduced? Is balanced attention given to needs of the self and requirements of communities? If a therapeutic critique of traditional morality is undertaken, is the critique based on a sound moral perspective, or do the therapeutic attitudes degenerate into ethical subjectivism and egoism?

Second, regarding responsibilities for health: Are these responsibilities taken seriously and yet coordinated with other responsibilities? Is sickness being used to excuse? If so, is the excuse based on a reasonable interpretation of the special obstacles confronting the individual, or is there an unspoken and unwarranted assumption that sickness automatically excuses? Is attention paid to different aspects of disorders—to their causes, cures, defining features, and harm caused under the influence of the disorder? And is due care taken in adjusting to different health-related contexts, such as preventing sickness, assigning financial liabilities for health care costs, giving meaning to suffering, and interacting with health care professionals?

Third, regarding the embeddedness of moral values in mental health: Exactly which moral values are being assumed in defining mental disorders and positive mental health? Are the values so fundamental that we might expect all reasonable persons to share them, or do they represent controversial moral revisions? Even if the values are elemental ones such as vitality, self-worth, and self-mastery, are they interpreted narrowly, in the egoistic directions charted by Freud and Nietzsche? Is it understood that moral judgments can and should be supported by sound moral reasons, that morality includes self-respect and duties to ourselves as well as to others, and that health-oriented critiques of morality are themselves subject to rational scrutiny?

The culture wars impede answers to these questions whenever a morality-therapy dichotomy is invoked, but responsible political discourse can stimulate helpful answers. I am not calling for de-politicizing the therapeutic trend. The trend is far too important to avoid interacting with political ideals which in a democracy will always be contested. My hope is simply that disagreements become less about the legitimacy of the therapeutic trend and more about specific areas of promise and peril. As Dewey envisioned, an integrated, moral-therapeutic understanding can help us to "locate the points of effective endeavor," "focus available resources upon them," and exercise "creative intelligence" in uniting the needs of individuals with the requirements of community.[1]

NOTES

Introduction

1. Rem B. Edwards, "The Medical Model and Disvalues in Psychiatric Classification," in Rem B. Edwards, ed., *Ethics of Psychiatry* (Amherst, Mass.: Prometheus Books, 1997), p. 103.

2. Gabriel Fackre, ed., *Judgment Day at the White House* (Grand Rapids, Mich.: William B. Eerdmans, 1999).

3. John J. Goldman, "Swan Song for Jules Feiffer's Satiric Dancer," *Los Angeles Times* (June 17, 2000), pp. F1, F22.

4. Jerome D. Levin, *The Clinton Syndrome: The President and the Self-Destructive Nature of Sexual Addiction* (Rocklin, Calif.: Prima, 1998).

5. Of course, those who admire Clinton's sexual bravado will deny he is either sick or immoral.

6. Greg Krikorian and Beth Shuster, "L.A. Mayor Calls for Hernandez to Quit Council," *Los Angeles Times* (Oct. 28, 1997), pp. A1, A24; and Betty Wyman, "Applaud Hernandez for Courage," *Los Angeles Times*, editorial page (Nov. 6, 1997).

7. Carl Elliott, *Better Than Well: American Medicine Meets the American Dream* (New York: W.W. Norton, 2003).

8. Ronald Bayer, *Homosexuality and American Psychiatry* (Princeton, N.J.: Princeton University Press, 1987).

9. A. W. Richard Sipe, *Sex, Priests, and Power: Anatomy of a Crisis* (New York: Brunner/Mazel, 1995); and Frank Bruni and Elinor Burkett, *A Gospel of Shame: Children, Sexual Abuse, and the Catholic Church* (New York: Perennial, 2002).

10. Johanna McGeary, "Can the Church Be Saved?," *Time*, 159, no. 13 (Apr.1, 2002), pp. 29–40.

11. James Gilligan, "Beyond Morality: Psychoanalytic Reflections on Shame, Guilt, and Love," in Thomas Lickona, ed., *Moral Development and Behavior* (New York: Holt, Rinehart and Winston, 1976), p. 145.

12. Philip Rieff, The *Triumph of the Therapeutic* (Chicago: University of Chicago, 1987 [1966]).

13. C. R. Snyder and Shane J. Lopez, eds., *Handbook of Positive Psychology* (New York: Oxford University Press, 2002), pp. 6–7, 45, 53.

14. Mildred Blaxter, *Health* (Cambridge, Mass.: Polity Press, 2004).

15. American Psychiatric Association, *Diagnostic and Statistical Manual of Mental Disorders,* Fourth Edition, Text Revision (Washington, D.C.: American Psychiatric Association, 2000). (Cited as *DSM* in the text.)

16. Robert L. Woolfolk, *The Cure of Souls: Science, Values, and Psychotherapy* (San Francisco: Jossey-Bass, 1998), p. 116.

17. Eva S. Moskowitz, *In Therapy We Trust: America's Obsession with Self-Fulfillment* (Baltimore: Johns Hopkins University Press, 2001).

18. Ibid., pp. 2–3, 6–7.

19. Ibid., p. 284.

20. William James, *Essays on Faith and Morals*, ed. Ralph Barton Perry (New York: Meridian Books, 1962), p. 160.

21. Ibid., pp. 131, 89.

22. Ibid., p. 241.

23. William James, *The Principles of Psychology* (New York: Dover, 1950 [1890]), vol. 1, p. 122.

24. John Dewey, *Human Nature and Conduct* (New York: Modern Library, 1957), pp. 37, 47.

25. Ibid., p. 25.

26. Ibid., p. 4.

27. Ibid., p. 292.

28. John Dewey, *Reconstruction in Philosophy* (Boston: Beacon Press, 1957), p. 172.

29. Dewey, *Human Nature and Conduct*, p. 5.

30. Ibid., pp. 12–13.

31. For example, Erich Fromm, *Man for Himself: An Inquiry into the Psychology of Ethics* (New York: Fawcett Publications, 1965 [1947]). Humanistic psychologists deserve praise, however, for integrating morality and mental health.

32. Dewey, *Human Nature and Conduct*, pp. 181–186; and Dewey, *The Theory of the Moral Life* (New York: Holt, Rinehart and Winston, 1960), p. 141. James D. Wallace insightfully discusses Dewey in *Moral Relevance and Moral Conduct* (Ithaca, N.Y.: Cornell University Press, 1988).

33. Dewey, *Reconstruction in Philosophy*, p. 167. Cf. D. Micah Hester, *Community as Healing: Pragmatist Ethics in Medical Encounters* (Lanham, Md.: Rowman and Littlefield, 2001), pp. 71–73.

34. Dewey, *Human Nature and Conduct*, p. 130.

35. John Dewey, "A Sick World," in Jo Ann Boydston, ed., *John Dewey: The Middle Works* (Carbondale: Southern Illinois University Press, 1983), vol. 15, pp. 43–44.

36. Of special interest, see Arthur E. Murphy, "The Moral Self in Sickness and in Health," in A. I. Melden, ed., *The Theory of Practical Reason* (La Salle, Ill.: Open Court, 1965), pp. 134–161.

37. Plato, *Republic*, trans. F. M. Cornford (New York: Oxford University Press, 1945), 444e.

38. Lawrence C. Becker, *A New Stoicism* (Princeton, N.J.: Princeton University Press, 1998), p. 104; italics deleted.

39. Ibid.

40. Cf. James Rachels, *Elements of Moral Philosophy*, 4th ed. (Boston: McGraw-Hill, 2003), pp. 188–189.

41. Neal O. Weiner, *Harmony of the Soul: Mental Health and Moral Virtue Reconsidered* (Albany, N.Y.: State University of New York Press, 1993), p. 16.

Chapter 1: Moral sickness

1. Plato, *Republic*, trans. F. M. Cornford (New York: Oxford University Press, 1945), 444e.

2. For example, Anthony Kenny, *The Anatomy of the Soul* (London: Basil Blackwell, 1973), pp. 1–27.

3. Darcy O'Brien, *Power to Hurt* (New York: HarperCollins, 1997), p. 454.

4. Jonathan Jacobs, *Choosing Character: Responsibility for Virtue and Vice* (Ithaca, N.Y.: Cornell University Press, 2001).

5. Cf. Arthur E. Murphy, "The Moral Self in Sickness and in Health," in Arthur E. Murphy, *The Theory of Practical Reason*, ed. A. I. Melden (La Salle, Ill.: Open Court, 1965), pp. 134–161.

6. Mary Midgley, *Wickedness* (London: Routledge and Kegan Paul, 1984), p. 147.

7. Martha C. Nussbaum, *The Therapy of Desire: Theory and Practice in Hellenistic Ethics* (Princeton, N.J.: Princeton University Press, 1994), p. 13.

8. Richard Norman, *The Moral Philosophers*, 2d ed. (New York: Oxford University Press, 1998), pp. 11–26.

9. Plato, *Republic*, 571–572.

10. American Psychiatric Association, *Diagnostic and Statistical Manual of Mental Disorders,* Fourth Edition, Text Revision (Washington, D.C.: American Psychiatric Association, 2000), pp. 147–171.

11. American Psychiatric Association, *Diagnostic and Statistical Manual of Mental Disorders*, p. xxxi.

12. Ibid.

13. Cf. Neal O. Weiner, *The Harmony of the Soul: Mental Health and Moral Virtue Reconsidered* (Albany: State University of New York Press, 1993); John Z. Sadler, Osborne P. Wiggins, and Michael A. Schwartz, eds., *Philosophical Perspectives on Psychiatric Diagnostic Classification* (Baltimore: Johns Hopkins University Press, 1994); and Herb Kutchins and Stuart A. Kirk, *Making Us Crazy* (New York: Free Press, 1997).

14. That might change in future editions of the *DSM*, as powerful new drugs and brain research reshape psychiatry and psychology. See Allan V. Horwitz, *Creating Mental Illness* (Chicago: University of Chicago Press, 2002), pp. 132–157; and Valerie Gray Hardcastle, ed., *Where Biology Meets Psychology: Philosophical Essays* (Cambridge, Mass.: MIT Press, 1999).

15. American Psychiatric Association, *Diagnostic and Statistical Manual of Mental Disorders*, p. 197.

16. Ibid., p. 663.

17. Ibid., p. 685.

18. Ibid., p. xxxvii.

19. Thomas S. Szasz, *The Myth of Mental Illness*, rev. ed. (New York: Harper and Row, 1974).

20. Robert B. Baker, "Pathologizing Homosexuality," in Robert B. Baker, Kathleen J. Wininger, and Frederick A. Elliston, eds., *Philosophy and Sex*, 3d ed. (Amherst, N.Y.: Prometheus Books, 1998), p. 379.

21. Peter Conrad and Joseph W. Schneider, *Deviance and Medicalization: From Badness to Sickness* (Philadelphia: Temple University Press, 1992), p. 1 fn.

22. For example, see Nicholas Kittrie, *The Right to Be Different: Deviance and Enforced Therapy* (Baltimore: Johns Hopkins Press, 1971); Ivan Illich, *Medical Nemesis* (New York: Bantam, 1976); and Michel Foucault, *Madness and Civilization*, trans. Richard Howard (New York: Vintage, 1988).

23. Kenny, *Anatomy of the Soul*, pp. 24–25.

24. Ian Hacking, *Rewriting the Soul* (Princeton, N.J.: Princeton University Press, 1995); and Hacking, "The Looping Effects of Human Kinds," in D. Sperber, D. Premack, and A. J. Premack, eds., *Causal Cognition: A Multidisciplinary Approach* (Oxford: Clarendon, 1994), pp. 351–394.

25. Margaret Olivia Little calls this "cultural complicity" in "Cosmetic Surgery, Suspect Norms and the Ethics of Complicity," in Erik Parens, ed., *Enhancing Human Traits* (Washington, D.C.: Georgetown University Press, 1998), pp. 162–176.

26. Carl Elliott, *Better Than Well: American Medicine Meets the American Dream* (New York: W.W. Norton, 2003), p. 230.

27. Rem B. Edwards, ed., *Ethics of Psychiatry* (Amherst, Mass.: Prometheus Books, 1997), p. 17. Also see Robert L. Woolfolk, "The Concept of Mental Illness: An Analysis of Four Pivotal Issues," *Journal of Mind and Behavior*, 22, no. 2 (2001): 161–178.

28. Cf. Bernard Gert and Charles M. Culver, "Defining Mental Disorder," in Jennifer Radden, ed., *The Philosophy of Psychiatry: A Companion* (New York: Oxford University Press, 2004), pp. 415–425.

29. Kenny, *Anatomy of the Soul*, pp. 25, 26.

30. Thomas S. Szasz, "The Myth of Mental Illness," in Rem B. Edwards, ed., *Ethics of Psychiatry* (Amherst, N.Y.: Prometheus Books, 1997); quotations from pp. 27, 31, 26 (italics removed). First published in *American Psychologist*, 15 (1960): 113–118.

31. Mark Pestana, *Moral Virtue or Mental Health?* (New York: Peter Lang, 1998); quotations from pp. 95, 103, 96.

32. Pestana attempts to bolster his view by citing Marie Jahoda's conception of positive health, but in doing so he misinterprets her criteria as mere potentialities instead of actual tendencies. See my discussion of Jahoda in chapter 2.

33. Influenced by Pestana, Per-Anders Tengland equates (positive) mental health with individuals' "mental abilities to reach [their] vital goals." This leads him to the odd conclusion that a person can be fully healthy while adopting abhorrent goals such as those of the pedophile or sadist. Tengland, *Mental Health: A Philosophical Analysis* (Dordrecht: Kluwer Academic, 2001), pp. 94 (italics removed), 92–93, 170.

34. Rem B. Edwards, "Mental Health as Rational Autonomy," in Rem B. Edwards, ed., *Ethics of Psychiatry* (Amherst, N.Y.: Prometheus Books, 1997), pp. 52–53.

35. Jerome C. Wakefield, "The Concept of Mental Disorder," *American Psychologist*, 47 (March 1992): 374.

36. Ruth Benedict, "Anthropology and the Abnormal," *Journal of General Psychology* 10 (1934): 59–82 .

37. Foucault, *Madness and Civilization*.

38. Conrad and Schneider, *Deviance and Medicalization*, pp. 2, 223.

Chapter 2: Moral Health

1. Preamble to the Constitution of the World Health Organization, *Official Record of the World Health Organization* (Geneva: World Health Organization, 1946), vol. 2, p. 100.

2. Daniel Callahan, "The WHO Definition of 'Health,'" *Hastings Center Studies*, 1, no. 3 (1973).

3. Marie Jahoda, *Current Concepts of Mental Health* (New York: Basic Books, 1958), p. 3.

4. Ibid., p. 23. I rename and refocus some of Jahoda's categories. For example, I use "self-esteem" to refer to "attitudes of an individual toward his own self," under which she includes self-esteem, self-acceptance, self-confidence, self-respect, and self-reliance (pp. 23–24).

5. Shelley E. Taylor, *Positive Illusions: Creative Self-Deception and the Healthy Mind* (New York: Basic Books, 1989), p. 227.

6. David Sachs, "How to Distinguish Self-Respect from Self-Esteem," *Philosophy and Public Affairs*, 10 (1981): 346–360.

7. John Rawls, *A Theory of Justice*, rev. ed. (Cambridge: Harvard University Press, 1999), p. 386.

8. Stephen J. Massey, "Is Self-Respect a Moral or a Psychological Concept?" *Ethics*, 93 (1983). Cf. Robert N. Campbell, *The New Science: Self-Esteem Psychology* (Lanham, Md.: University Press of America, 1984), pp. 7–8.

9. Alan Gewirth, *Self-Fulfillment* (Princeton, N.J.: Princeton University Press, 1998), pp. 94–95.

10. Nathaniel Branden, *The Psychology of Self-Esteem* (New York: Bantam, 1969), p. 110. Although Branden's conception is not wholly subjective, it has a self-interested bent linked to his ethical egoism—morality as maximizing one's self-interest. See his essays in Ayn Rand, *The Virtue of Selfishness* (New York: New American Library, 1964).

11. Richard L. Bednar and Scott R. Peterson, *Self-Esteem: Paradoxes and Innovations in Clinical Theory and Practice*, 2d ed. (Washington, D.C.: American Psychological Association, 1995), p. 4.

12. Thomas Hill, *Autonomy and Self-Respect* (New York: Cambridge University Press, 1991); quotations from pp. 5–6. Also see p. 11.

13. Theodore Rubin, *Through My Own Eyes* (New York: Macmillan, 1982), pp. 171–172.

14. American Psychiatric Association, *Diagnostic and Statistical Manual of Mental Disorders,* Fourth Edition, Text Revision (Washington, D.C.: American Psychiatric Association, 2000), p. 725.

15. Rubin, *Through My Own Eyes*, p. 172.

16. American Psychiatric Association, *Diagnostic and Statistical Manual of Mental Disorders*, pp. 714–717.

17. Hill, *Autonomy and Self-Respect*, pp. 156–157.

18. Stephen L. Darwall, "Two Kinds of Respect," *Ethics*, 88 (1977).

19. Immanuel Kant, *Lectures on Ethics*, trans. Louis Infield (New York: Harper Torchbooks, 1963).

20. Linda Tschirhart Sanford and Mary Ellen Donovan, *Women and Self-Esteem* (New York: Penguin, 1984), pp. 9–10.

21. Neil J. Smelser, "Self-Esteem and Social Problems: An Introduction," in Andrew M. Mecca, Neil J. Smelser, and John Vasconcellos, eds., *The Social Importance of Self-Esteem* (Berkeley: University of California Press, 1989), p. 11.

22. Jahoda, *Current Concepts of Mental Health*, p. 36.

23. Amelie Rorty, "Integrity: Political, Not Psychological," in Alan Montefiore and David Vines, eds., *Integrity in the Public and Private Domains* (New York: Routledge, 1999), p. 113.

24. Jahoda, *Current Concepts of Mental Health*, pp. 39–40

25. Margaret Cohen, "A Psychoanalytic View of the Notion of Integrity," in Alan Montefiore and David Vines, eds., *Integrity in the Public and Private Domains* (New York: Routledge, 1999), p. 88.

26. Amelie Oksenberg Rorty, "Integrity: Political, Not Psychological," in Alan Montefiore and David Vines, eds., *Integrity in the Public and Private Domains* (New York: Routledge, 1999), pp. 108–109.

27. A similar criticism can be raised against John Rawls, who thinks of the virtues of integrity as purely formal, with minimal content. Rawls, *A Theory of Justice*, p. 456.

28. Edward Erwin, *Philosophy and Psychotherapy* (London: Sage Publications, 1997), pp. 1, 30.

29. Jahoda, *Current Concepts of Mental Health*, p. 45.

30. Diana T. Meyers, *Self, Society, and Personal Choice* (New York: Columbia University Press, 1989), p. 76.

31. Ibid., pp. 19, 63.

32. Abraham H. Maslow, "Comments on Dr. Frankl's Paper," in Anthony J. Sutich and Miles A. Vich, eds., *Readings in Humanistic Psychology* (New York: Free Press, 1969), pp. 128–129.

33. Charles Taylor, *The Ethics of Authenticity* (Cambridge, Mass.: Harvard University Press, 1992), p. 39.

34. Robert J. Lifton, *The Protean Self* (New York: Basic Books, 1993); and Kenneth J. Gergen, *The Saturated Self* (New York: Basic Books, 1991).

35. Susan Harter, "Authenticity," in C. R. Snyder and Shane J. Lopez, eds., *Handbook of Positive Psychology* (New York: Oxford University Press, 2002), p. 392.

36. Abraham H. Maslow, *The Farther Reaches of Human Nature* (New York: Penguin, 1976), p. 41.

37. Alan Gewirth, *Self-Fulfillment*, p. 160.

38. Ibid., p. 32.

39. Jahoda, *Current Concepts of Mental Health*, p. 53.

40. C. R. Snyder and Beth L. Dinoff, "Coping: Where Have You Been?," in C. R. Snyder, ed., *Coping: The Psychology of What Works* (New York: Oxford University Press, 1999), p. 5.

41. "Slide to subjectivism" is used by Charles Taylor in *The Ethics of Authenticity* (Cambridge, Mass.: Harvard University Press, 1992).

42. See, for example, C. R. Snyder and Shane J. Lopez, eds., *Handbook of Positive Psychology* (New York: Oxford University Press, 2002).

43. Michael E. McCullough and C. R. Snyder, "Classical Sources of Human Strength: Revisiting an Old Home and Building a New One," *Journal of Social and Clinical Psychology*, 19 (2000): 1–10. The authors draw on I. A. M. Nicholson, "Gordon Allport, Character, and the 'Culture of Personality,'" *History of Psychology*, 1 (1998): 52–68.

44. Carol D. Ryff and Burton Singer, "The Contours of Positive Human Health," *Psychological Inquiry*, 9 (1998): 2.

45. Carol D. Ryff and Burton Singer, "From Social Structure to Biology: Integrative Science in Pursuit of Human Health and Well-Being," in C. R. Snyder and Shane J. Lopez, eds., *Handbook of Positive Psychology* (New York: Oxford University Press, 2002), pp. 540–555.

46. Carol D. Ryff, "Happiness Is Everything, or Is It? Explorations on the Meaning of Psychological Well-Being," *Journal of Personality and Social Psychology*, 57 (1989): 1072.

47. Carol D. Ryff and Burton Singer, "Human Health: New Directions for the Next Millennium," *Psychological Inquiry*, 9 (1998): 73.

48. Similar comments apply to Martin E. P. Seligman's discussion of the scientific study of values in *Authentic Happiness* (New York: Free Press, 2002), p. 129.

Chapter 3: Sick Morality

1. Edwin R. Wallace, "Freud as Ethicist," in Paul E. Stepansky, ed., *Freud: Appraisals and Reappraisals* (New York: Analytic Press, 1986), p. 84.

2. Friedrich Nietzsche, *On the Genealogy of Morality*, trans. Maudemarie Clark and Alan J. Swensen (Indianapolis: Hackett, 1998 [1887]), p. 56; and Sigmund Freud, *Civilization and Its Discontents*, trans. James Strachey (New York: W.W. Norton, 1989 [1930]), p. 97.

3. Irvin D. Yalom, "'The Wrong One Died,'" in *Love's Executioner and Other Tales of Psychotherapy* (New York: HarperPerennial, 1989), pp. 118–143.

4. R. Jay Wallace, *Responsibility and the Moral Sentiments* (Cambridge, Mass.: Harvard University Press, 1996), pp. 40–50. Herbert Morris objects to the therapeutic eclipse of guilt, but his objection applies only to replacement projects, not integrative projects. Morris, "The Decline of Guilt," in John Deigh, *Ethics and Personality: Essays in Moral Psychology* (Chicago: University of Chicago Press, 1992), p. 126.

5. Freud, "Mourning and Melancholia," in *General Psychological Theory* (New York: Collier Books, 1963), p. 167.

6. Freud, *Civilization and Its Discontents*, p. 99.

7. Ibid., p. 108.

8. Ibid., pp. 55, 57, 66.

9. Philip Reiff, *Freud: The Mind of the Moralist*, 3d ed. (Chicago: University of Chicago Press, 1979), p. 354. See also Richard H. Price, *Abnormal Behavior* (New York: Holt, Rinehart and Winston, 1972), p. 44.

10. Freud, *Civilization and Its Discontents*, p. 110.

11. Sigmund Freud, *New Introductory Lectures on Psychoanalysis*, trans. James Strachey (New York: W.W. Norton, 1965), p. 162.

12. Ibid., pp. 108–109.

13. Ibid., p. 56.

14. Morris Ginsberg, "Psycho-Analysis and Ethics," in Brian A. Farrell, ed., *Philosophy and Psychoanalysis* (New York: Macmillan, 1994), p. 130.

15. Friedrich Nietzsche, *The Gay Science*, trans. Walter Kaufmann (New York: Vintage Books, 1974), p. 35.

16. Nietzsche says surprisingly little about sex, however. See Eric Blondel, "Nietzsche and Freud, or: How to Be within Philosophy While Criticizing It from Without," in Jacob Golomb, Weaver Santaniello, and Ronald Lehrer, eds., *Nietzsche and Depth Psychology* (Albany: State University of New York Press, 1999), p. 178.

17. Nietzsche, *On the Genealogy of Morality*, pp. 4, 2, 102.

18. Friedrich Nietzsche, *Daybreak*, trans. R. J. Hollingdale, ed. Maudemarie Clark and Brian Leiter (New York: Cambridge University Press, 1997), sec. 103.

19. Cf. David Couzens Hoy, "Nietzsche, Hume, and the Genealogical Method," in Richard Schacht, ed., *Nietzsche, Genealogy, Morality* (Berkeley: University of California Press, 1994), p. 265; Daniel R. Ahern, *Nietzsche as Cultural Physician* (University Park: Pennsylvania State University Press, 1995), p. 4; and Friedrich Nietzsche, *Twilight of the Idols*, trans. Duncan Large (New York: Oxford University Press, 1998), p. 59.

20. Nietzsche, *The Gay Science*, secs. 120, 349, 382; Friedrich Nietzsche, *Ecco Homo* in Walter Kaufmann, ed., *Basic Writings of Nietzsche* (New York: Modern Library, 1968), p. 680; and David Farrell Krell, *Infectious Nietzsche* (Bloomington: Indiana University Press, 1996).

21. Friedrich Nietzsche, *The Will to Power*, trans. Walter Kaufmann and R. J. Hollingdale (New York: Vintage Books, 1968), sec. 1013.

22. Nietzsche, *On the Genealogy of Morality*, pp. 16, 66. The tension between honesty and health-promoting illusions is most fully explored in Friedrich Nietzsche, *On the Advantage and Disadvantage of History for Life*, trans. Peter Preuss (Indianapolis: Hackett, 1980).

23. Richard Norman, *The Moral Philosophers*, 2d ed. (New York: Oxford University Press, 1998), p. 142; cf. Robert C. Solomon, "One Hundred Years of *Ressentiment*: Nietzsche's *Genealogy of Morals*," in Richard Schacht, ed., *Nietzsche, Genealogy, Morality* (Berkeley: University of California Press, 1994), p. 112. Brian Leiter suggests that health, for Nietzsche, is "something closer to resilience, to how one deals with ordinary (physical) sickness and setbacks." Leiter, *Nietzsche on Morality* (New York: Routledge, 2002), p. 119.

24. Ahern, *Nietzsche as Cultural Physician*, p. 19.

25. David Owen and Aaron Ridley, "Dramatis Personae: Nietzsche, Culture, and Human Types," in Alan D. Schrift, ed., *Why Nietzsche Still?* (Berkeley: University of California Press, 2000), p. 142.

26. Graham Parkes, *Composing the Soul: Reaches of Nietzsche's Psychology* (Chicago: University of Chicago Press, 1994), p. 377.

27. Nietzsche, *The Gay Science*, sec. 335; Friedrich Nietzsche, *Thus Spoke Zarathustra*, trans. Walter Kaufmann (New York: Penguin, 1978), pp. 58–60.

28. Nietzsche, *The Gay Science*, sec. 349; and Nietzsche, *On the Genealogy of Morality*, p. 42.

29. Friedrich Nietzsche, *Beyond Good and Evil*, trans. Walter Kaufmann (New York: Vintage Books, 1966), sec. 208; Nietzsche, *On the Genealogy of Morality*, p. 4.

30. Nietzsche, *The Gay Science*, secs. 305, 290.

31. Nietzsche, *The Will to Power*, sec. 778; cf. Nietzsche, *Daybreak*, sec. 109.

32. Nietzsche, *Thus Spoke Zarathustra*, p. 193.

33. Nietzsche, *The Gay Science*, sec. 334.

34. Nietzsche, *The Genealogy of Morality*, pp. 87–88.

35. Cf. Simon May, *Nietzsche's Ethics and His War on "Morality"* (Oxford: Clarendon Press, 1999).

36. Nietzsche, *The Genealogy of Morality*, pp. 19, 16, 30, 28, 21.

37. Ibid., p. 63.

38. Ibid., p. 116.

39. In *Thus Spoke Zarathustra*, the snake that chokes Zarathustra is the need to accept mass humanity in affirming the eternal recurrence of the world in all its "details."

40. Jonathan Glover, *Humanity: A Moral History of the Twentieth Century* (New Haven, Conn.: Yale University Press, 2000), p. 11.

41. Nietzsche, *Beyond Good and Evil*, sec. 259.

42. Max Scheler, *Ressentiment*, trans. William W. Holdheim (New York: Schocken Books, 1972).

43. Cf. Michael S. Moore, "The Moral Worth of Retribution," in Ferdinand Schoeman, ed., *Responsibility, Character, and the Emotions* (New York: Cambridge University Press, 1987), pp. 179–219.

44. Michael Friedman, "Toward a Reconceptualization of Guilt," *Contemporary Psychoanalysis*, 21 (1985): pp. 503–504. Cf. Herbert Morris, *On Guilt and Innocence* (Berkeley: University of California, 1976). John Dewey critiques Freud's theory of instincts in *Human Nature and Conduct* (New York: Modern Library, 1957 [1922]), pp. 140–156.

45. Erich Fromm, *Man for Himself: An Inquiry into the Psychology of Ethics* (New York: Fawcett Publications, 1965 [1947]), p. 17.

46. Erich Fromm, *The Art of Loving* (New York: Harper and Row, 1956).

47. Erich Fromm, *Man For Himself: An Inquiry into the Psychology of Ethics*, pp. 148–175.

48. Erich Fromm, *The Sane Society* (New York: Fawcett, 1965 [1955]), pp. 33–66. Also see Richard Norman, *The Moral Philosophers* (Oxford: Clarendon Press, 1983), pp. 202–224.

49. Bernard Williams, *Shame and Necessity* (Berkeley: University of California, 1993), p. 93.

50. Ibid., pp. 177, 174.

51. Ibid., pp. 93, 102.

52. For an illustration, see Virginia Woolf's story "The New Dress," in *A Haunted House and Other Short Stories* (New York: Harcourt Brace Jovanovich, 1972). Also, as discussed in chapter 11, James Gilligan offers a therapeutic critique of shame that is no less sweeping than Freud's and Nietzsche's critiques of guilt.

53. Cf. Michael Lewis, *Shame: The Exposed Self* (New York: Free Press, 1995); and Thomas J. Scheff and Suzanne M. Retzinger, *Emotions and Violence: Shame and Rage in Destructive Conflicts* (Lexington, Mass.: Lexington Books, 1991).

54. Gabriele Taylor, *Pride, Shame, and Guilt* (Oxford: Clarendon Press, 1985), p. 132.

55. R. Fitzgibbons, "Anger and the Healing Power of Forgiveness: A Psychiatrist's View," in R. D. Enright and J. North, eds., *Exploring Forgiveness* (Madison: University of Wisconsin Press, 1998), p. 63. See also Mary Sherrill Durham, *The Therapist's Encounters with Revenge and Forgiveness* (London: Jessica Kingsley, 2000), p. 7; Beverly Flanigan, *Forgiving Yourself* (New York: Macmillan, 1996); Michael E. McCullough, Kenneth I. Pargament, and Carl E. Thoresen, eds., *Forgiveness: Theory, Research, and Practice* (New York: Guilford Press, 2000). Forgiveness is also receiving renewed attention in philosophy: for example, Jeffrie G. Murphy and Jean Hampton, *Forgiveness and Mercy* (New York: Cambridge University Press, 1988); and Joram Graf Haber, *Forgiveness: A Philosophical Study* (Lanham, Md.: Rowman and Littlefield, 1991.

56. An example of this excess is Marietta Jaeger, "The Power and Reality of Forgiveness: Forgiving the Murderer of One's Child," in R. D. Enright and J. North, eds., *Exploring Forgiveness* (Madison: University of Wisconsin Press, 1998), p. 10.

57. Cf. John Dewey, *Human Nature and Conduct* (New York: Modern Library, 1957), pp. 292–293.

58. Cf. Gregory Kavka, *Hobbesian Moral and Political Theory* (Princeton, N.J.: Princeton University Press, 1986).

Chapter 4: Responsibility in Therapy

1. Brief quotations are from Samuel Butler, *Erewhon* (New York: New American Library, 1960 [1872]), pp. 78–101. In an afterword (pp. 233–240), Kingsley Amis discusses the multilayered satire in the novel.

2. Butler, *Erewhon*, p. 87.

3. Ibid, p. 80.

4. Ibid, p. 89.

5. Allan M. Brandt and Paul Rozin, eds., *Morality and Health* (New York: Routledge, 1997).

6. The idea of responsibilities for health has a long lineage. See S. J. Reiser, "Responsibility for Personal Health: A Historical Perspective," *Journal of Medicine and Philosophy*, 10 (1985): 7–17; Meredith Minkler, "Personal Responsibility for Health: Contexts and Controversies," in Daniel Callahan, ed., *Promoting Healthy Behavior: How Much Freedom? Whose Responsibility?* (Washington, D.C.: Georgetown University Press, 2002), pp. 1–22; Daniel Callahan, "Freedom, Healthism, and Health Promotion: Finding the Right Balance," in the same volume, pp. 138–152; and Daniel Callahan, *False Hopes* (New York: Simon and Schuster, 1998), pp. 173–207.

7. Tibor R. Machan, "Morality and Smoking," in David Benatar, ed., *Ethics for Everyday* (Boston: McGraw-Hill, 2002), pp. 627–637.

8. John Stuart Mill, *On Liberty* (Indianapolis: Hackett, 1978), p. 80.

9. John H. Knowles, "The Responsibility of the Individual," Daedelus, 106 (1977): 59.

10. Ibid., p. 75.

11. Edmund L. Pincoffs, *Quandaries and Virtues* (Lawrence: University Press of Kansas, 1986).

12. Immanuel Kant, *Lectures on Ethics*, trans. Louis Infield (New York: Harper and Row, 1963), p. 123.

13. Cf. Robin S. Dillon, "Toward a Feminist Conception of Self-Respect," *Hypatia*, 7 (1992): 52–69.

14. E. D. Pellegrino, and D. C. Thomasma, *The Virtues of Medical Practice* (New York: Oxford University Press, 1993), p. 58; and Robert M. Veatch, *Basics of Bioethics* (Upper Saddle River, N.J.: Prentice Hall, 2000), p. 41.

15. Gerald Dworkin, "Paternalism," in Richard A. Wasserstrom, ed., *Morality and the Law* (Belmont, Calif.: Wadsworth, 1971).

16. Talcott Parsons, "Definitions of Health and Illness in the Light of American Values and Social Structure," in E. G. Jaco, ed., *Patients, Physicians and Illness*, 3d ed. (London: Free Press, 1979), p. 117; and Parsons, "The Sick Role and the Role of the Physician Reconsidered," *MMFQ: Health and Society*, 53 (Summer 1975), p. 262. Despite acknowledging patients' responsibility, critics of the sick role model believe its emphasis on "the good patient" fosters passivity toward health professionals, especially in hospital settings. See Shelley E. Taylor, *Health Psychology*, 4th ed. (Boston: McGraw-Hill, 1999), p. 259; and Robert M. Veatch, "The Medical Model: Its Nature and Problems," *Hastings Center Studies*, 1 (1976): 59–76.

17. Allen Frances and Michael B. First, *Am I Okay?: A Layman's Guide to the Psychiatrist's Bible* (New York: Touchstone, 1998), p. 416.

18. American Psychiatric Association, *Diagnostic and Statistical Manual of Mental Disorders*, Fourth Edition, Text Revision (Washington, D.C.: American Psychiatric Association, 2000), p. xxxvii.

19. Frances and First, *Am I Okay?* p. 416.

20. R. Jay Wallace, *Responsibility and the Moral Sentiments* (Cambridge, Mass.: Harvard University Press), p. 76.

21. Irvin D. Yalom, *The Gift of Therapy* (New York: HarperCollins, 2002), pp. 139–140.

22. Edward Erwin, *Philosophy and Psychotherapy* (London: Sage Publications, 1997, p. 30; cf. pp. 18, 24. Also see Ethel S. Person, *Feeling Strong* (New York: William Morrow, 2002).

23. Willard Gaylin, *How Psychotherapy Really Works* (Chicago: Contemporary Books, 2001), pp. 266–267.

24. More exactly, my view is soft determinism: compatibilism is true *and* all events and actions are determined. For the distinction, see Robert Kane, "Introduction" to Robert Kane, ed., *Free Will* (Malden, Mass., 2002), p. 22.

25. Daniel C. Dennett, *Elbow Room: The Varieties of Free Will Worth Wanting* (Cambridge, Mass.: MIT Press, 1984); and Dennett, *Freedom Evolves* (New York: Viking, 2003).

26. Owen Flanagan, *The Problem of the Soul: Two Visions of Mind and How to Reconcile Them* (New York: Basic Books, 2002), pp. 104–105.

27. See P. F. Strawson's reflections on his essay in, "P. F. Strawson Replies," in Zak Van Straaten, ed., *Philosophical Subjects: Essays Presented to P. F. Strawson* (Oxford: Clarendon Press, 1980), pp. 265, 8, 12, 8, 19. Strawson says, without elaboration, that the attitude of psychotherapists toward their patients "straddles" the opposition between participation and objectivity (p. 20). To the contrary, therapists and their patients share a moral and therapeutic relationship. See Jonathan Bennett, "Accountability," in Zak van Straaten, ed., *Philosophical Subjects: Essays Presented to P. F. Strawson* (Oxford: Clarendon Press, 1980), p. 35.

28. P. F. Strawson, "Freedom and Resentment," in *Freedom and Resentment and Other Essays* (London: Methuen and Co, 1974), p. 22.

29. In this he might have been influenced by the emotivism and noncognitivism popular at the time he wrote—that is, the view that moral judgment is little more than expressing attitudes. See T. M. Scanlon, "The Significance of Choice," in Sterling M. McMurrin, ed., *The Tanner Lecture on Human Values* (Salt Lake City: University of Utah Press, 1988), vol. 8, pp. 149–216; and Wallace, *Responsibility and the Moral Sentiments*, p. 74.

30. Wallace, *Responsibility and the Moral Sentiments*, p. 69.

31. Many others make this assumption, as well. They include Wallace in *Responsibility and the Moral Sentiments*, p. 155; and Susan Wolf, *Freedom within Reason* (New York: Oxford University Press, 1990), p. 71 (cf. p. 90, but also see p. 151 fn. 7).

32. Jonathan Jacobs, *Choosing Character: Responsibility for Virtue and Vice* (Ithaca, N.Y.: Cornell University Press, 2001), p. 1.

Chapter 5: Responsibility in Community

1. See also James L. Nolan Jr., *The Therapeutic State* (New York: New York University Press, 1998); Eva S. Moskowitz, *In Therapy We Trust* (Baltimore: Johns Hopkins University Press, 2001); and Christina Hoff Sommers and Sally Satel, *One Nation under Therapy: How the Helping Culture Is Eroding Self-Reliance* (New York: St. Martin's Press, 2005). Despite their generally polemical tone against what Sommers and Satel call "therapism," or what I call shallow versions of the therapeutic trend in ethics, in places these books gesture toward an integrated view. For example, see Sommers and Satel's discussion of addiction as both a moral and therapeutic matter (pp. 107–109).

2. James Davison Hunter, *The Death of Character* (New York: Basic Books, 2000), p. xiii.

3. Quoted by Caryn James, "Addicted to a Mob Family Potion," in *The New York Times on The Sopranos* (New York: ibooks, 2001), p. 119.

4. Glen O. Gabbard, *The Psychology of The Sopranos* (New York: Basic Books, 2002), p. 48. Gabbard is editor in chief of the *International Journal of Psychoanalysis*.

5. Quoted by Charles Strum, "Even a Mobster Needs Someone to Talk To," in *The New York Times on* The Sopranos, (New York: ibooks, 2001), pp. 105–106.

6. Robert N. Bellah, Richard Madsen, William M. Sullivan, Ann Swidler, and Steven M. Tipton, *Habits of the Heart* (Berkeley: University of California Press, 1985), pp. 99, 163.

7. Ibid., p. 122.

8. Philip Rieff, *The Triumph of the Therapeutic* (Chicago: University of Chicago Press, [1966] 1987), p. 235. Cf. p. 36.

9. Harriett G. Lerner, *The Dance of Deception* (New York: HarperCollins, 1994), p. 3.

10. Rieff, *Triumph of the Therapeutic*, p. 58.

11. Cf. Alasdair MacIntyre, *After Virtue*, 2d ed. (Notre Dame, Ind.: University of Notre Dame Press, 1984), pp. 30–31.

12. Bellah et al., *Habits of the Heart*, p. 101.

13. Rieff, *Triumph of the Therapeutic*, pp. 13, 74.

14. Christopher Lasch, *The Culture of Narcissism* (New York: Warner Books, 1979), p. 33.

15. Russell Shorto, *Saints and Madmen* (New York: Henry Holt, 1999); and James K. Boehnlein, ed., *Psychiatry and Religion: The Convergence of Mind and Spirit* (Washington, D.C.: American Psychiatric Press, 2000).

16. Bellah et al., *Habits of the Heart*, p. 290.

17. *Ibid.*, pp. 139, 129.

18. In his insightful study of these deeper forces, Robert D. Putnam makes no mention of the therapeutic trend. See Putnam, *Bowling Alone: The Collapse and Revival of American Community* (New York: Touchstone, 2000).

19. In a few unelaborated asides overlooked by his followers, Rieff allows that therapeutic culture is not inherently corrupt and that it is too early to know what it might contribute to human fulfillment. Rieff, *Triumph of the Therapeutic*, pp. xiii, 12.

20. Wade Clark Roof, *Spiritual Marketplace* (Princeton, N.J.: Princeton University Press, 1999).

21. Charles J. Sykes, *A Nation of Victims* (New York: St. Martin's Press, 1992), pp. 3, 22, 136.

22. Albert Camus explores this theme in *The Fall*, trans. Justin O'Brien (New York: Vintage Books, 1956), p. 81.

23. For example, see Paula J. Caplan, *They Say You're Crazy: How the World's Most Powerful Psychiatrists Decide Who's Normal* (Reading, Mass.: Addison-Wesley, 1995); Herb Kutchins and Stuart A. Kirk, *Making Us Crazy: DSM—The Psychiatric Bible and the Creation of Mental Disorders* (New York: Free Press, 1997); Tana Dineen, *Manufacturing Victims*, 3d ed. (Montreal: Robert Davies Multimedia, 2000); and Thomas S. Szasz, *The Myth of Mental Illness*, rev. ed. (New York: Harper and Row, 1974).

24. Alan Wolfe, *Moral Freedom* (New York: W.W. Norton, 2001), p. 183.

25. Wendy Kaminer, *I'm Dysfunctional, You're Dysfunctional* (New York: Vintage Books, 1993), p. 6. See also Gary Greenberg's *The Self on the Shelf: Recovery Books and the Good Life* (Albany: State University of New York Press, 1994); Tom Tiede, *Self-Help Nation* (New York: Atlantic Monthly Press, 2001); and John Steadman Rice, *A Disease of One's Own* (New Brunswick, N.J.: Transaction, 1996).

26. *Alcoholics Anonymous*, 3d ed. (New York: Alcoholics Anonymous World Services, 1976), p. 59.

27. At one point (pp. 71–72) Kaminer seems to admit as much, at least with regard to AA, and says she is merely expressing her personal distaste for religious (or quasi-religious) groups. But if that were true, I doubt she would have written such a one-sided critique.

28. Robert Wuthnow, *Sharing the Journey: Support Groups and America's New Quest for Community* (New York: Free Press, 1994), pp. 375–378.

29. Elayne Rapping, like Wuthnow, provides a balanced assessment of self-help groups in *The Culture of Recovery* (Boston: Beacon Press, 1996). She expresses feminist concerns that the preoccupation with individual sickness in self-help groups deflects attention from the wider social causes of individual suffering.

30. Thomasina Jo Borkman, *Understanding Self-Help/Mutual Aid: Experiential Learning in the Commons* (New Brunswick N.J.: Rutgers University Press, 1999), pp. xi, 13–14.

31. Robert Jay Lifton, *The Protean Self: Human Resilience in an Age of Fragmentation* (New York: Basic Books, 1993), p. 103.

32. Hunter, *The Death of Character*, p. 201.

33. Ibid., pp. 122, 100.

34. Ibid., pp. 127, 129.

35. Ibid., p. 188.

36. William Damon, *Greater Expectations: Overcoming the Culture of Indulgence in America's Homes and Schools* (New York: Free Press, 1995), pp. 79, 72.

37. California Task Force to Promote Self-Esteem and Personal and Social Responsibility, *Toward a State of Esteem: The Final Report of the California Task Force to Promote Self-esteem and Personal and Social Responsibility* (Sacramento: California Department of Education, 1990), p. 4. Also see Nathaniel Branden, *The Six Pillars of Self-Esteem* (New York: Bantam, 1994), p. xv.

38. William B. Swann, *Self-Traps: The Elusive Quest for Higher Self-Esteem* (New York: W.H. Freeman, 1996); and Roy F. Baumeister, Jennifer D. Campbell, Joachim I. Krueger, and Kathleen D. Vohs, "Does High Self-Esteem Cause Better Performance, Interpersonal Success, Happiness, or Healthier Lifestyles?," *Psychological Science in the Public Interest*, 4, no. 1 (May 2003): 1–44.

39. Neil J. Smelser, "Self-Esteem and Social Problems: An Introduction," in Andrew M. Mecca, Neil J. Smelser, and John Vasconcellos, eds., *The Social Importance of Self-Esteem* (Berkeley: University of California Press, 1989), p. 15.

40. Lauren Slater, "The Trouble with Self-Esteem," *New York Times Magazine* (Feb. 3, 2002), pp. 44–47.

41. The overemphasis on self-esteem that erodes academic standards is discussed by Maureen Stout in *The Feel-Good Curriculum: The Dumbing Down of America's Kids in the Name of Self-Esteem* (Cambridge, Mass.: Perseus, 2000); and John P. Hewitt, *The Myth of Self-Esteem* (New York: St. Martin's Press, 1998).

42. Charles Taylor, *Sources of The Self* (Cambridge: Cambridge University Press, 1989), pp. 507–509.

43. Charles Taylor, *The Ethics of Authenticity* (Cambridge, Mass.: Harvard University Press, 1992), p. 16.

44. Ibid., pp. 28–29.

45. Taylor, *Sources of the Self*, p. 511.

46. John P. Hewitt, "The Social Construction of Self-Esteem," in C. R. Snyder and Shane J. Lopez, eds., *Handbook of Positive Psychology* (New York: Oxford University Press, 2002), pp. 135–147.

47. Roy Schafer, *Retelling a Life: Narration and Dialogue in Psychoanalysis* (New York: Basic Books, 1992).

48. Owen Flanagan, *The Problem of the Soul: Two Visions of Mind and How to Reconcile Them* (New York: Basic Books, 2002), p. 251.

49. Calvin O. Schrag, *The Self after Postmodernity* (New Haven, Conn.: Yale University Press, 1997), p. 88.

Chapter 6: Blaming Victims

1. In this chapter I am concerned with both mental disorders and organic diseases, especially in areas where they overlap.

2. Audre Lorde, *The Cancer Journals* (San Francisco: Aunt Lute Books, 1980), p. 74.

3. Claudia Card, *The Unnatural Lottery: Character and Moral Luck* (Philadelphia: Temple University Press, 1996), p. 28.

4. In an extended usage of "blame," which refers to simple causation rather than moral agency, we blame animals and machines.

5. Barbara Houston, "In Praise of Blame," *Hypatia*, 7 (1992): 128–147.

6. R. Janoff-Bulman, "Characterological versus Behavioral Self-Blame: Inquiries into Depression and Rape," *Journal of Personality and Social Psychology*, 37 (1979): 1798–1809.

7. Ferdinand Schoeman, "Alcohol Addiction and Responsibility," in Mary I. Bockover, ed., *Rules, Rituals, and Responsibility* (La Salle, Ill.: Open Court, 1991), pp. 11–36.

8. Peter Strawson, "Freedom and Resentment," *Proceedings of the British Academy*, 48 (1962): 187–211.

9. Joseph Butler, "Upon Resentment," in W. R. Matthews, ed., *Fifteen Sermons* (London: G. Bell. 1964), p. 123.

10. John P. Allegrante, and Lawrence W. Green, "When Health Policy Becomes Victim Blaming," *New England Journal of Medicine*, 305 (1991): 1528–1529.

11. John H. Knowles, "The Responsibility of the Individual," *Daedelus*, 106 (1977): 57–80; and Leon R. Kass, "Regarding the End of Medicine and the Pursuit of Health," *Public Interest*, 40 (1975): 41.

12. Meredith Minkler, "Personal Responsibility for Health: Contexts and Controversies," in Daniel Callahan, ed., *Promoting Healthy Behavior: How Much Freedom? Whose Responsibility?* (Washington, D.C.: Georgetown University Press, 2002), pp. 13–14.

13. Robert Crawford, "Individual Responsibility and Health Politics," in Peter Conrad, ed., *The Sociology of Health and Illness: Critical Perspectives*, 5th ed. (New York: St. Martin's Press, 1997), p. 393. See also William Ryan, *Blaming the Victim*, rev. ed. (New York: Vintage, 1976).

14. Lorde, *Cancer Journals*, p. 74.

15. Howard M. Leichter, "Lifestyle Correctness and the New Secular Morality," in Allan M. Brandt and Paul Rozin, eds., *Morality and Health* (New York: Routledge, 1997), pp. 359–378.

16. Daniel Callahan, *False Hopes* (New York: Simon and Schuster, 1998), pp. 199, 191.

17. Gerald Dworkin, "Taking Risks, Assessing Responsibility," *Hastings Center Report*, 11 (1981): 31. Cf. Daniel Wikler, "Who Should Be Blamed for Being Sick?," *Health Education Quarterly*, 14 (1987): 11–25.

18. Mildred Blaxter, "Why Do the Victims Blame Themselves?," in Alan Radley, ed., *Worlds of Illness* (New York: Routledge, 1993), pp. 124–142.

19. Richard A. Shweder, Nancy C. Much, Manamohan Mahapatra, and Lawrence Park, "The 'Big Three' of Morality (Autonomy, Community, Divinity) and the 'Big Three' Explanations of Suffering," in Allan M. Brandt and Paul Rozin, eds., *Morality and Health* (New York: Routledge, 1997), pp. 161–162.

20. Keith Thomas, "Health and Morality in Early Modern England," in Allan M. Brandt and Paul Rozin, eds., *Morality and Health* (New York: Routledge, 1997), p. 17.

21. Shweder et al., "The 'Big Three' of Morality (Autonomy, Community, Divinity)," p. 161.

22. Friedrich Nietzsche, *On the Genealogy of Morality*, trans. Maudemarie Clark and Alan J. Swensen (Indianapolis: Hackett, 1998), p. 44.

23. Lorde, *Cancer Journals*, p. 10.

24. Susan Sontag, *Illness as Metaphor and AIDS and Its Metaphors* (New York: Doubleday, 1990), pp. 58, 3, 57.

25. Linda Gordon, "Teenage Pregnancy and Out-of-Wedlock Birth: Morals, Moralism, Experts," in Allan M. Brandt and Paul Rozin, eds., *Morality and Health* (New York: Routledge, 1997), p. 253.

26. Lorde, *Cancer Journals*, p. 60.

27. Arthur Frank, *At the Will of the Body: Reflections on Illness* (New York: Houghton Mifflin, 1991), pp. 122–123.

28. S. Poirier, "Expressing Illness: Review Essay of Arthur W. Frank, *The Wounded Storyteller*," *Medical Humanities Review*, 10 (1996): 74–79.

29. The same comment applies to David B. Morris, *The Culture of Pain* (Berkeley: University of California Press, 1991), p. 289.

30. Cf. Anatole Broyard, *Intoxicated by My Illness* (New York: Fawcett Columbine, 1992).

31. Kat Duff, *The Alchemy of Illness* (New York: Bell Tower, 1993), p. 42.

32. Cf. Michele L. Crossley, *Rethinking Health Psychology* (Philadelphia: Open University Press, 2000), p. 94.

33. Arthur Kleinman, *The Illness Narratives: Suffering, Healing, and the Human Condition* (New York: Basic Books, 1988), p. 171.

34. Talcott Parsons, "Definitions of Health and Illness in the Light of American Values and Social Structure," in E. G. Jaco, ed., *Patients, Physicians and Illness*, 3d ed. (London: Free Press, 1979), p. 117.

35. F. P. McKegney and P. Lange, "The Decision to No Longer Live on Chronic Hemodialysis," *American Journal of Psychiatry*, 128 (1971), p. 271. Cf. Linda Alexander, "The Double-Bind between Dialysis Patients and Their Health Practitioners," in

L. Eisenberg and A. Kleinman, eds., *The Relevance of Social Science for Medicine* (Dordrecht, Holland: D. Reidel, 1980), pp. 307–329.

36. Felton and Ornish quoted in Bill Moyers, *Healing the Mind* (New York: Doubleday, 1993), pp. 227, 102.

37. Moyers, *Healing the Mind*, p. 32.

38. Sharon Lamb, *The Trouble with Blame* (Cambridge: Harvard University Press, 1996), p. 31.

Chapter 7: Alcoholism

1. Cf. J. Ogden, *Health Psychology* (Philadelphia: Open University Press, 1996); and Michele L. Crossley, *Rethinking Health Psychology* (Philadelphia: Open University Press, 2000), p. 40. Sadly, Caroline Knapp, discussed next, died at age 42 from lung cancer, probably due to her addiction to cigarettes.

2. Carolyn Knapp, *Drinking: A Love Story* (New York: Dell, 1996), pp. 5, 1–2, 128, 261, 263.

3. "A Debate: 'We Should Reject the Disease Concept of Alcoholism,' by Herbert Fingarette, and 'We Should Retain the Disease Concep of Alcoholism,' by George E. Vaillant," in L. Grinspoon, and J. B. Bakalar, eds., *Alcohol Abuse and Dependence, Harvard Medical School Mental Health Review*, no. 2 (1990):11–15.

4. J. A. Corlett, "Fingarette on the Disease Concept of Alcoholism," *Theoretical Medicine*, 11 (1990): 243–249; Stanton Peele, "Herbert Fingarette, Radical Revisionist: Why Are People So Upset with This Retiring Philosopher?," in Mary I. Bockover, ed., *Rules, Rituals, and Responsibility* (La Salle, Ill.: Open Court, 1991), pp. 37–53; and Robert E. Haskell, "Realpolitic in the Addictions Field: Treatment-Professional, Popular-Culture Ideology, and Scientific Research," *Journal of Mind and Behavior*, 14, no. 3 (1993): 257–276.

5. Aristotle, *Nicomachean Ethics*, trans. Terence Irwin (Indianapolis: Hackett, 1985); and John Dewey, *Human Nature and Conduct* (New York: Modern Library, 1957), pp. 25–41. Surprisingly, Fingarette does not refer to these thinkers.

6. Jim Orford, *Excessive Appetites: A Psychological View of Addictions* (New York: John Wiley, 1985), p. 315.

7. Vince Fox, *Addiction, Change and Choice: The New View of Alcoholism* (Tucson: See Sharp Press, 1993).

8. American Psychiatric Association, *Diagnostic and Statistical Manual of Mental Disorders,* Fourth Edition, Text Revision (Washington, D.C.: American Psychiatric Association, 2000), p. 199.

9. Ibid., p. 197.

10. Knapp, *Drinking: A Love Story*, p. 17.

11. Ibid., pp. 58, 80.

12. J. H. Kupfer, *Autonomy and Social Interaction* (Albany: State University of New York Press, 1990), pp. 14–22.

13. Alfred A. Mele, *Irrationality: An Essay on Akrasia, Self-Deception, and Self-Control* (New York: Oxford University Press, 1987), p. 26.

14. George E. Vaillant, *The Natural History of Alcoholism Revisited* (Cambridge: Harvard University Press, 1995), p. 19.

15. Peter Conrad and Joseph W. Schneider, *Deviance and Medicalization: From Badness to Sickness*, rev. ed. (Philadelphia: Temple University Press, 1992).

16. In personal correspondence (July 17, 1999), Fingarette indicated openness to applying the looser notion of sickness to alcoholism. He also emphasized that the term "disease" has no clear meaning in this context. Hence, technically he is not asserting that alcoholism is not a disease—an assertion that would use a word lacking a clear meaning.

17. Herbert Fingarette, *Heavy Drinking* (Berkeley: University of California Press, 1988), p. 100.

18. Conrad and Schneider, *Deviance and Medicalization*, pp. 73–109.

19. Vaillant, *Natural History of Alcoholism Revisited*, p. 376; cf. pp. 19–23.

20. Dorothy Nelkin and M. S. Lindee, *The DNA Mystique* (New York: W.H. Freeman, 1995), p. 92.

21. Vaillant, *Natural History of Alcoholism Revisited,* pp. 19, 118–119.

22. Francis F. Seeburger, *Addiction and Responsibility* (New York: Crossroad, 1995); and Jefferson A. Singer, *Message in a Bottle: Stories of Men and Addiction* (New York: Free Press, 1997).

23. Fingarette, *Heavy Drinking*, p. 103.

24. Pete Hamill, *A Drinking Life* (Boston: Little, Brown, 1994).

25. Vaillant, *Natural History of Alcoholism Revisited*, pp. 21, 384, 385.

26. Fingarette, *Heavy Drinking*, p. 115.

27. Knapp, *Drinking: A Love Story*, pp. 256, 281.

28. Fingarette, *Heavy Drinking*, pp. 128–129. Cf. Ferdinand Schoeman, "Alcohol Addiction and Responsibility," in Mary I. Bockover, ed., *Rules, Rituals, and Responsibility* (La Salle, Ill.: Open Court, 1991), pp. 20–21.

29. Vaillant, *Natural History of Alcoholism Revisited*, pp. 377–378.

30. Fingarette, *Heavy Drinking*, p. 129; and Fingarette, *The Self in Transformation* (New York: Basic Books, 1963).

31. Fingarette, *Heavy Drinking*, p. 4.

32. K. Liska*, Drugs and the Human Body, With Implications for Society*, 3d ed. (New York: Macmillan, 1990); and Grinspoon and Bakalar, *Alcohol Abuse and Dependence*.

33. Alcoholics Anonymous, *Twelve Steps and Twelve Traditions* (New York: Alcoholics Anonymous World Services, 1953).

34. Klaus Makela et al., *Alcoholics Anonymous as a Mutual-Help Movement: A Study in Eight Societies* (Madison: University of Wisconsin Press, 1996), p. 124. Cf. H. A. M. J. Ten Have, "Drug Addiction, Society and Health Care Ethics," in Raanan Gillon, ed., *Principles of Health Care Ethics* (New York: Wiley, 1994), pp. 896, 900.

35. Fingarette, *Heavy Drinking*, p. 91.

36. Ferdinand Schoeman, "Alcohol Addiction and Responsibility," in Mary I. Bockover, ed., *Rules, Rituals, and Responsibility* (La Salle, Ill.: Open Court, 1991), p. 28.

37. Ibid., p. 33.

38. Cf. James Q. Wilson, *Moral Judgment* (New York: Basic Books, 1997), p. 31; and Stanton Peele, "A Moral Vision of Addiction: How People's Values Determine Whether They Become and Remain Addicts," in Stanton Peele, ed., *Visions of Addiction: Major Contemporary Perspectives on Addiction and Alcoholism* (Lexington, Ky: D.C. Heath, 1988), pp. 201–233; and Peele, *Diseasing of America* (New York: Lexington Books, 1995).

39. K. Matson, *Short Lives: Portraits in Creativity and Self-Destruction* (New York: William Morrow, 1980).

40. Robin S. Dillon, ed., *Dignity, Character, and Self-Respect* (New York: Routledge, 1995).

41. Knapp, *Drinking: A Love Story*, pp. 128, 269.

Chapter 8: Pathological Gambling

1. Joshua Green, "The Bookie of Virtue," *Washington Monthly* (June 2003); available at http://www.washingtonmonthly.com/features/2003/9006.green.html

2. William J. Bennett, ed., *The Book of Virtues: A Treasury of Great Moral Stories* (New York: Simon and Schuster, 1993), pp. 88, 53.

3. Quoted by Katharine Q. Seelye, "Moral Crusader Says He Will Gamble No More," *New York Times* (May 6, 2003).

4. On these and related distinctions, see Michael B. Walker, *The Psychology of Gambling* (Oxford: Pergamon Press, 1992), p. 151.

5. Most philosophical discussions of gambling center on questions about its moral status and economic justice. For example, Lisa Newton, "Gambling: A Preliminary Inquiry," *Business Ethics Quarterly*, 3 (1993): 405–418; Michael Scriven, "The Philosophical Foundations of Las Vegas," *Journal of Gambling Studies*, 11 (1995): 61–75; Richard L. Lippke, "Should States Be in the Gambling Business?" *Public Affairs Quarterly*, 11 (1997): 57–73; Jeffrie G. Murphy, "Indian Casinos and the Morality of Gambling," *Public Affairs Quarterly*, 12 (1988): 119–136; and Peter Collins, "Is Gambling Immoral?" in David Benatar, ed., *Ethics for Everyday* (Boston: McGraw-Hill, 2002), pp. 570–583.

6. R. Jay Wallace offers an insightful discussion along this line in "Addiction as Defect of the Will: Some Philosophical Reflections," *Law and Philosophy*, 18/6 (1999): 621–654. See also Gary Watson, "Disordered Appetites," in *Addiction: Entries and Exits*, ed. Jon Elster (New York: Russell Sage, 1999), pp. 3–28.

7. Richard J. Rosenthal, "The Psychodynamics of Pathological Gambling: A Review of the Literature," in T. Galski, ed., *Handbook of Pathological Gambling* (Springfield, Ill.: Charles C. Thomas, 1987), pp. 41–70.

8. Parenthetical page references are to Fyodor Dostoevsky, *The Gambler*, trans. A. R. MacAndrew (New York: W.W. Norton, 1964). Bettina L. Knapp insightfully discusses the novel in *Gambling, Game, and Psyche* (Albany: State University of New York, 2000), pp. 97–125.

9. Sheila B. Blume, "Compulsive Gambling and the Medical Model," *Journal of Gambling Behavior*, 3 (1987): 237–247; quotation on p. 243.

10. American Psychiatric Association, *Diagnostic and Statistical Manual of Mental Disorders,* Fourth Edition, Text Revision (Washington, D.C.: American Psychiatric Association, 2000), p. 674. In labeling and summarizing the criteria, I draw on H. R. Lesieur and R. J. Rosenthal's "Pathological Gambling and the New Criteria: DSM IV," presented at the Eighth International Conference on Risk and Gambling (London, August 1990); cited in Walker, *Psychology of Gambling*, p. 172. For doubts about viewing problem gambling as an addiction, see Jon Elster, "Gambling and Addiction," in Jon Elster and Ole-Jorgen Skog, eds., *Getting Hooked: Rationality and Addiction* (New York: Cambridge University Press, 1999), pp. 208–234; and Elster, *Strong Feelings: Emotion, Addiction, and Human Behavior* (Cambridge, Mass.: MIT Press, 1999).

11. Blume, "Compulsive Gambling and the Medical Model," p. 245.

12. Herbert Fingarette, *Heavy Drinking* (Berkeley: University of California Press, 1988). John Dewey, *Human Nature and Conduct* (New York: Modern Library, 1957), pp. 55, 25. This appreciation of the identity- and agency-shaping power of habits also permeates many psychologists' approach to addictions. See Jim Orford, *Excessive Appetites: A Psychological View of Addictions* (New York: Wiley, 1985); and Stanton Peele, "A Moral Vision of Addiction: How People's Values Determine Whether They Become and Remain Addicts," in Stanton Peele, ed., *Visions of Addiction* (Lexington, Ky.: D.C. Heath, 1988), pp. 201–233.

13. Blume, "Compulsive Gambling and the Medical Model," pp. 243, 246.

14. Richard J. Rosenthal, "The Pathological Gambler's System for Self-Deception," *Journal of Gambling Behavior*, 2 (1986): 108–120.

15. Richard Geha, "Dostoevsky and 'The Gambler': A Contribution to the Psychogenesis of Gambling," *Psychoanalytic Review*, 57 (1970): 95–123, 289–302.

16. Durand F. Jacobs, "A General Theory of Addictions: A New Theoretical Model," *Journal of Gambling Behavior*, 2 (1986): 15–31.

17. Peter L. Carlton and Paul Manowitz, "Physiological Factors as Determinants of Pathological Gambling," *Journal of Gambling Behavior*, 3 (1987): 274–285.

18. Ellen J. Langer, "The Illusion of Control," *Journal of Personality and Social Psychology*, 32 (1975): 311–328; and M. D. Griffiths, "The Cognitive Psychology of Gambling," *Journal of Gambling Studies*, 6 (1990): 31–42.

19. Walker, *Psychology of Gambling*, p. 136.

20. Dewey, *Human Nature and Conduct*, p. 292; and Sharon Lamb, *The Trouble with Blame: Victims, Perpetrators, and Responsibility* (Cambridge: Harvard University Press, 1996), p. 11.

21. Robert Goodman, *The Luck Business* (New York: Free Press, 1995).

22. I. Nelson Rose, "Compulsive Gambling and the Law: From Sin to Vice to Disease," *Journal of Gambling Behavior*, 4 (1988): 240–260.

23. Dewey, *Human Nature and Conduct*, p. 29.

24. Alfred R. Mele, *Irrationality: An Essay on Akrasia, Self-Deception, and Self-Control* (New York: Oxford University Press, 1987), p. 26.

25. Blume, "Compulsive Gambling and the Medical Model," p. 246.

26. Martin C. McGurrin, "Diagnosis and Treatment of Pathological Gambling," in Judith A. Lewis, ed., *Addictions: Concepts and Strategies for Treatment* (Gaithersburg, Md.: Aspen, 1994), p. 126.

27. J. Ingersoll Taber and Richard A. McCormick, "The Pathological Gambler in Treatment," in T. Galski, ed., *The Handbook of Pathological Gambling* (Springfield, Ill.: Charles C. Thomas, 1987).

28. Blume, "Compulsive Gambling and the Medical Model," p. 246.

Chapter 9: Crime and Punishment

1. There are other forms of major crime, of course, such as a single instance of grand larceny, that should not be pathologized.

2. Plato, *Gorgias*, trans. W.W. Woodhead, in Edith Hamilton and Huntington Cairns, eds., *The Collected Dialogues of Plato* (Princeton, N.J.: Princeton University Press, 1961), pp. 229–307, secs. 476–480.

3. Karl Menninger, *The Crime of Punishment* (New York: Viking Press, 1968), p. 17.

4. Ibid., pp. 203, 262.

5. Ibid., p. 96.

6. Paul Chodoff, "Misuse and Abuse of Psychiatry: An Overview," in Sidney Bloch, Paul Chodoff, and Stephen A. Green, eds., *Psychiatric Ethics*, 3d ed. (New York: Oxford University Press, 1999), pp. 49–66; and Nicholas N. Kittrie, *The Right to Be Different: Deviance and Enforced Therapy* (Baltimore: Johns Hopkins University Press, 1971).

7. See especially Jeffrie G. Murphy, "Criminal Punishment and Psychiatric Fallacies," in Jeffrie G. Murphy, ed., *Punishment and Rehabilitation* (Belmont, Calif.: Wadsworth, 1973), pp. 197–210.

8. Paul S. Appelbaum, "Psychopathology, Crime, and the Law," in Andrew E. Skodol, ed., *Psychopathology and Violent Crime* (Washington, D.C.: American Psychiatric Press, 1998), p. 141.

9. Herbert Morris, *On Guilt and Innocence* (Berkeley: University of California Press, 1976), pp. 36–37, 43.

10. Antony Flew, *Crime or Disease?* (New York: Harper and Row, 1973), pp. 66, 20. The book is reprinted under the title *Crime, Punishment and Disease* (New Brunswick, N.J.: Transaction, 2002).

11. Ibid., p. 67.

12. See Richard Moran, "The Search for the Born Criminal and the Medical Control of Criminality," in Peter Conrad and Joseph W. Schneider, eds., *Deviance and*

Medicalization: From Badness to Sickness, exp. ed. (Philadelphia: Temple University Press, 1992), pp. 215–240.

13. Cf. Friedrich Nietzsche, *On the Genealogy of Morality*, trans. Maudemarie Clark and Alan J. Swensen (Indianapolis: Hackett, 1998), p. 53.

14. Restorative justice is also called reparative or restitution justice.

15. Wesley Cragg, *The Practice of Punishment: Towards a Theory of Restorative Justice* (New York: Routledge, 1992); and John Braithwaite, *Restorative Justice and Responsive Regulation* (New York: Oxford, 2002).

16. For example, Conrad G. Brunk promulgates the false stereotypes of therapeutic outlooks in "Restorative Justice and the Philosophical Theories of Criminal Punishment," in Michael L. Hadley, ed., *The Spiritual Roots of Restorative Justice* (Albany: State University of New York Press), pp. 31–56.

17. Marcus J. Goldman, *Kleptomania* (Far Hills, N.J.: New Horizon Press, 1998), pp. 109–118.

18. Ibid., p. 67.

19. American Psychiatric Association, *Diagnostic and Statistical Manual of Mental Disorders,* Fourth Edition, Text Revision (Washington, D.C.: American Psychiatric Association, 2000), p. 669.

20. Ibid., p. xxxvii.

21. Goldman, *Kleptomania*, p. 72.

22. David Musto, *The American Disease* (New York: Oxford University Press, 1987).

23. Jonathan Alter, "The War on Addiction," *Newsweek* (Feb. 12, 2001), pp. 37–39.

24. "Drug Courts, for Hard Cases," *Los Angeles Times* (Apr. 25, 2002), p. B-12.

25. Seema Mehta, "Low Funds Imperil Prop. 36 Rehab," *Los Angeles Times* (Apr. 7, 2003), pp. B1, B8.

26. John Terrence A. Rosenthal, "Therapeutic Jurisprudence and Drug Treatment Courts: Integrating Law and Science," in James L. Nolan, ed., *Drug Courts in Theory and in Practice"* (New York: Aldine De Gruyter, 2002), pp. 145–171.

27. Janet Reno, Comments before the Convention of the American Bar Association, Atlanta, Georgia, August 10, 1999. Quoted by James J. Chriss, "The Drug Court Movement: An Analysis of Tacit Assumptions," in James L. Nolan, ed., *Drug Courts in Theory and in Practice* (New York: Aldine De Gruyter, 2002), p. 193. See also James L. Nolan, *Reinventing Justice: The American Drug Court Movement* (Princeton, N.J.: Princeton University Press, 2001), p. 39.

28. Susan Meld Shell, "Drug Treatment Courts: A Traditional Perspective," in James L. Nolan, ed., *Drug Courts in Theory and in Practice* (New York: Aldine De Gruyter, 2002), p. 174. After using this dichotomy to criticize drug courts, Shell moves toward an integrated view stressing responsibility for addictions.

29. American Psychiatric Association, *Diagnostic and Statistical Manual of Mental Disorders*, p. 197.

30. Charles L. Glenn, *The Ambiguous Embrace: Government and Faith-Based Schools and Social Agencies* (Princeton, N.J.: Princeton University Press, 2000), p. 66.

31. Dave Batty, *Philosophy of Teen Challenge* (Springfield, Mo.: Teen Challenge National Office, 1994), p. 2.

32. On the importance of matching, see Edward Gottheil, A. McLellan, and Keith A. Druley, eds., *Matching Patient Needs and Treatment Methods in Alcoholism and Drug Abuse* (Springfield, Ill.: Charles C. Thomas, 1981).

33. Howard Spiro, *The Power of Hope: A Doctor's Perspective* (New Haven, Conn.: Yale University Press, 1998).

34. Eva Bertram, Morris Blachman, Kenneth Sharpe, and Peter Andreas, *Drug War Politics* (Berkeley: University of California Press, 1996), p. 185.

35. James Q. Wilson, *Thinking about Crime*, rev. ed. (New York: Vintage Books, 1985), p. 196; cf. p. 173.

36. It is noteworthy, however, that drug courts are becoming a model for how to deal with domestic violence and juvenile crime. R. C. Boldt, "Rehabilitative Justice and the Drug Court Movement," *Washington University Law Quarterly*, 76 (1998): 1205–1306; and Philip Bean, "Drug Courts, the Judge, and the Rehabilitative Ideal," in James L. Nolan, ed., *Drug Courts in Theory and in Practice* (New York: Aldine De Gruyter, 2002), pp. 235–254.

37. Adrian Raine, *The Psychopathology of Crime: Criminal Behavior as a Clinical Disorder* (San Diego, Calif.: Academic Press, 1993), p. 2. See especially pp. 1–26 and 287–314.

38. Ibid., p. 208.

39. Ibid., p. 310.

40. Cf. Paul S. Appelbaum, "Psychopathology, Crime, and Law," in Andrew E. Skodol, ed., *Psychopathology and Violent Crime* (Washington, D.C.: American Psychiatric Press, 1998), pp. 138–139.

41. Raine, *Psychopathology of Crime*, p. 307.

42. James W. Clarke, *On Being Mad or Merely Angry: John W. Hinckley, Jr., and Other Dangerous People* (Princeton, N.J.: Princeton University Press, 1990).

43. M'Naghten's Case, 8 *English Reports* 718 (1843).

44. Carl Elliott, *The Rules of Insanity: Moral Responsibility and Mentally Ill Offenders* (Albany: State University of New York Press, 1996), p. 63.

45. American Psychiatric Association Statement on the Insanity Defense," in Rem B. Edwards, ed., *Ethics of Psychiatry* (Amherst, N.Y.: Prometheus Books, 1997), p. 502. First published in *American Journal of Psychiatry*, 140, no. 6 (June 1983).

46. Alan M. Dershowitz, *The Abuse Excuse* (Boston: Little, Brown, 1994), p. 3.

47. James Q. Wilson, *Moral Judgment: Does the Abuse Excuse Threaten Our Legal System?* (New York: Basic Books, 1997). Cf. Peter Arenella, "Demystifying the Abuse Excuse: Is There One?" *Harvard Journal of Law and Public Policy*, 19, no. 3 (Spring 1996). [Partly reprinted in Richard P. Halgin, ed., *Taking Sides: Clashing Views on Controversial Issues in Abnormal Psychology*, 2d ed. (New York: McGraw-Hill, 2003), pp. 363–368.]

48. Michael Stocker, "Responsibility and Abuse Excuse," in Ellen Frankel Paul, Fred D. Miller Jr., and Jeffrey Paul, eds., *Responsibility* (New York: Cambridge University Press, 1999), p. 182.

Chapter 10: Violence and Evil

1. I set aside religious meanings of evil as satanic forces and rebellion against God. On how these meanings resonate in public debates, see Andrew Delbanco, *The Death of Satan: How Americans Have Lost the Sense of Evil* (New York: Farrar, Straus & Giroux, 1995).

2. Trudy Govier, *A Delicate Balance: What Philosophy Can Tell Us about Terrorism* (Cambridge, Mass.: Westview Press, 2002), p. 30.

3. Parenthetical page references are to James Gilligan, *Violence: Reflections on a National Epidemic* (New York: Vintage Books, 1997). See also Gilligan, *Preventing Violence* (New York: Thames and Hudson, 2001).

4. Lou Michel and Dan Herbeck, *American Terrorist: Timothy McVeigh and the Oklahoma City Bombing* (New York: Regan Books, 2001).

5. Cf. James Q. Wilson, *Thinking about Crime*, rev. ed. (New York: Vintage Books, 1985), p. 252; and Paul S. Appelbaum, "Psychopathology, Crime, and Law," in Andrew

E. Skodol, ed., *Psychopathology and Violent Crime* (Washington, D.C.: American Psychiatric Press, 1998), p. 141.

6. See, for example, Michael S. Moore, "The Moral Worth of Retribution," in Ferdinand Schoeman, ed., *Responsibility, Character, and the Emotions* (New York: Cambridge University Press, 1987), pp. 179–219.

7. Cf. Carl Goldberg, *Speaking with the Devil: Exploring Senseless Acts of Evil* (New York: Penguin Books, 1996); and Thomas J. Scheff and Suzanne M. Retzinger, *Emotions and Violence: Shame and Rage in Destructive Conflicts* (Lexington, Mass.: Lexington Books, 1991).

8. James Gilligan, "Beyond Morality: Psychoanalytic Reflections on Shame, Guilt, and Love," in Thomas Lickona, ed., *Moral Development and Behavior* (New York: Holt, Rinehart and Winston, 1976), p. 145.

9. Whereas James Gilligan equates justice with morality and caring with therapy, his wife Carol Gilligan famously contrasts an ethics of caring with an ethics of justice. Carol Gilligan, *In a Different Voice* (Cambridge: Harvard University Press, 1993).

10. Philip Hallie, "Response to Jeffrey Burton Russell," in Paul Woodruff and Harry A. Wilmer, eds., *Facing Evil* (La Salle, Ill.: Open Court, 1988), p. 62.

11. Donald W. Black, *Bad Boys, Bad Men: Confronting Antisocial Personality Disorder* (New York: Oxford University Press, 1999); Ann Rule, *The Stranger beside Me* (New York: Signet, 1989); Walter Glannon, "Psychopathy and Responsibility," *Journal of Applied Philosophy*, 14 (1997): 263–275; John Deigh, "Empathy and Universalizability," *Ethics*, 105 (July 1995): 743–763; and Antony Duff, "Psychopathy and Moral Understanding," *American Philosophical Quarterly*, 14 (1977): 189–200.

12. American Psychiatric Association, *Diagnostic and Statistical Manual of Mental Disorders,* Fourth Edition, Text Revision (Washington, D.C.: American Psychiatric Association, 2000), p. 706.

13. Peter Strawson "Freedom and Resentment," in *Freedom and Resentment and Other Essays* (London: Methuen and Co., 1974), pp. 16–17. In *Responsibility and Control* (New York: Cambridge University Press, 1998), Fischer and Ravizza distinguish between psychopaths who do not recognize moral reasons and those who recognize moral reasons but do not act on them, and they suggest the former are not responsible and the latter are. See also R. Jay Wallace, *Responsibility and the Moral Sentiments* (Cambridge: Harvard University Press, 1994), p. 178. Vinit Haksar calls sociopaths morally sick and infers they are not morally accountable: Haksar, "Aristotle and the Punishment of Psychopaths," *Philosophy*, 39 (1964): 323–340; and Haksar, "The Responsibility of Psychopaths," *Philosophical Quarterly*, 15 (1965): 135–145. I challenge all these views.

14. American Psychiatric Association, *Diagnostic and Statistical Manual of Mental Disorders,* p. 704.

15. Herbert Fingarette, *On Responsibility* (New York: Basic Books, 1967), p. 27.

16. Wallace, *Responsibility and the Moral Sentiments*, p. 69.

17. Jeffrie G. Murphy, "Moral Death: A Kantian Essay on Psychopathy," *Ethics*, 82 (1972): 291, 294–295.

18. Hervey Cleckley, *The Mask of Sanity*, 5th ed. (Saint Louis: C.V. Mosby, 1976), p. 346.

19. Cf. Jane English, "Abortion and the Concept of a Person," *Canadian Journal of Philosophy*, 5 (1975).

20. American Psychiatric Association, *Diagnostic and Statistic Manual of Mental Disorders*, p. 704.

21. Cleckley, *Mask of Sanity*, 46–55.

22. Robert J. Smith, "The Psychopath as Moral Agent," *Philosophy and Phenomenological Research*, 45 (1984): 193.

23. Robert W. Rieber, *Manufacturing Social Distress: Psychopathy in Everyday Life* (New York: Plenum Press, 1997), p. 5.

24. Cf. Deigh, "Empathy and Universalizability," p. 743; and Richard Tithecott, *Of Men and Monsters* (Madison: University of Wisconsin Press, 1997).

25. Raymond B. Flannery, *Violence in America* (New York: Continuum, 1997). See also Elizabeth Kandel Englander, *Understanding Violence* (Mahwah, N.J.: Lawrence Erlbaum Associates, 1997).

26. James Waller, *Becoming Evil: How Ordinary People Commit Genocide and Mass Killing* (New York: Oxford University Press, 2002), p. 87. The same theme is insightfully explored in the essays in Arthur G. Miller, ed., *The Social Psychology of Good and Evil* (New York: The Guilford Press, 2004).

27. Steven E. Barkan and Lynne L. Snowden, *Collective Violence* (Boston: Allyn and Bacon, 2001), pp. 80–81; and Peter C. Sederberg, "Explaining Terrorism," in B. Schechterman and M. Slann, eds., *Violence and Terrorism* (Guilford, Conn.: Dushkin, 2003), p. 25.

28. Jonathan Glover, *Humanity: A Moral History of the Twentieth Century* (New Haven, Conn.: Yale University Press, 1999), p. 33.

29. Friedrich Nietzsche, *On the Genealogy of Morality*, trans. Maudemarie Clark and Alan J. Swensen (Indianapolis: Hackett, 1998), p. 42.

30. Hannah Arendt, *Eichmann in Jerusalem* (New York: Penguin, 1963), p. 276.

31. For example, Stanley Milgram, *Obedience to Authority* (New York: Harper and Row, 1974).

32. Robert Jay Lifton, *The Nazi Doctors* (New York: Basic Books, 1986), p. 418.

33. Ibid., p. 442.

34. Robert Jay Lifton, *Destroying the World to Save It* (New York: Henry Holt, 1999).

35. In discussing Lifton, Berel Lang is a critic of therapeutic approaches, in *Act and Idea in the Nazi Genocide* (Chicago: University of Chicago Press, 1990), p. 48. Laurence Mordekhai Thomas is a defender, in *Vessels of Evil* (Philadelphia: Temple University Press, 1993), p. 102.

36. Donald G. Dutton, *The Batterer: A Psychological Profile* (New York: Basic Books, 1995), esp. pp. 22–38, 166.

37. M. Scott Peck, *People of the Lie: The Hope for Healing Human Evil* (New York: Simon and Schuster, 1983), p. 118; and see p. 129.

38. Ibid., p. 126.

39. Gary Watson, "Responsibility and the Limits of Evil: Variations on a Strawsonian Theme," in Gary Watson, *Agency and Answerability* (Oxford: Clarendon Press, 2004), p. 239.

40. Miles Corwin, "Icy Killer's Life Steeped in Violence," *Los Angeles Times* (May 16, 1982).

41. Watson, "Responsibility and the Limits of Evil," p. 249.

42. Ibid., p. 244.

43. Cf. John Kekes, *Facing Evil* (Princeton, N.J.: Princeton University Press, 1990), pp. 96–99.

44. Watson, "Responsibility and the Limits of Evil," p. 258.

45. Owen Flanagan, *Varieties of Moral Personality: Ethics and Psychological Realism* (Cambridge: Harvard University Press, 1991).

46. Robert C. Solomon, *A Passion for Justice* (Reading, Mass.: Addison-Wesley, 1990); and Peter French, *The Virtues of Vengeance* (Lawrence: University Press of Kansas, 2001).

Chapter 11: Are Bigots Sick?

1. For example, Wendell Berry, *The Hidden Wound* (Boston: Houghton Mifflin, 1970); Harlon L. Dalton, *Racial Healing* (New York: Doubleday, 1995); and Meri

Nana-Ama Danquah, "Writing the Wrongs of Identity," in Nell Casey, ed., *Unholy Ghost: Writers on Depression* (New York: William Morrow, 2001), p. 175. The term "antisemitism" was popularized by a racist ideologue who believed there are two distinct racial groups, Aryan and Semitic. This unsavory etymology leads some writers to abandon the term in favor of "anti-Jew" and "anti-Judaism." See Richard L. Rubenstein and John K. Roth, *Approaches to Auschwitz: The Holocaust and Its Legacy* (Atlanta: John Knox Press, 1987), pp. 27–28.

2. I borrow the term from Irving Thalberg in "Visceral Racism," *Monist* 56 (1972): 43–63. The distinction between shallow and visceral bigotry is only rough, marking opposite ends of a continuum.

3. Jeff Pearlman, "At Full Blast," *Sports Illustrated*, 91, no. 35 (Dec. 27, 1999–Jan. 3, 2000), pp. 60–64.

4. Alvin F. Poussaint, "What a Rorschach Can't Gauge," *New York Times* (Jan. 9, 2000), p. WK-19N; and see Emily Eakin, "Bigotry as Mental Illness or Just Another Norm," *New York Times* (Jan. 15, 2000), pp. A21 and A23.

5. Nora Zamichow, "First a Loner, Then a Separatist," *Los Angeles Times* (Aug. 22, 1999), pp. A1, 32–33.

6. Peter Wolson, "Strange to Say, but Neurotics Are Preferable," *Los Angeles Times* (Aug. 22, 1999), pp. M2, M6.

7. American Psychiatric Association, *Diagnostic and Statistical Manual of Mental Disorders,* Fourth Edition, Text Revision (Washington, D.C.: American Psychiatric Association, 2000), p. xxxi.

8. Alvin F. Poussaint and Amy Alexander, *Lay My Burden Down* (Boston: Beacon Press, 2000), p. 125.

9. Ibid.

10. Letter from Robert Spitzer to the Committee of Black Psychiatrists (Dec. 29, 1975). Quoted by Stuart A. Kirk and Herb Kutchins, *The Selling of DSM* (New York: Aldine De Gruyter, 1992), p. 102.

11. Rem B. Edwards, ed., *Ethics of Psychiatry* (Amherst, N.Y.: Prometheus Books, 1997), p. 53.

12. Martin P. Golding, "On the Idea of Moral Pathology," in Alan Rosenberg and Gerald E. Myers, eds., *Echoes from the Holocaust: Philosophical Reflections in a Dark Time* (Philadelphia: Temple University Press, 1988), p. 135. See also E. Mansell Pattison, "The Holocaust as Sin: Requirements in Psychoanalytic Theory for Human Evil and Mature Morality," in Steven A. Luel and Paul Marcus, eds., *Psychoanalytic Reflections on the Holocaust: Selected Essays* (New York: KTAV, 1984), pp. 71–91.

13. Ruth Benedict, "Anthropology and the Abnormal," *Journal of General Psychology*, 10 (1934): 59–82.

14. Gordon W. Allport, *The Nature of Prejudice* (Reading, Mass.: Addison-Wesley, 1979), p. 12. Research has also refuted the generalizations set forth in T. W. Adorno, Else Frenkel-Brunswik, Daniel J. Levinson, and R. Nevitt Sanford, *The Authoritarian Personality* (New York: Harper and Brothers, 1950). See William F. Stone, Gerda Lederer, and Richard Christi, eds., *Strength and Weakness: The Authoritarian Personality Today* (New York: Springer-Verlag, 1993).

15. Hannah Arendt, *Eichmann in Jerusalem: A Report on the Banality of Evil* (New York: Penguin Books, 1977 [1963]), pp. 252, 276.

16. Stanley Milgram, *Obedience to Authority* (New York: Harper and Row, 1974), p. 6.

17. George M. Kren, "The Holocaust: Moral Theory and Immoral Acts," in Alan Rosenberg and Gerald E. Myers, eds., *Echoes from the Holocaust: Philosophical Reflections in a Dark Time* (Philadelphia: Temple University Press, 1988), p. 254.

18. Robert Jay Lifton, *The Nazi Doctors* (New York: Basic Books, 1986).

19. Albert Lee, *Henry Ford and the Jews* (New York: Stein and Day, 1980), p. 146. For sample antisemitic articles, see Richard S. Levy, ed., *Antisemitism in the Modern World* (Lexington, Ky.: D.C. Heath, 1991), pp. 166–177.

20. Sigmund Freud, *Civilization and Its Discontents*, trans. James Strachey (New York: W.W. Norton, 1961), p. 91. Cf. Erich Fromm, *The Sane Society* (New York: Fawcett, 1955).

21. Nathan W. Ackerman and Marie Jahoda, *Anti-Semitism and Emotional Disorder: A Psychoanalytic Interpretation* (New York: Harper and Brothers, 1950), p. 5.

22. Theodore Isaac Rubin, *Anti-Semitism: A Disease of the Mind* (New York: Continuum, 1990), p. 23.

23. Ibid., pp. 17 and 31.

24. Ackerman and Jahoda, in *Anti-Semitism and Emotional Disorder*, also make both correlation and constitutive claims on, respectively, p. 4 and p. 2.

25. Elisabeth Young-Bruehl, *The Anatomy of Prejudices* (Cambridge: Harvard University Press, 1996), pp. 32–33. Mortimer Ostow also adopts a relativistic definition of health in *Myth and Madness: The Psychodynamics of Antisemitism* (New Brunswick: Transaction, 1996).

26. Young-Bruehl, *Anatomy of Prejudices,* pp. 32, 209.

27. Ibid., p. 28; cf. p. 185.

28. Ibid., p. 34.

29. Naomi Zack, *Thinking about Race* (Belmont, Calif.: Wadsworth, 1998), pp. 41–42.

30. Ibid., p. 42.

31. Ann E. Cudd, "Psychological Explanations of Oppression," in Cynthia Willett, *Theorizing Multiculturalism: A Guide to the Current Debate* (Malden, Mass.: Blackwell, 1998), pp. 192–193.

32. Gordon W. Allport, *The Nature of Prejudice* (Reading, Mass.: Addison-Wesley, 1979), pp. 495–496.

33. Quoted from an interview with Lynell George, "Facing the Problem," *Los Angeles Times* (Feb. 27, 2000), p. E2. See also Jody David Armour, *Negrophobia and Reasonable Racism* (New York: New York University Press, 1997).

34. Philip Lichtenberg, Janneke van Beusekom, and Dorothy Gibbons, *Encountering Bigotry* (Northvale, N.J.: Jason Aronson, 1997). Unfortunately, the authors embrace a morality-therapy dichotomy; see p. xi.

35. Cudd, "Psychological Explanations of Oppression," pp. 192–193.

36. Paul Wachtel, *Race in the Mind of America* (New York: Routledge, 1999), pp. 97–141.

37. Jean-Paul Sartre, *Anti-Semite and Jew*, trans. George J. Becker (New York: Schocken Books, 1948), pp. 21–22, 53.

38. John Dewey, *Human Nature and Conduct* (New York: Modern Library, 1957 [1922]).

Chapter 12: Depression and Identity

1. Michael Miller, "Foreword" to Jacques Hassoun, *The Cruelty of Depression* (Reading, Mass.: Addison-Wesley, 1997), p. vii. For especially insightful studies, see Lewis Wolpert, *Malignant Sadness: The Anatomy of Depression* (New York: Free Press, 1999); and Andrew Solomon, *The Noonday Demon: An Atlas of Depression* (New York: Scribner, 2001).

2. John Stuart Mill, *Autobiography* (New York: Penguin, 1989 [1873]), p. 112. Brief quotations are to pp. 111–121.

3. Richard Garrett speaks of "project-specific despair" in "The Problem of Despair," in George Graham and G. Lynn Stephens, eds. *Philosophical Psychopathology* (Cambridge, Mass.: MIT Press, 1994), p. 74.

4. Elizabeth E. Anderson, "John Stuart Mill and Experiments in Living," *Ethics*, 102 (1991): 4–26.

5. Mill, *Autobiography*, pp. 113, 116, 121, 113, 119.

6. American Psychiatric Association, *Diagnostic and Statistical Manual of Mental Disorders,* Fourth Edition, Text Revision (Washington, D.C.: American Psychiatric Association, 2000), p. 356.

7. Mill, *Autobiography*, p. 116.

8. Kay Redfield Jamison insightfully explores bipolar disorder in *An Unquiet Mind* (New York: Vintage Books, 1995).

9. Sigmund Freud, "Mourning and Melancholia," trans. Joan Rivière, in Philip Rieff, ed., *General Psychological Theory* (New York: Collier Books, 1917), p. 169.

10. Sigmund Freud, *Civilization and Its Discontents*, trans. James Strachey (New York: W.W. Norton, 1961).

11. A. W. Levi, "The 'Mental Crisis' of John Stuart Mill," *Psychoanalytic Review*, 32 (1945): 98. Cf. Clinton Machann, "John Stuart Mill's 'Mental Crisis': Adlerian Interpretation," *Journal of Individual Psychology*, 29 (1973): 76–87; and Peter Glassman, *J. S. Mill: The Evolution of a Genius* (Gainesville: University of Florida Press, 1985).

12. Robert T. Fancher, *Cultures of Healing* (New York: W.H. Freeman, 1995).

13. Stanley W. Jackson, "Acedia: The Sin and Its Relationship to Sorrow and Melancholia," in Arthur Kleinman and Byron Good, eds., *Culture and Depression* (Berkeley: University of California Press, 1985), pp. 43–62. Had he been Protestant, he might have cited Kierkegaard's ruminations about the sick soul. See Abrahim H. Khan, "Melancholy: An Elusive Dimension of Depression?" *Journal of Medical Humanities*, 15 (1994): 113–122.

14. Peter C. Whybrow, *A Mood Apart* (New York: HarperPerennial, 1997), p. 95.

15. Ibid., p. 145.

16. Ibid., p. 189.

17. Ibid., pp. 234, 193.

18. Robert Solomon, *The Passions* (New York: Anchor Books, 1977), pp. 294–295.

19. A variety of historical perspectives on depression and melancholy are anthologized in Jennifer Radden, ed., *The Nature of Melancholy: From Aristotle to Kristeva* (New York: Oxford University Press, 2000).

20. George Graham, "Melancholic Epistemology," *Synthese*, 82 (1990): 417. Also see Allan D. Nelson, "John Stuart Mill: The Reformer Reformed," *Interpretation*, 13 (1985): 360.

21. Graham, "Melancholic Epistemology," p. 401.

22. Arthur Kleinman, *The Illness Narratives: Suffering, Healing, and the Human Condition* (New York: Basic Books, 1988); Frederick K. Goodwin and Kay Redfield Jamison, eds., *Manic-Depressive Illness* (New York: Oxford University, 1990); William Styron, *Darkness Visible* (New York: Random House, 1990); and Nell Casey, *Unholy Ghost: Writers on Depression* (New York: William Morrow, 2001).

23. Graham, "Melancholic Epistemology, p. 406.

24. James C. Coyne, "Ambiguity and Controversy: An Introduction," in James C. Coyne, ed., *Essential Papers on Depression* (New York: New York University Press, 1986), p. 16.

25. Dorothy Rowe, *Depression: The Way out of Your Prison*, 2nd ed. (New York: Routledge, 1996).

26. Aaron Beck, *Depression: Causes and Treatment* (Philadelphia: University of Pennsylvania Press, 1967), p. 7. The same occurs in Martin E. P. Seligman's *Learned Optimism* (New York: Alfred A. Knopf, 1991).

27. Peter Kramer, *Listening to Prozac* (New York: Penguin, 1997).

28. Carl Elliott, *A Philosophical Disease: Bioethics, Culture, and Identity* (New York: Routledge, 1999), p. 95. See also Carl Elliott and Tod Chambers, eds., *Prozac as a Way of Life* (Chapel Hill: University of North Carolina Press, 2004).

29. Kramer, *Listening to Prozac*, pp. 274, 257.

30. Ibid., p. 268.

31. Ibid., p. 270.

32. A. M. Weisberger, "The Ethics of the Broader Usage of Prozac: Social Choice or Social Bias?" *International Journal of Applied Philosophy*, 10 (1995): 69–74.

33. David A. Karp, *Speaking of Sadness: Depression, Disconnection, and the Meanings of Illness* (New York: Oxford University Press, 1996), pp. 54, 80 (italics removed), 79.

34. M. M. Weissman, R. C. Bland, G. J. Canino, C. Faravelli, S. Greenwald, et al., "Cross-National Epidemiology of Major Depression and Bipolar Disorder," *Journal of the American Medical Association*, 276, no. 4, (1996): 293–299.

35. L. B. Alloy and L.Y. Abramson, "Judgment of Contingency in Depressed and Nondepressed Students," *Journal of Experimental Psychology: General*, 108 (1979): 441–485; S. Golin, F. Terrell, and B. Johnson, "Depression and the Illusion of Control," *Journal of Abnormal Psychology*, 86 (1997): 440–442.

36. Garrett, "Problem of Despair," pp. 73–89.

37. William James, *The Varieties of Religious Experience* (New York: Modern Library, 1902).

Chapter 13: Self-Deception and Hope

1. By honesty I mean truthfulness, as distinct from trustworthiness. Bernard Williams explores the two meanings in *Truth and Truthfulness* (Princeton, N.J.: Princeton University Press, 2002).

2. Henrik Ibsen, *The Wild Duck*, in Henrik Ibsen, *Four Major Plays*, trans. Rolf Fjelde (New York: New American Library, 1965), p. 202.

3. Ibid., p. 203.

4. Several anthologies provide a good sampling of approaches: Mike W. Martin, ed., *Self-Deception and Self-Understanding: New Essays in Philosophy and Psychology* (Lawrence: University Press of Kansas, 1985); Brian P. McLaughlin and Amelie Oksenberg Rorty, eds., *Perspectives on Self-Deception* (Berkeley: University of California Press, 1988); Joan S. Lockard and Delroy L. Paulhus, eds., *Self-Deception: An Adaptive Mechanism?* (Englewood Cliffs, N.J.: Prentice Hall, 1988); Roger T. Ames and Wimal Dissanayake, eds., *Self and Deception* (Albany: State University of New York Press, 1996); and Jean-Pierre Dupuy, ed., *Self-Deception and Paradoxes of Rationality* (Stanford, Calif.: Center for the Study of Language and Information, 1998).

5. Stanley Paluch, "Self-Deception," *Inquiry*, 10 (1967): 268–278.

6. Alfred R. Mele, *Self-Deception Unmasked* (Princeton, N.J.: Princeton University Press, 2001), pp. 50–51.

7. Raphael Demos, "Lying to Oneself," *Journal of Philosophy*, 57 (1960): 588–595.

8. Jean-Paul Sartre, *Being and Nothingness*, trans. Hazel E. Barnes (New York: Washington Square Press, 1966), p. 113. And see Ronald E. Santoni, *Bad Faith, Good Faith, and Authenticity in Sartre's Early Philosophy* (Philadelphia: Temple University Press, 1995).

9. Herbert Fingarette, *Self-Deception* (Berkeley: University of California Press, 2000), p. 164. This edition contains a new essay, "Self-Deception Needs No Explaining," in which Fingarette refines his position. The first edition was published in 1969 by Routledge and Kegan Paul and the Humanities Press.

10. Ibid., pp. 172, 170.

11. See also Mike W. Martin, *Self-Deception and Morality* (Lawrence: University Press of Kansas, 1986), pp. 109–137; and Jerome Neu, "Life-Lies and Pipe Dreams: Self-Deception in Ibsen's *The Wild Duck* and O'Neill's *The Iceman Cometh*," *Philosophical Forum*, 19 (1988): 241–269.

12. Lockard and Paulhus, *Self-Deception*, p. 2.

13. Jonathon D. Brown, *The Self* (Boston: McGraw-Hill, 1998), p. 268. Also see Timothy D. Wilson, *Strangers to Ourselves: Discovering the Adaptive Unconscious* (Cambridge, Mass.: Belknap Press, 2002).

14. Shelley E. Taylor, *Positive Illusions: Creative Self-Deception and Healthy Mind* (New York: Basic Books, 1989), p. 7. See also Shelley E. Taylor and Jonathon D. Brown's essay, "Illusion and Well-Being: A Social Psychological Perspective on Mental Health," *Psychological Bulletin*, 103 (1988): 193–210.

15. Taylor, *Positive Illusions*, pp. 228, 48.

16. "Positive" means optimistic. It does not mean healthy, for that would make it tautological that "positive illusions are healthy," whereas Taylor regards the claim as empirical.

17. Ibid., pp. 10–11.

18. Ibid., pp. 126, 198.

19. Sigmund Freud, *The Future of an Illusion*, trans. James Strachey (New York: W.W. Norton, 1961), p. 39.

20. Marie Jahoda, *Current Concepts of Mental Health* (New York: Basic Books, 1958), pp. 49, 51.

21. Taylor, *Positive Illusions*, p. 219.

22. R. D. Laing, *The Divided Self* (Baltimore: Penguin Books, 1965); Jules Henry, *Pathways to Madness* (New York: Vintage Books, 1973); and Erving Goffman, *Frame Analysis* (New York: Harper and Row, 1974).

23. Abraham J. Twerski, *Addictive Thinking: Understanding Self-Deception*, 2d ed. (Center City, Minn.: Hazelden, 1997). Also see Herbert Fingarette, "Alcoholism and Self-Deception," in Mike W. Martin (ed.), *Self-Deception and Self-Understanding: New Essays in Philosophy and Psychology* (Lawrence: University Press of Kansas, 1985), pp. 52–67.

24. See, for example, Eugene O'Neill, *Long Days' Journey into Night* (New Haven, Conn.: Yale University Press, 1973), p. 93.

25. Willard Gaylin, *How Psychotherapy Really Works* (Chicago: Contemporary Books, 2001), pp. 174, 190. Freud caused confusion when he sometimes portrayed all psychological defense as pathological, as in *The Psychopathology of Everyday Life*.

26. Morris Eagle, "Psychoanalysis and Self-Deception, in Joan S. Lockard and Delroy L. Paulhus, eds., *Self-Deception: An Adaptive Mechanism?* (Englewood Cliffs, N.J.: Prentice Hall, 1988), p. 78. Like Herbert Fingarette, Roy Schafer interprets psychological defense as (often) self-deception; see Schafer, *A New Language for Psychoanalysis* (New Haven, Conn.: Yale University Press, 1976).

27. Marcia Cavell, *The Psychoanalytic Mind* (Cambridge: Harvard University Press, 1996), p. 186. Also see Jerome L. Singer, ed., *Repression and Dissociation: Implications for Personality Theory, Psychopathology, and Health* (Chicago: University of Chicago Press, 1990).

28. Cavell, *Psychoanalytic Mind*, p. 81.

29. Jonathan Glover, "Freud, Morality and Responsibility," in Jonathan Miller, ed., *Freud: The Man, His World, His Influence* (Boston: Little, Brown, 1972), pp. 152–163.

30. Immanuel Kant, *The Doctrine of Virtue*, trans. Mary J. Gregor (Philadelphia: University of Pennsylvania Press, 1964), pp. 94–95.

31. Jean-Paul Sartre, "Existentialism Is a Humanism," trans. Philip Mairet, in Walter Kaufmann, ed., *Existentialism from Dostoevsky to Sartre* (New York: New American Library, 1975), p. 366. In a nonabsolutist vein, Annette Barnes sees "epistemic cowardice" as the primary vice of self-deceivers; Barnes, *Seeing through Self-Deception* (Cambridge: Cambridge University Press, 1997), pp. 158–175.

32. Daniel A. Putman, "Virtue and Self-Deception," *Southern Journal of Philosophy*, 25, no. 4 (1987), p. 549. Robert Brown provides a nuanced discussion of how integrity and integration are related in "Integrity and Self-Deception," *Critical Review*, 25 (1983): 115–131.

33. John King-Farlow, "Review of Herbert Fingarette's *Self-Deception*," *Metaphilosophy*, 4 (1973): 76–84; and Amelie Oksenberg Rorty, "Belief and Self-Deception," *Inquiry*, 15 (1972): 387–410.

34. Mike W. Martin, "Honesty with Oneself," in Mary I. Bockover, ed., *Rules, Rituals, and Responsibility* (La Salle, Ill.: Open Court, 1991), pp. 115–136; and Robert Solomon, *The Joy of Philosophy* (New York: Oxford University Press, 1999), pp. 198–217.

Chapter 14: Philosophical Counseling

1. Gerd B. Aschenbach has since come to see the relationship between psychotherapy and philosophical counseling as a "relationship of cooperation and competition." See Aschenbach, "Philosophy, Philosophical Practice, and Psychotherapy," in Ran Lahav and Maria da Venza Tillmanns, eds., *Essays on Philosophical Counseling* (Lanham, Md.: University Press of America, 1995), pp. 61–74. In a similar vein, see Peter B. Raabe, *Philosophical Counseling: Theory and Practice* (Westport, Conn.: Praeger, 2001); and Elliot D. Cohen, *What Would Aristotle Do?: Self-Control through the Power of Reason* (Amherst, N.Y.: Prometheus Books, 2003).

2. Parenthetical page references are to Lou Marinoff, *Plato, Not Prozac!: Applying Philosophy to Everyday Problems* (New York: HarperCollins, 1999).

3. Ben Mijuskovic, "Some Reflections on Philosophical Counseling and Psychotherapy," in Ran Lahav and Maria da Venza Tillmanns, eds., *Essays on Philosophical Counseling* (Lanham, Md.: University Press of America, 1995), p. 94. Marinoff says the man had been a monk for ten years.

4. Marinoff's flawed discussion of depression suggests philosophical counselors should be given some training in psychotherapy and psychiatry. Cf. Mijuskovic, "Some Reflections on Philosophical Counseling and Psychotherapy," p. 96; and Karl Pfeifer, "Philosophy outside the Academy: The Role of Philosophy in People-Oriented Professions and the Prospects for Philosophical Counseling," *Inquiry: Critical Thinking across the Disciplines*, 14 (1994): 58–69.

5. American Psychiatric Association, *Diagnostic and Statistical Manual of Mental Disorders,* Fourth Edition, Text Revision (Washington, D.C.: American Psychiatric Association, 2000), p. 356.

6. Similar remarks apply to Roger Paden in "Defining Philosophical Counseling," *International Journal of Applied Philosophy*, 12, no. 1 (1998).

7. Rem B. Edwards, "Introduction" to Rem B. Edwards, ed., *Ethics of Psychiatry* (Amherst, N.Y.: Prometheus Books, 1997), p. 17.

8. Howard Kirschenbaum and Valerie Land Henderson, eds., *Carl Rogers: Dialogues* (Boston: Houghton Mifflin, 1989).

9. Jerome D. Frank and Julia B. Frank, *Persuasion and Healing: A Comparative Study of Psychotherapy*, 3d ed. (Baltimore: Johns Hopkins University Press, 1991), pp. 40–43.

10. Cf. David A. Jopling, " 'First Do No Harm': Over-Philosophizing and Pseudo-Philosophizing in Philosophical Counseling," *Inquiry: Critical Thinking across the*

Disciplines, 17, no. 3 (1997): 100–112. Even Marinoff comes close to acknowledging as much on p. 34.

11. Cf. Ran Lahav, "A Conceptual Framework for Philosophical Counseling: Worldview Interpretation," in Ran Lahav and Maria Da Venza Tillmanns, eds., *Essays on Philosophical Counseling* (Lanham, Md.: University Press of America, 1995), pp. 11–12.

12. Albert Ellis and W. Dryden, *The Practice of Rational Emotive Behaviour Therapy* (New York: Springer, 1997).

13. Deborah Anna Luepnitz, *Schopenhauer's Porcupines: Intimacy and Its Dilemmas* (New York: Basic Books, 2002), p. 125.

14. Alan C. Tjeltveit, *Ethics and Values in Psychotherapy* (London: Routledge, 1999), pp. 35, 157.

15. See especially Irvin D. Yalom, *Existential Psychotherapy* (New York: Basic Books, 1980).

16. Eckart Ruschmann, "Foundations of Philosophical Counseling," *Inquiry: Critical Thinking across the Disciplines*, 17, no. 3 (1997): 24.

17. Ran Lahav, "Philosophical Counseling and Taoism: Wisdom and Lived Philosophical Understanding," *Journal of Chinese Philosophy*, 23, no. 3 (1996): 266.

18. Martha C. Nussbaum, *The Therapy of Desire: Theory and Practice in Hellenistic Ethics* (Princeton, N.J.: Princeton University Press, 1994), esp. pp. 58–75.

19. Ibid., p. 49; italics removed.

20. Ran Lahav, "What Is Philosophical Counseling?," *Journal of Applied Philosophy*, 13 (1996): 268. See also David A. Jopling, "Philosophical Counselling, Truth and Self-Interpretation," *Journal of Applied Philosophy*, 13 (1996): 297–310.

Chapter 15: Healthy Love

1. Plato, *Symposium*, trans. Alexander Nehamas and Paul Woodruff (Indianapolis: Hackett, 1989), sec. 191D.

2. Judith Shklar, *Ordinary Vices* (Cambridge: Harvard University Press, 1984).

3. William Shakespeare, *Othello*, ed. David Bevington (New York: Bantam Books, 1988), sec. 5.2.354.

4. American Psychiatric Association, *Diagnostic and Statistical Manual of Mental Disorders,* Fourth Edition, Text Revision (Washington, D.C.: American Psychiatric Association, 2000), p. 325.

5. Barry Morenz and Richard D. Lane, "Morbid Jealousy and Criminal Conduct," in Louis B. Schlesinger, ed., *Explorations in Criminal Psychopathology* (Springfield, Ill.: Charles C. Thomas, 1996), p. 80; also Paul E. Mullen, "Jealousy: The Pathology of Passion," *British Journal of Psychiatry*, 158 (1991): 593–601.

6. Mary Midgley, *Wickedness* (London: Routledge and Kegan Paul, 1984), pp. 135–152.

7. Arthur Kirsch, *Shakespeare and the Experience of Love* (Cambridge: Cambridge University Press, 1981), p. 32; and Evelyn Gajowski, *The Art of Loving: Female Subjectivity and Male Discursive Traditions in Shakespeare's Tragedies* (Newark, N.J.: University of Delaware Press, 1992), pp. 53–54.

8. Plato, *Symposium*, sec. 186B.

9. Jerome Neu, "Jealous Thoughts," in Amelie Oksenberg Rorty, ed., *Explaining Emotions* (Berkeley: University of California Press, 1980), p. 432.

10. Paul E. Mullen, "Jealousy: The Pathology of Passion," *British Journal of Psychiatry*, 158, (1991): 600. See also Jessie Bernard, "Jealousy and Marriage," in Gordon Clanton and Lynn G. Smith, eds., *Jealousy* (Lanham, Md.: University Press of America, 1986), pp. 141–150; and Peter N. Stearns, *Jealousy: The Evolution of an Emotion in*

American History (New York: New York University Press, 1989). An attack on jealousy is a linchpin in Richard Taylor's defense of extramarital affairs in *Having Love Affairs* (New York: Prometheus Books, 1982).

11. Oscar Wilde, *Salome*, in Richard Aldington and Stanley Weintraub, eds., *The Portable Oscar Wilde* (New York: Penguin, 1981), p. 428.

12. Helen K. Gediman, *Fantasies of Love and Death in Life and Art: A Psychoanalytic Study of the Normal and the Pathological* (New York: New York University Press, 1995), pp. 68, 69.

13. D. H. Lawrence, *Women in Love* (New York: Penguin, 1982); quotations from pp. 430, 542.

14. Denis de Rougemont, *Love in the Western World*, rev. ed., trans. Montgomery Belgion (New York: Harper and Row, 1956); quotations from pp. 46, 277.

15. Deborah Anna Luepnitz, *Schopenhauer's Porcupines: Intimacy and Its Dilemmas* (New York: Basic Books, 2002), pp. 2–3, 21–65.

16. I develop this conception of love in Martin, *Love's Virtues* (Lawrence: University Press of Kansas, 1996).

17. For example, Laurence R. Barnhill, "Healthy Family Systems," *Family Coordinator*, 28 (1979): 94–100; Myron F. Weiner, "Healthy and Pathological Love," in Kenneth S. Pope, ed., *On Love and Loving* (San Francisco: Jossey-Bass, 1980), pp. 114–132; Hilda Kessler, ed., *Treating Couples* (San Francisco: Jossey-Bass, 1996); Otto F. Kernberg, *Love Relations: Normality and Pathology* (New Haven, Conn.: Yale University Press, 1995); Florence W. Kaslow, ed., *Handbook of Relational Diagnosis and Dysfunctional Family Patterns* (New York: Wiley, 1996); and Adrian B. Kelly and Frank D. Fincham, "Marital Health," *Encyclopedia of Mental Health* (San Diego, Calif.: Academic Press, 1998), pp. 605–619.

18. Martin, *Love's Virtues*, p. 105 ff.

19. Susan Moller Okin, *Justice, Gender, and the Family* (New York: Basic Books, 1989).

20. Peter D. Kramer, *Should You Leave?* (New York: Penguin Books, 1997), pp. 245–246.

21. Thelma Jean Goodrich, Cheryl Rampage, Barbara Ellman, and Kris Halstead, *Feminist Family Therapy* (New York: W.W. Norton, 1988).

22. Hilda Kessler and Margaret Thaler Singer, "Myths in Couples Therapy," in Hilda Kessler, ed., *Treating Couples* (San Francisco: Jossey-Bass, 1996), p. 45. See also Elaine E. Englehardt, ed., *Ethical Issues in Interpersonal Communication* (Fort Worth, Tex.: Harcourt, 2001).

23. Carol Gilligan develops an integrated, moral-therapeutic perspective on mature love in *In a Different Voice* (Cambridge: Harvard University Press, 1982), and Gilligan, *The Birth of Pleasure* (New York: Alfred A. Knopf, 2002).

24. Robert Nozick, "Love's Bond," in *The Examined Life* (New York: Simon and Schuster, 1989), p. 71.

25. Michael P. Nichols and Richard C. Schwartz, *Family Therapy: Concepts and Methods*, 4th ed. (Boston: Allyn and Bacon, 1998), p. 330.

26. V. Goldner, "Feminism and Family Therapy," *Family Process*, 24 (1985): 31. Cited in Michael P. Nichols and Richard C. Schwartz, *Family Therapy: Concepts and Methods*, 4th ed. (Boston: Allyn and Bacon, 1998), p. 327.

27. Annette C. Baier, *Moral Prejudices* (Cambridge: Harvard University, 1994), p. 49.

28. Robert Solomon, *Love: Emotion, Myth, and Metaphor* (New York: Anchor, 1981); Solomon, *About Love* (New York: Simon and Schuster, 1988); and Robert Nozick, *The Examined Life* (New York: Simon and Schuster, 1989), p. 70.

29. Parenthetical page references are to Robert N. Bellah, Richard Madsen, William M. Sullivan, Ann Swidler, and Steven M. Tipton, *Habits of the Heart: Individualism and*

Commitment in American Life (Berkeley: University of California Press, 1985). Ann Swidler is the primary contributor to the chapter on love and marriage.

30. Cf. Jeffrey Stout, *Ethics after Babel* (Princeton, N.J.: Princeton University Press, 2001), pp. 191–200.

31. Anne Wilson Schaef, *Co-Dependence: Misunderstood-Mistreated* (San Francisco: Harper and Row, 1986), p. 35. For insightful critiques of the co-dependency movement, see Gary Greenberg, *The Self on the Shelf: Recovery Books and the Good Life* (Albany: State University of New York Press, 1994); and John Steadman Rice, *A Disease of One's Own: Psychotherapy, Addiction, and the Emergence of Co-Dependency* (New Brunswick, N.J.: Transaction, 1986).

32. Hilda Kessler and Margaret Thaler Singer, "Myths in Couples Therapy," in Hilda Kessler, ed., *Treating Couples* (San Francisco: Jossey-Bass, 1996), pp. 35–60.

33. Ann Swidler, *Talk of Love* (Chicago: University of Chicago Press, 2001), p. 143.

34. Ibid., pp. 17–18.

35. Barbara Ehrenreich and Deirdre English, *For Her Own Good: 150 Years of the Experts' Advice to Women* (New York: Anchor, 1978), p. 271.

Chapter 16: Meaningful Work

1. Richard Schacht, *The Future of Alienation* (Urbana: University of Illinois Press, 1994), pp. 20–21, 45–47; and Kai Nielsen, "Alienation and Work," in Gertrude Ezorsky, ed., *Moral Rights in the Workplace* (Albany: State University of New York Press, 1987), pp. 28–34.

2. Karl Marx, *Economic and Philosophical Manuscripts*, in Erich Fromm, *Marx's Concept of Man*, trans. T. B. Bottomore (New York: Ungar, 1966), p. 98.

3. Parenthetical page references are to Herman Melville, "Bartleby," in *Billy Budd and Other Tales by Herman Melville* (New York: New American Library, 1961).

4. See Howard P. Vincent, ed., *Bartleby the Scrivener* (Kent, Ohio: Kent State University Press, 1966); and M. Thomas Inge, ed., *Bartleby the Inscrutable* (Hamden, Conn.: Archon Books, 1979).

5. Dan McCall, *The Silence of Bartleby* (Ithaca, N.Y.: Cornell University Press), p. 113.

6. Maurice Friedman, "Bartleby and the Modern Exile," in Howard P. Vincent, ed., *Bartleby the Scrivener* (Kent, Ohio: Kent State University Press, 1966), pp. 79–80.

7. Ibid., pp. 33–58.

8. American Psychiatric Association, *Diagnostic and Statistical Manual of Mental Disorders, Fourth Edition, Text Revision* (Washington, D.C.: American Psychiatric Association, 2000), pp. 694–697.

9. Cf. Adam Cohen, "When Life Offers a Choice between the White Wall and the Brick Wall," *New York Times* (Aug. 29, 2003), p. A 22.

10. Alan A. Cavaiola and Neil J. Lavender, *Toxic Coworkers* (Oakland, Calif.: New Harbinger, 2000), p. 166.

11. On professional distance, see Mike W. Martin, *Meaningful Work: Rethinking Professional Ethics* (New York: Oxford University Press, 2000), pp. 82–100.

12. Daniel Goleman, *Working with Emotional Intelligence* (New York: Bantam, 1999), p. 7. John D. Mayer and Peter Salovey, who first articulated emotional intelligence as specific intelligences concerning the emotions, criticize Goleman for inflating the term's reference and meaning to include motivation. John D. Mayer, Peter Salovey, and David R. Caruso, "Emotional Intelligence as Zeitgeist, as Personality, and as Mental Ability," in Reuven Bar-On and James D. A. Parker, eds., *The Handbook of Emotional Intelligence* (San Francisco: Jossey-Bass, 2000), pp. 92–117.

13. Goleman, *Working with Emotional Intelligence*, pp. 26–27. The list is shortened in Daniel Goleman, Richard Boyatzis, and Annie McKee, *Primal Leadership: Realizing the Power of Emotional Intelligence* (Boston: Harvard Business School Press, 2002), p. 39.

14. Daniel Goleman, *Emotional Intelligence* (New York: Bantam, 1995), p. 285.

15. Without this moral explicitness, Goleman is vulnerable to the charge that he merely provides a trendy new way for employers to manipulate workers. See James Davison Hunter, *The Death of Character: Moral Education in an Age without Good or Evil* (New York: Basic Books, 2000), p. 85.

16. Arlie Russell Hochschild, *The Managed Heart: Commercialization of Human Feeling* (Berkeley: University of California Press, 1983), p. 197.

17. Goleman, *Working with Emotional Intelligence*, pp. 80–81.

18. Martin E. P. Seligman, *Authentic Happiness* (New York: Free Press, 2002), pp. 125–184.

19. Ibid., p. 177.

20. Joanne B. Ciulla, *The Working Life: The Promise and Betrayal of Modern Work* (New York: Random House, 2000), pp. 217, 212.

21. Ilene Philipson, *Married to the Job* (New York: Free Press, 2002), p. 1.

22. Cf. Gilbert C. Meilaender, *Friendship: A Study in Theological Ethics* (Notre Dame, Ind.: University of Notre Dame Press, 1981), p. 97.

23. Marilyn Machlowitz, *Workaholics: Living with Them, Working with Them* (New York: New American Library, 1980), pp. 7–8.

24. Juliet B. Schor, *The Overworked American: The Unexpected Decline of Leisure* (New York: Basic Books, 1991).

25. For an example of creative obsession with work, see Donald Hall, *Life Work* (Boston: Beacon Press, 1993), p. 8.

26. An example of health-oriented studies is Eleanor Langer, "Inside the New York Telephone Company," in Richard C. Edwards et al., eds., *The Capitalist System*, 2d ed. (Englewood Cliffs, N.J.: Prentice Hall), pp. 4–11. Discussed by Kai Nielsen, "Alienation and Work," in Gertrude Ezorsky, ed., *Moral Rights in the Workplace* (Albany: State University of New York Press, 1987), pp. 28–34.

27. John De Graaf, David Wann, and Thomas H. Naylor, *Affluenza: The All-Consuming Epidemic* (San Francisco: Berrett-Koehler, 2001), p. 2. Cf. Philip Slater, *Wealth Addiction* (New York: E.P. Dutton, 1980).

28. Juliet B. Schor, *The Overspent American: Why We Want What We Don't Need* (New York: HarperPerennial, 1998), p. 158; Jeffrey A. Kottler, *Exploring and Treating Acquisitive Desire* (London: Sage Publications, 1999); Tim Kasser and Allen D. Kanner, eds., *Psychology and Consumer Culture* (Washington, D.C.: American Psychological Association, 2004); and Peter C. Whybrow, *American Mania: When More Is Not Enough* (New York: W.W. Norton, 2005).

29. Robert Holman Coombs, *Drug-Impaired Professionals* (Cambridge: Harvard University Press, 1997).

30. Howard Gardner, Mihaly Csikszentmihalyi, and William Damon, *Good Work: When Excellence and Ethics Meet* (New York: Basic Books, 2001), p. 13. See also Mihaly Csikszentmihalyi, *Good Business: Leadership, Flow, and the Making of Meaning* (New York: Viking, 2003).

31. Gardner et al., *Good Work*, pp. 30–31.

32. Richard Sennett, *The Corrosion of Character* (New York: W.W. Norton, 1998), p. 146.

33. Ibid., p. 130.

34. Ibid., p. 135.

35. See Roy Schafer, *Retelling a Life: Narration and Dialogue in Psychoanalysis* (New York: Basic Books, 1992).

Chapter 17: Community Service

1. Mike W. Martin, *Virtuous Giving: Philanthropy, Voluntary Service, and Caring* (Bloomington: Indiana University Press, 1994). On the diversity of American philanthropy, see Robert H. Bremner, *American Philanthropy*, 2d ed. (Chicago: University of Chicago Press, 1988).

2. Robert D. Putnam reports a decline in philanthropy: "Total giving by living individuals as a fraction of national income fell from 2.26 percent in 1964 to 1.61 percent in 1998, a relative fall of 29 percent." Putnam, *Bowling Alone* (New York: Touchstone, 2000), p. 27. Putnam does not blame the therapeutic trend for contributing to this decline.

3. Jane Addams, *Twenty Years at Hull-House* (New York: New American Library, 1981), pp. 64, 91. See also Jean Bethke Elshtain, *Jane Addams and the Dream of American Democracy: A Life* (New York: Basic Books, 2002); Louise W. Knight, "Jane Addams's Views on the Responsibilities of Wealth," in Dwight F. Burlingame, ed., *The Responsibilities of Wealth* (Bloomington: Indiana University Press, 1992), pp. 118–137; and Christopher Lasch, "Jane Addams: The College Woman and the Family Claim," in Christopher Lasch, *The New Radicalism in America* (New York: Alfred A. Knopf, 1966), pp. 3–37.

4. Addams, *Twenty Years at Hull-House*, p. 73.

5. On wounded healers, see Arthur W. Frank, *The Wounded Storyteller: Body, Illness, and Ethics* (Chicago: University of Chicago Press, 1995).

6. Addams, *Twenty Years at Hull-House*, p. 92.

7. Parenthetic page references are to Robert Wuthnow, *Acts of Compassion* (Princeton, N.J.: Princeton University Press, 1991).

8. That is the problem with ethical emotivism, the view that moral judgments are nothing but expressions of emotions.

9. Simply taking a course in economics can significantly lower students' incoming beliefs about the extent of altruism. See R. H. Frank, T. Gilovich, and D. T. Regan, "Does Studying Economics Inhibit Cooperation?," *Journal of Economic Perspectives*, 7 (1993): 159–171.

10. D. T. Miller, "The Norm of Self-Interest," *American Psychologist*, 54 (1999): 1053–1060; and Shelley E. Taylor, *The Tending Instinct* (New York: Times Books, 2002), p. 182.

11. Bernard Williams, *Moral Luck* (Cambridge: Cambridge University Press, 1981), pp. 1–19.

12. Neera Badhwar, "Altruism versus Self-Interest: Sometimes a False Dichotomy," in Ellen Frankel Paul, Fred D. Miller Jr., and Jeffrey Paul, eds., *Altruism* (New York: Cambridge University Press, 1993), p. 105.

13. Fred R. Berger, "Gratitude," *Ethics*, 85 (1975): 298–309; Paul F. Caminisch, "Gift and Gratitude in Ethics," *Journal of Religious Ethics*, 9 (1981): 1–34; and Terrance McConnell, *Gratitude* (Philadelphia: Temple University Press, 1993).

14. James Brabazon, *Albert Schweitzer: A Biography*, 2d ed. (Syracuse, N.Y.: Syracuse University Press, 2000).

15. Albert Schweitzer, *Out of My Life and Thought*, trans. A. B. Lemke (New York: Henry Holt, 1990), p. 82.

16. Albert Schweitzer, *Reverence for Life: Sermons 1900–1919*, trans. Reginald H. Fuller (New York: Irvington, 1993), p. 141. See also Mike W. Martin, "Good Fortune Obligates: Gratitude, Philanthropy, and Colonialism," *Southern Journal of Philosophy*, 37 (1999): 57–75.

17. Albert Schweitzer, *Memoirs of Childhood and Youth*, trans. Kurt Bergel and Alice R. Bergel (New York: Syracuse University Press, 1997), p. 74.

18. Schweitzer, *Reverence for Life*, p. 141.

19. Robert A. Emmons and Charles M. Shelton, "Gratitude and the Science of Positive Psychology," in C. R. Snyder and Shane J. Lopez, eds., *Handbook of Positive Psychology* (New York: Oxford University Press, 2002), pp. 459–471.

20. Claudia Card, "Gratitude and Obligation," *American Philosophical Quarterly*, 25 (1988): 115–127.

21. Abraham Maslow, *Motivation and Personality*, 3d ed. (New York: Harper and Row, 1970), p. 136. Cited in Emmons and Shelton, "Gratitude and the Science of Positive Psychology," p. 460.

22. R. A. Emmons and C. A. Crumpler, "Gratitude as Human Strength: Appraising the Evidence," *Journal of Social and Clinical Psychology*, 19 (2000): 56–69.

23. For example, see William James, "The Sentiment of Rationality," in Ralph Barton Perry, ed., *Essays on Faith and Morals* (New York: Meridian Books, 1962). The other sense of "healthy-mindedness"—wrongly ignoring evil—is used in William James, *The Varieties of Religious Experience* (New York: Modern Library, 1002), p. 86, and see p. 160.

24. James, "The Sentiment of Rationality," p. 102.

25. C. R. Snyder, "Hypothesis: There Is Hope," in C. R. Snyder, ed., *Handbook of Hope* (San Diego, Calif.: Academic Press, 2000), p. 8.

26. Anne Colby and William Damon, *Some Do Care: Contemporary Lives of Moral Commitment* (New York: Free Press, 1992), p. 238.

27. Martin E. P. Seligman, *Learned Optimism* (New York: Alfred A. Knopf, 1991), pp. 286, 290, 52.

28. Betty Friedan, *Life So Far* (New York: Simon and Schuster, 2000); Judith Hennessee, *Betty Friedan: Her Life* (New York: Random House, 1999); and Marcia Cohen, *The Sisterhood* (New York: Simon and Schuster, 1988).

29. Betty Friedan, *The Feminine Mystique* (New York: W.W. Norton, 2001), p. 314.

30. Gloria Steinem, *Revolution from Within: A Book of Self-Esteem* (Boston: Little, Brown, 1992), pp. 17, 9–10.

31. Eva S. Moskowitz, *In Therapy We Trust: America's Obsession with Self-Fulfillment* (Baltimore: Johns Hopkins University Press, 2001), pp. 178–217; quotation from p. 284.

32. On the diversity of good lives, see Lawrence C. Becker, "Good Lives: Prolegomena," *Social Philosophy and Policy*, 9 (1992): 15–37.

Epilogue

1. John Dewey, *Human Nature and Conduct* (New York: Modern Library, 1957), pp. 12–13.

INDEX